Advances in Infectious Diseases and Clinical Microbiology during and after the COVID-19 Pandemic: 2nd Edition

Advances in Infectious Diseases and Clinical Microbiology during and after the COVID-19 Pandemic: 2nd Edition

Guest Editors

Yusra Habib Khan
Tauqeer Hussain Mallhi

MDPI

Basel • Beijing • Wuhan • Barcelona • Belgrade • Novi Sad • Cluj • Manchester

Guest Editors

Yusra Habib Khan
Department of Clinical Pharmacy
Jouf University
Sakaka
Saudi Arabia

Tauqeer Hussain Mallhi
Department of Clinical Pharmacy
Jouf University
Sakaka
Saudi Arabia

Editorial Office

MDPI AG
Grosspeteranlage 5
4052 Basel, Switzerland

This is a reprint of the Special Issue, published open access by the journal *Medicina* (ISSN 1648-9144), freely accessible at: https://www.mdpi.com/journal/medicina/special_issues/24I57G96AW.

For citation purposes, cite each article independently as indicated on the article page online and as indicated below:

Lastname, A.A.; Lastname, B.B. Article Title. *Journal Name* **Year**, *Volume Number*, Page Range.

ISBN 978-3-7258-4389-3 (Hbk)
ISBN 978-3-7258-4390-9 (PDF)
https://doi.org/10.3390/books978-3-7258-4390-9

Contents

About the Editors

Yusra Habib Khan

Dr. Yusra Habib Khan is a distinguished researcher and educator in clinical pharmacy, holding a Ph.D. and Master's in Clinical Pharmacy from Universiti Sains Malaysia. Her career encompasses diverse academic and research roles across Malaysia, Pakistan, Saudi Arabia, and now Australia, with significant contributions to the advancement of pharmaceutical sciences and healthcare.

Dr. Khan has authored more than 170 peer-reviewed articles in reputable scientific journals and is the author of the book, *Expanded Dengue Syndrome*. She has contributed over 35 chapters to academic volumes, further enriching the healthcare literature. Her research has been widely recognized, particularly in areas such as vaccine hesitancy, infectious diseases, nephrology, pharmacoepidemiology, pharmacovigilance, and patient care. Her work has notably advanced the understanding of clinical outcomes in chronic kidney disease and the complexities of infectious diseases.

Dr. Khan is listed among the top 2% of scientists globally, reflecting the international impact and recognition of her scholarly contributions. She has led funded projects in health sciences, supervised postgraduate students, and received multiple awards for research excellence and scientific presentations. Her commitment to evidence-based practice, pharmaceutical care, and public health, along with her active roles as an editorial board member and reviewer, make her a respected leader in clinical pharmacy and healthcare research.

Tauqeer Hussain Mallhi

Dr. Tauqeer Hussain Mallhi is a distinguished researcher and educator in clinical pharmacy practice, holding a Ph.D. and bringing a wealth of diverse experience in academia, clinical research, and healthcare management. Over the course of his career, he has held impactful roles as an Assistant Professor, Research Officer, Clinical Research Associate, and Field Marketing Manager, with professional contributions spanning Pakistan, Saudi Arabia, Malaysia, and now Australia.

With an extensive publication record of over 185 peer-reviewed research papers, Dr. Mallhi has made significant contributions to fields such as infectious diseases, drug safety, antimicrobial resistance, vaccine hesitancy, nephrology, and patient care. His dedication to knowledge dissemination also includes authoring two books and contributing twenty-four chapters to esteemed academic volumes, all aimed at advancing clinical pharmacy practices and improving healthcare outcomes. His work is internationally recognized, placing him among the top 2% of scientists globally, as noted by Stanford University. In acknowledgment of his remarkable achievements, he was awarded the prestigious Global Talent Visa by the Australian Department of Home Affairs.

Dr. Mallhi is also a dedicated mentor, having supervised numerous postgraduate students, guiding the next generation of healthcare professionals with a commitment to academic and professional excellence. His passion for expanding the role of clinical pharmacy practice is evident in his focus on practice innovations and research-driven approaches that elevate patient outcomes. Known as a distinguished researcher, he continues to advocate for advancing clinical pharmacy through evidence-based practices that support public health on a global scale.

Preface

The COVID-19 pandemic has profoundly transformed the landscape of infectious diseases and clinical microbiology, presenting both unprecedented challenges and remarkable opportunities for scientific advancement. This Special Issue, "Advances in Infectious Diseases and Clinical Microbiology during and after the COVID-19 Pandemic: 2nd Edition," was conceived to capture the breadth of research, clinical observations, and innovative strategies that have emerged during this pivotal era. Our aim was to provide a platform for investigators and clinicians worldwide to share their experiences, discoveries, and lessons learned, with the goal of advancing our collective understanding and preparedness for current and future infectious threats.

The scope of this reprint encompasses a diverse array of topics, including the epidemiology of emerging and re-emerging pathogens, advances in diagnostic technologies, antimicrobial resistance, and the evolving role of infection prevention and control. The included articles reflect the dedication of researchers, clinicians, and laboratory professionals who have worked tirelessly under the extraordinary circumstances of the pandemic.

This Special Issue is intended for a broad audience of healthcare professionals, microbiologists, public health experts, and researchers who seek to stay informed about the latest developments in infectious diseases and clinical microbiology. We extend our sincere gratitude to all contributing authors, reviewers, and editorial staff whose efforts have made this collection possible. Their commitment to scientific excellence and collaboration has been instrumental in shaping this timely and impactful reprint.

Yusra Habib Khan and Tauqeer Hussain Mallhi
Guest Editors

medicina

MDPI

Review

Atypical Complications during the Course of COVID-19: A Comprehensive Review

Tauqeer Hussain Mallhi [1,*], Aqsa Safdar [2], Muhammad Hammad Butt [3,*], Muhammad Salman [4], Sumbal Nosheen [5], Zia Ul Mustafa [6], Faiz Ullah Khan [7] and Yusra Habib Khan [1]

1 Department of Clinical Pharmacy, College of Pharmacy, Jouf University, Sakaka 72388, Saudi Arabia; yhkhan@ju.edu.sa
2 Faculty of Pharmaceutical Sciences, University of Central Punjab, Lahore 54000, Pakistan; l1f20mpch0005@ucp.edu.pk
3 Department of Medicinal Chemistry, Faculty of Pharmacy, Uppsala University, 75123 Uppsala, Sweden
4 Institute of Pharmacy, Faculty of Pharmaceutical and Allied Health Sciences, Lahore College for Women University, Lahore 54000, Pakistan; msk5012@gmail.com
5 Department of Pharmacy, The Children's Hospital and the University of Child Health Sciences, Lahore 54600, Pakistan; dr.sumbal@chich.edu.pk
6 Department of Pharmacy Services, District Headquarter (DHQ) Hospital, Pakpattan 57400, Pakistan; zia.ucp@gmail.com
7 Department of Pharmacy Administration and Clinical Pharmacy, School of Pharmacy, Xi'an Jiaotong University, Xi'an 710061, China; fkhan@bs.qau.edu.pk
* Correspondence: thhussain@ju.edu.sa (T.H.M.); muhammad-hammad.butt.7587@student.uu.se (M.H.B.)

Abstract: COVID-19 is primarily a respiratory disease, but numerous studies have indicated the involvement of various organ systems during the course of illness. We conducted a comprehensive review of atypical complications of COVID-19 with their incidence range (IR) and their impact on hospitalization and mortality rates. We identified 97 studies, including 55 research articles and 42 case studies. We reviewed four major body organ systems for various types of atypical complications: (i) Gastro-intestinal (GI) and hepatobiliary system, e.g., bowel ischemia/infarction (IR: 1.49–83.87%), GI bleeding/hemorrhage (IR: 0.47–10.6%), hepatic ischemia (IR: 1.0–7.4%); (ii) Neurological system, e.g., acute ischemic stroke/cerebral venous sinus thrombosis/cerebral hemorrhage (IR: 0.5–90.9%), anosmia (IR: 4.9–79.6%), dysgeusia (IR: 2.8–83.38%), encephalopathy/encephalitis with or without fever and hypoxia (IR: 0.19–35.2%); (iii) Renal system, e.g., acute kidney injury (AKI)/acute renal failure (IR: 0.5–68.8%); (iv) Cardiovascular system, e.g., acute cardiac injury/non-coronary myocardial injury (IR: 7.2–55.56%), arrhythmia/ventricular tachycardia/ventricular fibrillation (IR: 5.9–16.7%), and coagulopathy/venous thromboembolism (IR: 19–34.4%). This review encourages and informs healthcare practitioners to keenly monitor COVID-19 survivors for these atypical complications in all major organ systems and not only treat the respiratory symptoms of patients. Post-COVID effects should be monitored, and follow-up of patients should be performed on a regular basis to check for long-term complications.

Keywords: COVID-19; complications; gastro-intestinal system; neurological system; renal system; cardiovascular system

1. Introduction

Coronavirus disease 2019, or COVID-19, is an exceedingly transmissible viral illness that is acquired by severe acute respiratory syndrome coronavirus 2 (SARS-CoV-2). It has had a disastrous consequence on the world, culminating in over six million deaths around the globe. Succeeding the early cases of this dominating respiratory viral disease, which were reported in December 2019 in Wuhan, Hubei Province, China, SARS-CoV-2 swiftly promulgated around the globe in a brief period of time. As a result, the World Health Organization (WHO) was forced to announce it as a global pandemic on 11 March 2020, and trials for the first human vaccine for COVID-19 started with the modern mRNA vaccine. By April 2020, 1 million cases were reported, and the WHO released guidance for mask-wearing. The major countries affected included the USA, the UK, India, Russia, and Vietnam. By September 2020, 1 million deaths were recorded. In November 2020, vaccine trials of Pfizer and BioNTech showed 90% efficacy. By April 2021, one billion doses of COVID-19 vaccination were given all across the world. According to recent data, three million new cases and more than 23,000 deaths have been reported from 13 March to 9 April 2023, a decline of 28% and 30%, respectively, in comparison to the preceding 28 days. As of 9 April 2023, over 762 million confirmed cases and over 6.8 million deaths have been reported all over the world [1–3].

According to its structure and phylogenetics, SARS-CoV-2 is identical to MERS-CoV and SARS-CoV. It is made up of four major structural proteins: membrane protein (M), nucleocapsid (N), envelope (E), and spike (S), together with sixteen nonstructural proteins and five to eight accessory proteins [4]. The surface spike glycoprotein (S) consists of an S1 subunit, which is divided further into the receptor-binding domain (RBD) and the N-terminal domain (NTD), which aids the virus to enter into the host cell and acts as a prospective target for neutralization concerning vaccines or antisera [5]. SARS-CoV-2 gains access into the host cell once its spike (S protein) abundantly binds to angiotensin-converting enzyme 2 (ACE2) receptors present on the respiratory epithelium, for example, type II alveolar epithelial cells. The amino acid site of the spike RBD permits functional processing of a similar kind in the presence of the human enzyme furin, which allows the amalgamation of viral and cell membranes, a vital transit for the virus's entry into the cell. This is followed by the subsequent endocytosis and viral replication along with virion assembly [6]. In addition to the respiratory epithelium, ACE2 receptors are also present in other organs such as enterocytes and the proximal tubular cells present inside the kidney, ileum, upper esophagus, myocardial cells, and the urothelial cells that make up the bladder [7].

Primarily, COVID-19 is considered a viral respiratory as well as vascular disease, as SARS-CoV-2 principally targets the respiratory and vascular systems. In spite of the fact that the respiratory system is the main target of SARS-CoV-2, it causes atypical complications in systems such as the renal, cardiovascular, hepatobiliary, gastrointestinal tract (GI), and central nervous systems [8]. SARS-CoV-2-prompted organ dysfunction, by and large, is possibly described by one or a combination of the suggested mechanisms, such as dysregulation of the renin–angiotensin–aldosterone system (RAAS), direct viral toxicity, dysregulation of the immune system, ischemic injury resulting from thrombo-inflammation, thrombosis, and vasculitis [9].

Considering the large volume of research data on the atypical complications of COVID-19, it is crucial to perform an overview so that current literature can be organized and identified to underline the scope of priority for successful clinical management and effective decision making by healthcare practitioners to not only curb the impact of these atypical complications on the patient's quality of life but also to reduce the economic burden on the healthcare system. Previously, there have been a few reviews on extrapulmonary manifestations [8,10–13], but the types of complications and their overall effect on hospitalization and mortality rates have never been explored. In addition, a large number of reviews exist on manifestations in individual organ systems of the body [14–19], but no study has ever attempted to gather information in a single article through extensive research on major organ systems. Furthermore, there are other infections that can cause atypical complications, i.e., dengue and Varicella-Zoster virus infections are well known to cause dementia, chronic encephalitis, aseptic meningitis, multiple sclerosis, acute pancreatitis, and myopericarditis [20–25] and such complications further accelerate patient hospitalization and rates of morbidity and mortality, which, in turn, render a huge burden on the healthcare system.

2. Purpose of Article

This review was intended (1) to summarize a large number of research studies and case reports on various atypical complications of the COVID-19 virus in major organ systems, (2) to assemble the data on the range of their incidence, and (3) to gather information on the impact of these complications on hospitalization and mortality rates.

3. Review Method

This article is not subject to ethical approval as it includes the synthesis of qualitative data from publicly available information. Inclusion criteria included articles that were either research studies or case studies related to atypical complications during or after SARS-CoV-2 diagnosis in four major organ systems, i.e., the gastrointestinal and hepatobiliary system, renal system, neurological system, and cardiovascular system. Research studies reporting the types of complications in the aforementioned organ systems with either incidence rates, mortality/hospitalization rates, or both were included in this review. Articles reporting atypical complications in diagnosis other than SARS-CoV-2 infection (e.g., HIV, Dengue, Varicella-Zoster virus) were excluded as their mechanisms for organ complications synergize with those of the SARS-CoV-2 virus. Articles that were not concerned with the preceding organ systems or had repetitive complications were also excluded.

PubMed, Scopus, EMBASE Cochrane Library, Medline, and ProQuest databases were searched for studies published between January 2020 and May 2023. A search strategy utilizing an extensive range of Medical Subject Headings (MeSH) was employed: "Atypical and extrapulmonary manifestations" [Mesh] OR "Atypical and extrapulmonary features" [Mesh] OR "Atypical symptoms" [Mesh] OR "Atypical complications" [Mesh] OR "Extra-pulmonary complications" [Mesh] AND ("COVID 19" [Majr] OR "SARS-CoV-2" [Majr] OR "Coronavirus" [Majr] OR "Coronavirus pandemic" [Majr]) AND ("Atypical" [Mesh] OR "Multiple organ manifestations" [Mesh] OR "Extrapulmonary features" [Mesh]).

All records were checked by independent reviewers on the basis of titles and abstracts for the purpose of addition to this review. Studies that did not harmonize the inclusion criteria or those that harmonized the exclusion criteria were discarded. The remaining records with abstracts providing adequate information were taken into consideration after the evaluation of the full text, which was carried out by the same reviewers independently. The reference lists of full-text articles were also screened for additional studies. Disagreements were solved by a third reviewer.

In this review, only studies were included that provided variable results so that the range of incidence of the identified complications could be recorded. For example, if a study reported the incidence of acute kidney injury as 0.5% and another study reported 0.57%, in order to determine the lowest incidence, only one study was considered so as to avoid the repetition of studies providing similar information. A similar method was adopted for the highest limit of the incidence rate. Also, where a particular complication was reported in 2 or 3 studies only, the incidence is reported separately instead of the incidence range (IR). Since this review aims to cover many complications, it was not possible to cover the enormous literature available to date.

The studies that were selected were scrutinized by two investigators, and the information was extracted by using the standardized system. The information that was gathered from research studies is as follows: author name, year of publication, country, type of study, demographics, complications, number of complications, incidence rate, and hospitalization and mortality rate. The following data were extracted from case reports: author name, publication year, demographics, type of complication, past history, laboratory tests (latest test values were noted where available), treatment, days of illness before hospitalization, hospital stay, and outcome.

4. Summary of Included Studies

Of 65,179 total studies, 17,880 studies were initially selected. Of these, 4365 studies were excluded after abstract screening. A total of 1513 full-text articles were assessed for eligibility. Finally, 55 research studies and 42 case reports were included in this review. The current review has identified complications pertaining to four major organ systems: (1) Gastrointestinal/hepatobiliary system, (2) neurological system, (3) renal system, and (4) cardiovascular system. Details of complications identified from the selected studies along with underlying pathophysiology and management considerations are described below.

4.1. Gastrointestinal System

4.1.1. Complications

In this review, seven research studies have been identified in which GI complications were reported. There was a total of 14 GI complications identified from research studies. The major complications were bowel ischemia/infarction (IR: 1.49–4.00%), GI bleeding/hemorrhage (IR: 0.47–10.6%), and hepatic ischemia/injury/infarct due to thromboembolism of the portal system (IR: 1.0–7.4%). Other complications included acute pancreatitis (incidence: 0.3%, 1.0%), transaminitis (incidence: 55%, 67.3%), and ileus (incidence: 48.0%, 55.8%). The rare complications identified were luminal and pancreaticobiliary disease (incidence: 2.7%), pneumatosis or portal venous gas (incidence: 20%), yellow discoloration of the bowel (2.23%), bowel-wall abnormalities (31%), bile stasis (incidence: 54.0%), acute cholecystitis (incidence: 3.8%), gastric feeding intolerance (incidence: 46.2%), Ogilvie-like Syndrome (incidence: 1.9%), and *Clostridium difficile* colitis (incidence: 3.8%). The overall mortality rate among research studies reporting GI complications ranged from 25% to 34.1% (Table 1). In Figure 1, the prevalence in terms of the maximum percentage of GI complications among different studies is presented.

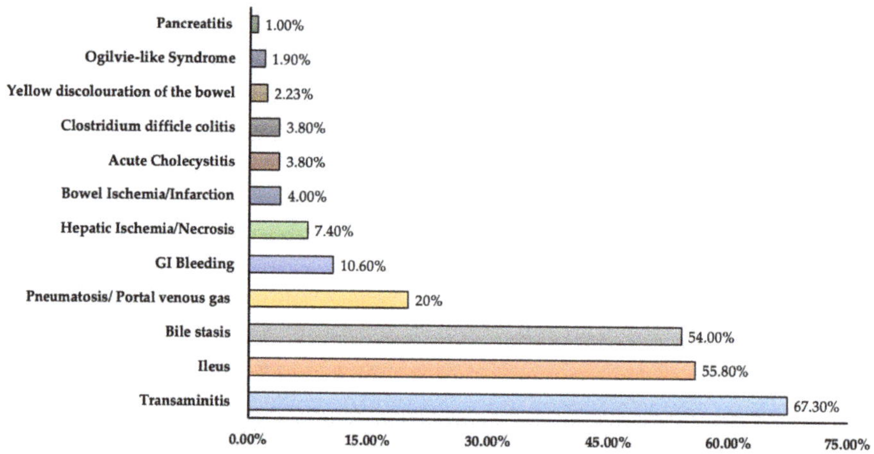

Figure 1. Prevalence of gastrointestinal complications among COVID-19 patients (prevalence represents the maximum percentage reported in the literature).

We included 14 case reports comprising 19 patients identified with GI complications. Of these, major complications were bowel ischemia/hepatic ischemia (38.88%), acute pancreatitis (22.22%), and bowel perforation (16.67%). Rare complications were Cytomegalovirus hemorrhagic enterocolitis (11.12%), paralytic ileus (11.12%), and intussusception (5.56%). Of case reports identifying GI complications, nine (50.0%) patients died, five (27.77%) patients were cured, and four (22.22%) patients were still hospitalized and undergoing treatment (Table 2).

4.1.2. Underlying Pathophysiology

The underlying pathophysiology related to GI damage among COVID-19 patients is most likely multifactorial. The most credible mechanism is direct virus-mediated tissue damage due to the existence of ACE2 receptors in the glandular cells of the intestine [26–29], in addition to the assimilation of the viral nucleocapsid protein among the epithelial cells of the stomach, duodenum, and rectum, as well as glandular enterocytes [27]. Additionally, diffused endothelial inflammation among the submucosal vessels of the small intestine in histopathological evidence and mesenteric ischemia suggest microvascular small-bowel injury [30]. The existence of infiltrating lymphocytes and plasma cells and interstitial edema in the gastric, duodenal, and rectal lamina propria of COVID-19 patients provides support for tissue damage mediated by inflammation [27]. It has also been suggested that the GI manifestations and severe disease progression are contributed by the modification of the intestinal flora caused by the virus [31].

4.1.3. Management Considerations

Specific management considerations should be considered by health practitioners, which should include differential diagnosis for COVID-19 among patients suffering from isolated GI symptoms in the non-appearance of respiratory symptoms [32]. Practitioners should prioritize testing for COVID-19 among patients presenting both GI and respiratory symptoms if testing resources are limited [33], and diagnostic endoscopy should only be utilized for emergency therapeutic reasons such as biliary obstruction or large-volume GI bleeding [34,35]. Hepatic transaminases should be monitored longitudinally, in particular among patients who are given investigational treatments. Decreased levels should not particularly be considered a contraindication when treating with tocilizumab, lopinavir, and remdesivir [36].

Table 1. Summary of research studies reporting gastrointestinal complications in COVID-19 patients.

Author Name, Year	Country	Type	Demographics	Complications Reported	Incidence	Mortality
El Moheb et al., 2020 [37]	United States	Retrospective cross-sectional	N = 92, Male: 52 (57%) Age: COVID-19 ARDS vs. non-COVID-19 ARDS: 64.5 (51.5–75.5) vs. 62 (48.5–71.5) (p = 0.24)	Transaminitis	COVID-19 ARDS vs. non-COVID-19 ARDS: 55% vs. 27% (p < 0.001)	COVID-19 ARDS vs. non-COVID-19 ARDS: 25% vs. 23% (p = 0.73)
				Severe ileus	48% vs. 22% (p < 0.001)	
				Bowel ischemia	4% vs. 0% (p = 0.04)	
Mauro et al., 2021 [38]	Italy	Retrospective cross-sectional	N = 23, Male: 18 (78.26%) Age: 75 years (IQR: 64–78).	Upper gastrointestinal bleeding (peptic ulcer)	0.47%	21.7%
Drake et al., 2021 [39]	United Kingdom	Prospective cohort	N = 41,025, Male: 21 758 (59.8%) Age: 71.1 years (SD: 18.7)	Gastrointestinal hemorrhage	1%	31.5%
				Pancreatitis	0.3%	
				Liver injury	7.4%	
Qayed et al., 2021 [40]	United States	Prospective cohort	N = 878 (Admitted to ICU), Male: 543 (61.8%) Age: 61.9 years (SD: 15.1)	Luminal and pancreaticobiliary	2.7%	34.1%
				Severe gastrointestinal bleeding	1.1%	
Bhayana et al., 2020 [41]	United States	Retrospective cross-sectional	N = 412 (224 abdominal imaging studies in 134 patients), Male: 241 (58%), Age: 57 years (Range 18–90)	Bowel-wall abnormalities	31% (Among CT images)	NA
				Pneumatosis or portal venous gas	Seen in 20% of CT images in ICU patients	
				Yellow discoloration of the bowel	2.23% of all abdominal imaging patients	
				Bowel infarction	1.49% of all abdominal imaging patients	
				Ischemic enteritis	1.49% of all abdominal imaging patients	
				Bile stasis	54% of ultrasound examinations in patients with liver laboratory findings	
Dane et al., 2020 [42]	United States	Retrospective cohort	N = 82 COVID-19 patients who underwent abdominopelvic ultrasound or CT), Male: 58 (71%), Mean age: 58.8 years (SD: 14.5)	Thromboembolic findings	11% (3 arterial, 1 venous, 4 infarcts, 1 portal vein thrombosis, and 2 lower extremity thrombosis)	NA

Table 1. *Cont.*

Author Name, Year	Country	Type	Demographics	Complications Reported	Incidence	Mortality
Kaafarani et al., 2020 [15]	United States	Retrospective cross-sectional	N= 141 (ICU patients), Male: 92 (65.2%), Median age: 57 (IQR: 47.70)	Transaminitis	67.3%	NA
				Acute cholecystitis	3.8%	
				Acute pancreatitis	1.0%	
				Hepatic ischemia and necrosis	1.0%	
				Gastric feeding intolerance	46.2%	
				Ileus	55.8%	
				Ogilvie like syndrome	1.9%	
				Bowel ischemia	3.8%	
				GI bleeding	10.6%	
				Clostridium difficile colitis	3.8%	

Abbreviations: ARDS, acute respiratory distress syndrome; CT, computed tomography; NA, Not available.

Table 2. Summary of case studies reporting gastrointestinal complications in COVID-19 patients.

Name of Author, Year, Ref	Demographics	Type of Complication	Past History	Laboratory Tests	Treatment	Days of Illness before Hospitalization	Hospital Stays	Outcome
De Nardi et al., 2020 [43]	53-year-old male patient	Bowel perforation	Hypertension and paroxysmal supraventricular tachycardia	Hb: 12.5, %, LDH: 313, WBC: 12.100, lymphocyte count: 6.5, CRP: 104 mg/L	At start: Antiretrovirals, hydroxychloroquine, anakinra, broad-spectrum antimicrobial treatment levofloxacin. During treatment: Low-molecular-weight heparin, anticoagulant therapy, and broad-spectrum antibiotic, piperacillin–tazobactam, and fluconazole	9 days	23 days	Cured
Del Hoyo et al., 2020 [44]	61 years, female	Extensive splanchnic vein thrombosis, liver, mesenteric and splenic ischemia	No	CRP: 9.43 mg/L, platelet count (46,000/µL), D-dimer levels: 43,998 µg/mL. AST 2728 U/L, ALT 1065 U/L	Enoxaparin 1 mg/kg SC q12h	NA	3 days	Died

Table 2. *Cont.*

Name of Author, Year, Ref	Demographics	Type of Complication	Past History	Laboratory Tests	Treatment	Days of Illness before Hospitalization	Hospital Stays	Outcome
Karna et al., 2020 [45]	61 years, female	Superior mesenteric artery thrombosis, gut ischemia	Hypertension	Hb: 7.1 mg/dL, TPC: 311,000 microliters, TLC: 23,000 per cubic millimeter, NLR: 18.5, monocyte: 5, CRP: 282 per cubic millimeter, aPTT: 32.9, PT/INR: 19/1.7	High-flow nasal oxygen (HFNO), cefoperazone-sulbactam, prophylactic enoxaparin, pantoprazole, vitamin C, and zinc	NA	Approximately 12 days	Died after surgery due to septic shock
Carll, Rady et al., 2021 [46]	Middle-aged woman	Cytomegalovirus hemorrhagic enterocolitis	No	Plasma interleukin (IL)-6: 14.1, elevated troponin-T, lymphocytopenia, and markedly elevated d-dimer, CRP and LDH	Remdesivir, two units of SARS-CoV-2 convalescent plasma, and systemic hydrocortisone IL-6 antagonist tocilizumab Ganciclovir Foscarnet systemic corticosteroids Ustekinumab	10 days	209 days	Cured
De Barry et al., 2020 [47]	79-year-old female	Arterial and venous abdominal thrombosis, extended bowel ischemia	No	CRP: 125 mg/L, hyperleukocytosis: (12,600/mm^3),	Laparotomy, thrombolysis and thrombectomy of the upper mesenteric artery	8 days	NA	Died
Chan et al., 2020 [48]	73-year-old male	Ischemic colitis	Hypertension and end-stage renal disease on hemodialysis	Hb: 5.6 g/dL, MCV: 86.1 fL, iron: 18 µg/dL, TIBC: 98 µg/dL, iron saturation: 18.4%, WBCs showed leucopenia 3.8 × 10^3/µL, lymphopenia with an absolute lymphocyte count of 600/µL, lactic acid level: 2 mmol/L, D-dimer: 3239 ng/mL, ferritin: 1713.5: ng/mL, CRP: 14.2 mg/dL.	Bowel rest, intravenous fluids, antibiotics (ciprofloxacin and metronidazole), and anticoagulants, Ciprofloxacin and metronidazole, anticoagulant	3 days	5 days	Died due to cardiac arrest
Corrêa Neto et al., 2020 [49]	80-year-old female	Acute perforated abdomen	Systemic arterial hypertension and ischemic heart disease	Leukocytosis: 19,950 mm^3, platelet count: 507,200 mm^3, GOT: 23.00 U/L, GPT: 41.00 U/L, creatinine: 5.54 mg/dL, urea: 139 mg/dL. D-dimer: 1466.8 ng/dL, ferritin: 1199 ng/dL, creatine phosphokinase: 239.00 U/L	Tazocin 4.5 g 3×/day and Azithromycin 500 mg/day, Rectosigmoidectomy with terminal colostomy	10 days	NA	Died
Hadi, Werge et al., 2020 [50]	47-years old woman	Acute pancreatitis	No	Pancreas-specific plasma amylase: 173 U/L	Fluid resuscitation and intravenous antibiotics	72 days	Patient was still admitted	N/A
Hadi, Werge et al., 2020 [50]	68-year-old woman	Acute pancreatitis	Hypertension, hypothyroidism, and osteoporosis	Amylase level: 85 U/L	Fluid resuscitation and intravenous antibiotics	2 days	Patient was still admitted	N/A

Table 2. *Cont.*

Name of Author, Year, Ref	Demographics	Type of Complication	Past History	Laboratory Tests	Treatment	Days of Illness before Hospitalization	Hospital Stays	Outcome
Hadi, Werge et al., 2020 [50]	71-year-old man	Acute pancreatitis	No	NA	Invasive mechanical ventilation, intravenous antibiotics, noradrenaline, and dopamine	3 days	NA	Died
Marchi, Vianello et al., 2020 [51]	73-year-old man	Cytomegalovirus-induced gastrointestinal bleeding and pancreatitis	Type 2 diabetes mellitus, hypertension, atrial fibrillation, multivessel coronary artery disease, and primary cutaneous large B-cell lymphoma leg type	CPR: 263 mg/L, leukocytosis: 16,610/mm^3, neutrophilia: 15,940/mm^3,	Empirical treatment was started with hydroxychloroquine, lopinavir/ritonavir, methylprednisolone	NA	43	Cured
Kangas-Dick, Prien et al., 2020 [52]	74-year-old male	Gastrointestinal perforation	No	Serum albumin 2.3 mg/dL WBCs: 15,900	Empirical treatment was started with hydroxychloroquine, azithromycin, and ceftriaxone	8–10 days	9 days	Dead
Farina, Rondi et al., 2020 [53]	70-year-old male	Acute bowel ischemia	No	WBCs: 15.3 × 10^3 µ/L, CRP: 149 mg/L	No	3 days	2 days	Dead
Moazzam, Salim et al., 2020 [54]	4 months, 25-day-old baby boy	Intussusception	No	CRP: 3.7 mg/L, Ferritin: 162.9, D-Dimer: 3.8 mcg/L	Co-amoxiclav, amikacin, metronidazole, paracetamol	2 days	2.5 days	Cured
Paul Joy et al., 2021 [55]	66-year-old male	Ischemic colitis	No	Rapid drop in Hb to 4.7 g/dL	Azithromycin, cefuroxime, hydroxychloroquine, methylprednisolone, tocilizumab and convalescent plasma	3 days	40 days	Cured
Ibrahim, Karuppasamy et al., 2020 [56]	33-year-old man	Paralytic ileus	No	ALT: 1589 U/L, AST: 1856 U/L	Ceftriaxone, azithromycin, hydroxychloroquine, methylprednisolone, and a dose of tocilizumab	2 days	NA	In ICU
Ibrahim, Karuppasamy et al., 2020 [56]	33-year-old man	Paralytic ileus	No	Blood urea: 55 78 mmol/L, creatinine: 1891 µmol/L, bicarbonate: 1.9 mmol/L, lipase: >1200 U/L, amylase: 390 U/L, ALT: 187 U/L, AST: 125 U/L	Prokinetic agents and intravenous potassium replacement	NA	NA	Patient is currently on renal replacement therapy

Abbreviations: WBCs, white blood cells; CRP, C-reactive protein; LDH, lactate dehydrogenase; AST, aspartate aminotransferase; ALT, alanine aminotransferase; Hb, hemoglobin; TPC, total platelet count; TLC, total leukocyte count; NLR, neutrophil-to-lymphocyte ratio; PT, prothrombin time; INR, international normalized ratio; aPTT, activated partial thromboplastin clotting time; MCV, mean corpuscular volume; TIBC, total iron-binding capacity; GOT, aspartate aminotransferase blood test; GPT, alanine aminotransferase blood test.

4.2. *Neurological System*

4.2.1. Complications

Our search identified 14 research studies reporting neurological complications during the course of COVID-19. These studies reported 26 neurological complications. Major complications in research studies were acute cerebrovascular disease including acute ischemic stroke, cerebral venous sinus thrombosis, cerebral hemorrhage (IR: 0.5–90.9%), anosmia (IR: 4.9–79.6%), dysgeusia (IR: 2.8–83.38%), encephalopathy/encephalitis with or without fever and hypoxia (IR: 0.19–35.2%), and seizures (IR: 0.5–27%). Other complications noted were impaired consciousness (IR: 7.5–9.6%), myalgia/myopathy/muscle pain (incidence: 9.3%, 17.2%/3.1%/15.1%), ataxia/movement disorders (incidence: 0.5%/0.7%), ageusia (incidence: 1.7%, 2.8%) and hyposmia (incidence: 5.1%, 20.4%). Rare complications included a combination of dysgeusia and hyposmia (incidence: 3.4%), dysgeusia and anosmia (incidence: 3.4%), ageusia and hyposmia (incidence: 3.4%), ageusia and insomnia (incidence: 8.5%), gustatory dysfunction (incidence: 88.8%), electrolyte disturbances (hypokalemia: 13%, hyponatremia: 11%, hypocalcemia: 7%), delayed recovery of mental status after sedation (2.5%), delirium (13.1%), dysautonomia (2.5%), Guillain–Barré Syndrome (0.19%), optic neuritis (0.19%), trigeminal neuralgia (3.3%), glossopharyngeal neuralgia (3.7%), vasglossopharyngeal neuralgia (0.8%), Restless Leg Syndrome (1.7%), and nerve pain (2.3%). All-cause mortality in research studies reporting neurological complications ranged from 0.46% to 24.60%. One study specified 54.5% mortality among patients with cerebrovascular disease, and one study reported 4.1% mortality among patients with all neurological complications (Table 3). In Figure 2, the prevalence in terms of the maximum percentage of neurological complications among different studies is presented.

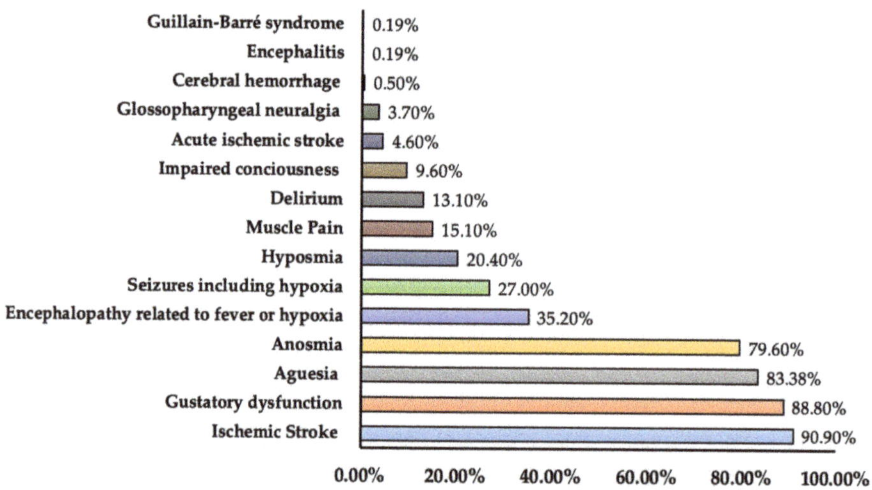

Figure 2. Prevalence of neurological complications among COVID-19 patients (prevalence represents maximum percentage reported in the literature).

We also included 10 case reports comprising 11 patients indicating the involvement of neurological complications. These reports identified a total of nine neurological complications. Major complications seen in case reports were encephalopathy/encephalitis (27.27%), Guillian–Barré Syndrome (27.27%), and epileptogenicity/focal seizures with impaired awareness (18.18%). Other complications included focal temporal lobe dysfunction (9.09%), meningitis (9.09%), intracranial hemorrhage (9.09%), acute myelitis (9.09%), Miller Fisher Syndrome (9.09%), and polyneuritis cranialis (9.09%). Among the case reports, seven (63.64%) patients were cured, and two (18.18%) patients were still hospitalized and undergoing treatment. No patient among 11 of them died (Table 4).

4.2.2. Underlying Pathophysiology

The underlying pathophysiological mechanisms proposed include direct invasion of neural parenchyma cells by the virus. The central nervous system is assessed by SARS-CoV-2 through the lamina cribrosa, olfactory bulb, and nasal mucosa or transport through the retrograde axonal. In the respiratory tree, ACE2 receptors are highly expressed in nasal epithelial cells [57,58], which may justify the symptoms of modified smell or taste mostly reported in outpatients retrospectively with SARS-CoV-2 [59–61]. The other complications are attributed to the neurovirulence of SARS-CoV-2, which reflects the prothrombotic and proinflammatory cascade resulting in cytokine storm [62], which in turn produces effects on the blood–brain barrier and brain vasculature. This has been particularly observed in critical patients experiencing toxic–metabolic prolongation of multi-organ dysfunction.

4.2.3. Management Considerations

Specific management considerations for health practitioners include continuous conformity to the guidelines established for acute ischemic stroke (thrombectomy and thrombolysis) [63]. Guidelines for the monitoring of post-acute care for pandemic restrictions should be adopted. A remote video assessment, whenever feasible, should be considered for hospitalized patients with symptoms that might be related to stroke [64]. A delayed or extended-interval dosing of long-term immunomodulatory therapies should be considered in diseases such as multiple sclerosis in SARS-CoV-2 patients [65].

Table 3. Summary of research studies reporting neurological complications in COVID-19 patients.

Author Name, Year, Ref	Country	Type of Study	Demographic	Complication	Incidence	Mortality
Klopfenstein et al., 2020 [66]	France	Retrospective Observational	N = 54, Female: 36 (67%), Mean Age: 47 years (SD: 16)	Anosmia	47%	4% (Overall hospitalization rate 37%)
Bagheri et al., 2020 [67]	Iran	Retrospective Cross-sectional study	N = 10,069, Female: 7162 (71.13%), Mean Age: 32.5 years (Range: 7–78)	Anosmia	76.24%	NA
				Aguesia	83.38%	
Giacomelli et al., 2020 [68]	China	Retrospective Cross-sectional study	N = 69, Male: 40 (67.8%) Median Age: 60 years (SD: 15.9)	Dysgeusia	8.5%	NA
				Ageusia	1.7%	
				Hyposmia	5.1%	
				Dysgeusia and hyposmia	3.4%	
				Dysgeusia and anosmia	3.4%	
				Ageusia and hyposmia	3.4%	
				Ageusia and anosmia	8.5%	
Li et al., 2020 [69]	China	Retrospective Observational Cohort	N = 219, Female: 130 (59.4%) Mean Age: 53.3 (57–91)	Acute ischemic stroke	4.6%	NA
				Cerebral venous sinus thrombosis	0.5%	
				Cerebral hemorrhage	0.5%	
Lu et al., 2020 [70]	China	Retrospective Observational Cohort	N = 304, Male: 182 (59.9%), Mean Age: 44 years	Encephalopathy	2.65%	3.31%
				Seizures including hypoxia	27%	
				Electrolyte disturbances including		
				Hypokalemia	13%	
				Hyponatremia	11%	
				Hypocalcemia	7%	
Ling Mao, 2020 [71]	China	Retrospective Observational Case Series	N = 214, Male: 87 (40.7%), Mean Age: 52.7 years (SD: 15.5)	Impaired consciousness	7.5%	0.46%
				Acute cerebrovascular disease	2.8%	
				Ataxia	0.5%	
				Seizure	0.5%	
Corrado Lodigiani, 2020 [72]	Italy	Retrospective Cross-Sectional	N = 388, Male: 68%, Median Age (range): 66 years (55–75)	Acute ischaemic stroke	2.5%	23.71%
Yanan Li, 2020 [69]	China	Retrospective Observational	N = 21, Male: 62.5%, Age: Mean (SD) 52.7 ± 15.5	Ischemic stroke	90.9%	54.5% (with cerebrovascular disease)
				Intracranial hemorrhage	9.1%	
Jerome R. Lechien, 2020 [59]	Europe	Prospective Cohort	N = 417, Female: 263 (63.1%), Mean Age: 36.9 years (SD: 11.4)	Anosmia	79.6%	NA
				Hyposmia	20.4%	
				Gustatory dysfunction	88.8%	

Table 3. *Cont.*

Author Name, Year, Ref	Country	Type of Study	Demographic	Complication	Incidence	Mortality
Fernando Daniel Flores-Silva, 2021 [73]	Mexico	Prospective Cross-Sectional Observational	N = 221, Male: 59.3%, Age: Mean (SD); 36.9 ± 11.4	Delayed recovery of mental status after sedation	2.5%	24.6%
				Seizures	0.8%	
				Stroke	0.8%	
				Encephalitis	0.2%	
				Delirium	13.1%	
Carlos Manuel Romero-Sánchez, 2020 [74]	Spain	Retrospective Observational	N = 841, Male: 473 (56.2%), Mean Age: 66.42 years (SD: 14.96)	Myalgia	17.2%	4.1% (with neurologic complications)
				Anosmia	4.9%	
				Dysgeusia	6.2%	
				Disorders of consciousness	19.6%	
				Myopathy	3.1%	
				Dysautonomia	2.5%	
				Cerebrovascular disease	1.7%	
				Seizures	0.7%	
				Movement disorders	0.7%	
				Encephalitis	0.19%	
				Guillain–Barre syndrome	0.19%	
				Optic neuritis	0.19%	
Ömer Karadaş, 2020 [75]	Turkey	Prospective Cross-Sectional	N = 239, Male: 133 (55.6%), Mean Age: 46.46 years (SD: 15.41)	Impaired consciousness-confusion	9.60%	NA
				Muscle pain	15.1%	
				Cerebrovascular disorders	3.8%	
				Trigeminal neuralgia	3.3%	
				Glossopharyngeal neuralgia	3.7%	
				Vasoglossopharyngeal neuralgia	0.8%	
				Restless Leg Syndrome	1.7%	

Table 3. *Cont.*

Author Name, Year, Ref	Country	Type of Study	Demographic	Complication	Incidence	Mortality
Mao et al. 2020 [71]	China	Retrospective Observational Case Series	N = 214, Male: 87 (40.7%), Mean Age: 52.7 years (SD: 15.5)	Impaired consciousness	7.50%	NA
				Seizures	0.50%	
				Acute cerebrovascular disease	2.80%	
				Anosmia	5.10%	
				Dysgeusia	5.60%	
				Nerve pain	2.3%	
Marco Luigetti, 2020 [76]	Italy	Retrospective Observational	N = 213, Male: 137 (64.32%), Mean Age: 70.2 (SD: 13.9)	Encephalopathy related to fever or hypoxia	35.2%	18.7%
				Encephalopathy not related to fever or hypoxia	5.1%	
				Ageusia/dysgeusia	2.8%	
				Anosmia/hyposmia	6.1%	
				Seizure	2.8%	
				Ischemic stroke	0.9%	
				Hemorrhagic stroke	0.9%	
				Encephalitis	0.5%	
				Myalgia	9.3%	

Table 4. Summary of case studies reporting neurological complications in COVID-19 patients.

Name of Author, Year, Ref	Demographics	Type of Complication	Past History	Laboratory Tests	Treatment	Days of Illness before Hospitalization	Hospital Stays	Outcome
Filatov et al., 2020 [17]	74-year-old male	Encephalopathy, focal temporal lobe dysfunction, and epileptogenicity	Chronic obstructive pulmonary disease (COPD), Parkinson's disease, cardioembolic stroke, atrial fibrillation, cellulitis	Chest X-ray showed small right pleural effusion as well as bilateral ground-glass opacities. CT of chest revealed patchy bibasilar consolidations and subpleural opacities. CT scan of head showed area of encephalomalacia in the left temporal region	Antiepileptic medication, vancomycin, meropenem, acyclovir, hydroxychloroquine and lopinavir/ritonavir	NA	NA	Patient was still in the ICU, Critically ill with poor prognosis

Table 4. *Cont.*

Name of Author, Year, Ref	Demographics	Type of Complication	Past History	Laboratory Tests	Treatment	Days of Illness before Hospitalization	Hospital Stays	Outcome
Moriguchi et al., 2020 [77]		Meningitis/encephalitis	No	Blood investigation demonstrated high levels of WBCs, neutrophil dominance, and increased CRP. The CSF cell count was 12/μL	Intravenous (IV) ceftriaxone, steroids, aciclovir, and vancomycin. Intravenous administration of Levetiracetam, Favipiravir was also administered	NA	NA	Treatment continued
Poyiadji et al., 2020 [78]	58-year-old female	Acute hemorrhagic necrotizing encephalopathy	No	CT scan of head showed bilateral medial thalami. Brain MRI showed hemorrhagic rim	Intravenous immunoglobulin	3 days	NA	NA
Gutiérrez-Ortiz et al., 2020 [79]	50-year-old male	Miller Fisher syndrome	Bronchial asthma	Neuro-ophthalmological testing showed right internuclear ophthalmoparesis along with right fascicular oculomotor palsy. Lymphopenia: 1000 cells/μL, CRP: 2.8 mg/dL, CSF examination opening pressure of 11 cm H_2O	IV immunoglobulin 0.4 g/kg for 5 days	2 days	2 weeks	Ataxia and cranial neuropathies improved, Discharged
Gutiérrez-Ortiz et al., 2020 [79]	39-year-old male	Polyneuritis cranialis	No	Neuro-ophthalmological exam showed fixed nystagmus. severe abduction deficits were also observed in both eyes	Treated symptomatically with acetaminophen	3 days	NA	Discharged, Complete recovery afterward
Sharifi-Razavi et al., 2020 [80]	79-year-old male	Intracranial hemorrhage	No	Lymphopenia: 590 cells/mm^2, ESR: 85 mm/h, CRP 10 mg/L, creatinine: 1.4 mg/dL, platelets: 210 × 10^9/L, PT: 12 s, INR: 1, PTT: 64 s	NA	3 days	NA	NA
Paybast et al., 2020 [81]	38-year-old male	Guillain–Barré Syndrome	Hypertension, upper respiratory tract infection	Nerve conduction study was performed which demonstrated considerable decrease in the amplitude of compound motor action potentials	Therapeutic plasma exchange, labetalol by intravenous bolus along with hydroxychloroquine sulfate orally	5 days	NA	Discharged

Table 4. *Cont.*

Name of Author, Year, Ref	Demographics	Type of Complication	Past History	Laboratory Tests	Treatment	Days of Illness before Hospitalization	Hospital Stays	Outcome
Bozzali et al., 2021 [82]	54-year-old female	Focal seizures with impaired awareness	No	Brain MRI scan which showed white matter hyperintensities on T2-weighted images. CSF examination showed a slight elevation of proteins (55 mg/dL) while cell count was normal	Levetiracetam therapy showed partial benefit so treatment was shifted to carbamazepine	NA	NA	Cured
H. Zhao et al., 2020 [83]	61-year-old female	Guillain–Barré Syndrome	No	Lymphocytopenia: 0· 52 × 10^9/L, thrombocytopenia: 113 × 10^9/L	Intravenous immunoglobulin, rbidol, lopinavir, and ritonavir	1 day	30 days	Cured and discharged
K. Zhao et al., 2020 [84]	66-year-old male	Acute myelitis	No	Decreased RBCs, Hb, serum total protein, serum albumin, elevated CRP, ALT, AST, and CK.	Ganciclovir, lopinavir/ritonavir, moxifloxacin, meropenem, glutathione, dexamethasone, human immunoglobulin, mecobalamin, and pantoprazole	2 days	NA	Cured and discharged
Sedaghat and Karimi 2020 [85]	65 years- old male	Guillain–Barré syndrome	Type 2 diabetes mellitus	Serum glucose: 159 mg/dL, BUN: 19 mg/dL, creatinine: 0.8 mg/dL, ALT: 35 IU/L, AST: 47 IU/L, WBC count: 14,700 cells per microliter; ESR: 72 mm/hour, CRP: 2+, Hb: 11.6 g/dL	Hydroxychloroquine, lopinavir/ritonavir (LPV/RTV), and azithromycin	5 days	9 days	Cured

Abbreviations: WBCs, white blood cells; RBCs, red blood cells; CRP, C-reactive protein; Hb, hemoglobin; BUN, bloodurea nitrogen; CT, computed tomography; AST, aspartate aminotransferase; ALT, alanine aminotransferase; CK, creatine kinase; ESR, erythrocyte sedimentation rate; MRI, magnetic resonance imaging; CSF, cerebrospinal fluid; PT, prothrombin time; PPT, partial thromboplastin time.

4.3. Renal System

4.3.1. Complications

We included 16 studies reporting renal complications among COVID-19 patients. A total of seven renal complications were noted in research studies. The major complication was acute kidney injury (AKI)/acute renal failure (IR: 0.5–68.8%). Other complications included electrolyte disturbances (incidence: 7.2%, 23%), acidosis (incidence: 9%, 12%), proteinuria (incidence: 6.5%, 43.9%), hematuria (incidence: 26.7%), alkalosis (incidence: 28%) and continuous renal replacement therapy clotting due to hypertriglyceridemia. All-cause mortality ranged from 1.4% to 52.4%, whereas 9% to 93.6% of patients were still hospitalized due to at least one complication. Mortality rates caused by AKI/kidney disease ranged between 16.1% and 66.35%, and patients still hospitalized due to them varied significantly. In one retrospective cohort study, 50% of non-survivors died due to acute kidney injury [86]. In one retrospective case series, mortality was observed among patients with acidosis (12%), alkalosis (28%), AKI (25%), and hyperkalemia (23%) [87] (Table 5). In Figure 3, the prevalence in terms of the maximum percentage of renal complications among different studies was presented.

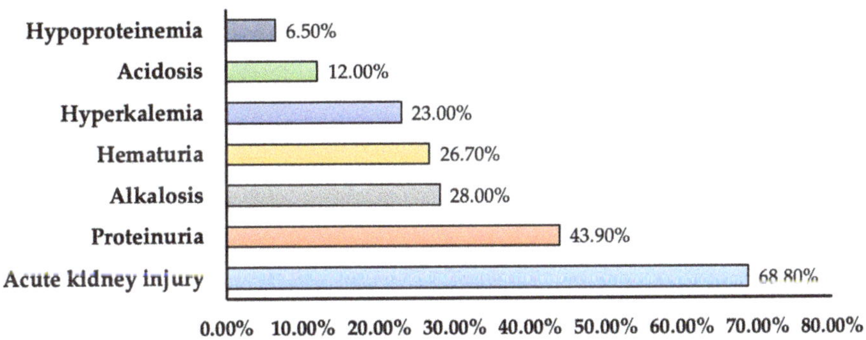

Figure 3. Prevalence of renal complications among COVID-19 patients (prevalence represents maximum percentage reported in the literature).

We included seven case reports comprising seven patients in the current review. These case reports reported a total of eight renal complications. The major complications identified were renal/splenic/cerebral infarct or aortic thrombosis (57.14%). Rare complications were catastrophic thrombotic syndrome (14.29%), glomerulonephritis (14.29%), polycystic kidney disease (14.29%), IgA neuropathy (14.29%), and spinal epidural abscess (14.29%). Of the seven patients in these case reports, 71.43% (n = 5/7) were cured/improved, one patient died, and one patient was discharged but not completely cured (Table 6).

4.3.2. Underlying Pathophysiology

Several possible pathophysiological mechanisms have been identified for renal abnormalities. Firstly, the virus may infect the renal cells directly, as evidenced by the existence of ACE2 receptors on them and histopathological findings [88–90]. Secondly, microvascular dysfunction is incidental to endothelial damage as demonstrated by renal lymphocytic endothelialitis, and moreover to the inclusion of particles of the virus in the endothelium of glomerular capillary cells [30]. Thirdly, cytokine storm may have a vital role in the immunopathology of AKI [91]. Another likely mechanism for glomerular injury is arbitrated by specific immunological effector mechanisms induced by the virus or viral antigen immunocomplexes [88]. In addition, proteinuria is not considered the classic manifestation of AKI; short-term heavy albuminuria might arise from direct podocyte injury or endothelial dysfunction. Other causative etiologies for renal injury include acute respiratory distress syndrome, interstitial nephritis, volume depletion, and rhabdomyolysis [92].

4.3.3. Management Considerations

Specific management considerations by health practitioners for managing renal complications should include evaluation of the albumin-to-creatinine ratio and complete urine analysis, providing the coalition of hematuria and proteinuria with the outcomes [93,94]. Empirical systemic low-dose anticoagulants, when initiating and also in the routine management of RRT extracorporeal circuits, should be considered [95]. Consideration should be taken to co-localize patients requiring RRT, and a shared protocol for RRT should be used [96]. Additionally, acute peritoneal dialysis among select patients should be considered so as to minimize the requirement of personnel [96].

Table 5. Summary of research studies reporting renal complications in COVID-19 patients.

Author Name, Year, Ref	Country	Type	Demographic	Complication	Incidence	Mortality
Hirsch, Ng et al., 2020 [97]	USA	Observational Cohort Study	N = 5449, Male 3317 (60.87%) Median Age: 6[illegible].0 years (IQR: 52–75)	AKI	36.6%	35% (Among AKI patients) 39% patients still admitted to hospital.
Guan, Ni et al., 2020 [98]	China	Observational Cohort Study	N = 1099, Male 637 (57.96%) Median Age: 5[illegible] years (IQR: 46–67)	AKI	0.5%	1.4% 93.6% patients still admitted to hospital
Yan, Zuo et al., 2021 [99]	China	Observational Cohort Study	N = 882, Male: 440 (49.89%) Median Age: 7[illegible] years (IQR: 68–77)	AKI	13%	59.1% (Among AKI cohort) 24.3% AKI patients were still admitted to hospital
Cheng, Luo et al., 2020 [93]	China	Prospective Cohort Study	N = 701, Male: 367 (52.35%) Median Age: 63 years (IQR: 50–71)	AKI Proteinuria Hematuria	5.1% 43.9% 26.7%	16.1% (with kidney disease)
Abramovitz et al., 2023 [100]	USA	Retrospective Case Series	N = 11	Continuous renal replacement therapy clotting due to hypertriglyceridemia	73% related to propofol use causing hypertriglyceridemia 27% due to total parenteral nutrition administration	NA
Aggarwal et al., 2020 [101,102]	USA	Retrospective Cross-Sectional	N = 16, Male: [illegible]2 (75%), Median Age: 67 years (Range: 38–95)	AKI	68.8%	19%
Arentz et al., 2020 [102]	USA	Retrospective Cross-Sectional	N = 21, Male: [illegible]2%, Mean Age: 70 years (Range: 43–92)	Acute kidney failure	19.1%	52.4%
Tao Guo et al., 2020 [103]	China	Retrospective Case Series	N = 187, Male 91 (48.7%) Mean Age: 58.50 years (SD: 14.66)	AKI	14.6%	23%
Chaolin Huang et al., 2020 [104]	China	Prospective Cross-Sectional	N = 41, Male: 30 (73%), Median Age: 49·0 years (IQR: 41·0–58·0)	AKI	7%	15% 17% patients still admitted to hospital
Richardson et al., 2020 [105]	USA	Retrospective Cross-Sectional	N = 5700, Male: 3437 (60.3%), Median Age: [illegible]3 years (IQR: 52–75)	AKI	22.2%	66.35% (Among AKI patients), 27.63% AKI patients still admitted to hospital
Chan et al., 2021 [106]	USA	Retrospective Observational	N = 3993, Female:1704 (43%), Median Age: [illegible]4 years (IQR: 56–78)	AKI	46%	50% (Among AKI patients)
Mohamed et al., 2020 [107]	USA	Prospective Observational	N = 575, Female: 263 (45.74%), Median Age: 65 years (IQR: 36–96)	AKI	28%	50% (Among AKI cohort)
Zhou et al., 2020 [86]	China	Retrospective Cohort	N = 191, Male: 119 (62%), Median Age: 56 years (IQR: 46–67)	AKI Acidosis	15% 9%	50% (Among non-survivors)
Argenziano et al., 2020 [108]	USA	Retrospective Case Series	N = 1000, Male: 596 (59.6%), Median Age: 63.0 (IQR: 50.0–75.0)	AKI	34%	9% 21.1% still admitted to hospital

Table 5. *Cont.*

Author Name, Year, Ref	Country	Type	Demographic	Complication	Incidence	Mortality
Chen et al., 2020 [87]	China	Retrospective Case Series	N = 274, Male: 171 (62%), Median Age; 62.0 years (IQR: 44.0–70.0)	Acidosis	12%	14% (Among acidosis patients)
				Alkalosis	28%	40% (Among alkalosis patients)
				AKI	11%	25% (Among AKI patients
				Hyperkalemia	23%	37% (Among hyperkalemia patients)
Shi et al., 2020 [109]	China	Retrospective Cohort	N = 416, Female: 211 (50.7%), Median Age: 64.0 years (Range: 21–95)	Electrolyte disturbance	7.2%	13.7%, 76.1% still admitted to hospital
				AKI	1.9%	
				Hypoproteinemia	6.5%	

Abbreviation: AKI, acute kidney injury.

Table 6. Summary of case studies reporting renal complications in COVID-19 patients.

Name of Author, Year, Ref	Country	Age, Gender	Type of Complication	Past History	Laboratory Tests	Treatment	Days of Illness before Hospitalization	Hospital Stays	Outcome
Moeinzadeh, Dezfouli et al., 2020 [110]	Iran	25 years, Male	Glomerulonephritis	No	Creatine: 4.2, CRP: 2+, ESR: 120 mm/h, Hb: 4.5 g/dL, WBC: 4500/mm^3, protein in urine analysis = 3+	1 g of methylprednisolone IV, plasmapheresis with PLASMART, Versatile™ PES, 3 doses intravenous immunoglobulin (IVIG), 20 g each time	2 days	17 days	Cured
Haque, Jahan et al., 2020 [111]	Bangladesh	68 years, Male	Polycystic kidney disease	Nephrolithotomy	Hb: 9.2 gm/dL, thrombocytopenia: 112,000/cm^2, serum creatinine: 3.3 mg/dL, urea: 90 mg/dL	Anticoagulation along with linagliptin, aspirin, atorvastatin	N/R	More than 30 days	Expired
Mavraganis et al., 2022 [112]	Greece	64 years, Male	Renal infarct, splenic infarct, aortic thrombosis	No	Lymphopenia: 950 lymphocytes), ALT: 130 U/L, AST: 135 U/L, D-dimers:0.57 mg/L, hs-CRP: 19.9 mg/dL, CK: 1215 U/L, LDH: 551 U/L	Low-molecular-weight heparin at prophylactic dose, intravenous dexamethasone and remdesivir, omeprazole, tocilizumab, and ceftaroline	2 weeks	19 days	Discharged, Not cured completely

Table 6. *Cont.*

Name of Author, Year, Ref	Country	Age, Gender	Type of Complication	Past History	Laboratory Tests	Treatment	Days of Illness before Hospitalization	Hospital Stays	Outcome
Göre et al., 2022 [113]	Turkey	56 years, Male	IgA neuropathy and spinal epidural abscess	No	Creatinine: 3.64 mg/dL, GFR: 18 mL/min/1.73 m^2, leukocytes: 9.9 × 10^{-9}/L, lymphocytes: 1.87× 10^{-9}/L, neutrophils: 7.12 × 10^{-9}/L, platelets: 382 × 10^{-9}/L, Hb: 6.9 g/dL	Teicoplanin and ciprofloxacin, methylprednisolone at dose of 1 mg/kg/day	Almost one month	25 days	Marked improvement in complications
Rigual et al., 2022 [114]	Spain	53 years, Male	Cerebral, splenic, and renal infarction	No	D-dimer: 850 ng/dL, IL-6: 8.60 pg/dL, ferritin: 499 ng/dL fibrinogen 541 mg/dL, CRP: 7.8 mg/dL,	LMWH 1 mg subcutaneous enoxaparin/kg/24 h along with ASA methylprednisolone 1 mg/kg/24 h	16 days	30 days	Cured
Brem et al., 2022 [115]	Morocco	59 years, Male	Renal and splenic infarct with catastrophic thrombotic syndrome	Diabetes mellitus	WBCs: 15,000 elements/mm^3, lymphopenia: 450 elements/mm^3, platelets: 120,000 elements/mm^3, D-dimer level: 33,620 ng/mL, fibrinogen: 4.5 g/L, CRP: 189.88 mg/L, ferritin: 4150 ng/mL, LDH: 1221 unit/L, CK level: 20,500 U/L, creatinine level: 9.59 mg/L	LMWH 60 mg twice a day after embolectomy. Infracondylar amputation of the right lower limb afterward	NA	NA	Cured
Gjonbalaj et al., 2020 [116]	Kosovo	50 years, Male	Renal artery thrombosis	No	CRP: 4.3 mg/dL, troponin: 2.3 pg/mL urea: 29.96 g/dL, creatinine: 1.2 mg/dL, D-dimer: 142 ng/mL, CK-MB: 2.2 ng/mL.	Thrombus aspiration plus bolus administration of tirofiban. Oral anticoagulant therapy	2 days	3 days	Cured

Abbreviations: CRP, C-reactive protein; LDH, lactate dehydrogenase; Hb, hemoglobin; ALT, alanine aminotransferase; AST, aspartate aminotransferase; hs-CRP, high-sensitivity C-reactive protein; GFR, glomerular filtration rate; CK, creatine kinase; CK-MB, creatine kinase–myoglobin binding; LMWH, low-molecular-weight heparin; ASA, acetyl salicylic acid.

4.4. Cardiovascular System

4.4.1. Complications

We have included 18 research studies reporting cardiovascular complications. In total, 15 complications were uncovered from these research studies. The major complications in research studies included acute cardiac injury/non-coronary myocardial injury (IR: 7.2–55.56%), arrhythmia/ventricular tachycardia/ventricular fibrillation (IR: 5.9–16.7%), coagulopathy/venous thromboembolism (IR: 19–34.4%), and myocardial infarction/heart failure (IR: 23.0–44.44%). Other complications included acute coronary syndrome and cardiac insufficiency (incidence: 0.96% and 17.4%). In one study, disseminated intravascular coagulation was seen in 71.4% of the non-survivors. All-cause mortality ranged from 4.3% to 45%, and among in-hospital patients, it ranged from 6.7% to 76.7%. In one retrospective case series, 77% of acute cardiac injury patients and 49% of heart failure patients did not survive [87] (Table 7). In Figure 4, the prevalence in terms of the maximum percentage of cardiovascular complications among different studies was presented.

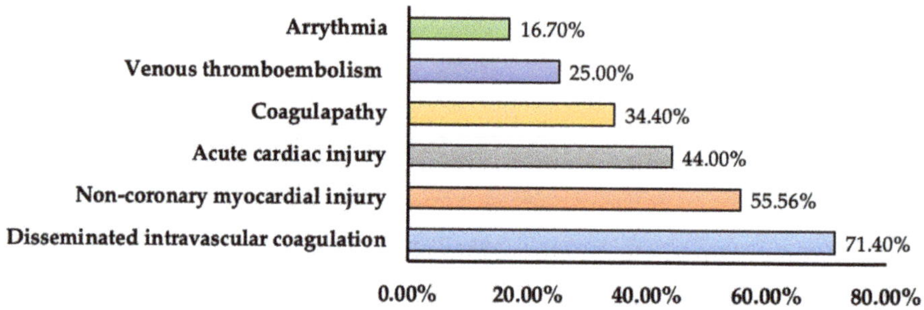

Figure 4. Prevalence of cardiovascular complications among COVID-19 patients (prevalence represents maximum percentage reported in the literature).

We have also included 11 case reports (11 patients) reporting cardiovascular complications. From case reports, a total of 10 cardiovascular complications were identified. Major complications in case reports were fulminant myocarditis (27.27%) and Takotsubo syndrome (18.18%). Other complications included myopericarditis complicated by cardiac tamponade (9.09%) and isolated hemorrhagic pericardial effusion with tamponade (9.09%). Of the twelve patients in case reports, five patients (33.33%) improved/were cured and were discharged from the hospitals, while two patients (16.67%) died (Table 8).

4.4.2. Underlying Pathophysiology

The underlying pathophysiology of CV complications is most likely multifactorial. ACE2 is highly expressed in endothelial cells, fibroblasts, and myocytes of the CV tissue [90,117], and direct viral injury is one possible mechanism. Myocarditis, MI, and circulatory failure may develop due to viral load and inflammatory infiltrates, as evidenced by some autopsy studies [118–120] and pathological reports [121,122]. In addition, endothelial damage mediated by viruses [30] and cytokine storms can be another assumed underlying mechanism for myocardial injury [123]. In general, viral infections further predispose patients to MI [124], and this risk is elevated in COVID-19 patients, with evidence of unjustifiably escalated hypercoagulability, which induces MI mediated by thrombotic events. Furthermore, isolated right ventricular malfunction may arise due to pulmonary thromboembolism [125,126] and increased pulmonary vascular pressures due to ARDS [127].

4.4.3. Management Considerations

Important management considerations for CV complications by health practitioners should not include the discontinuation of angiotensin-converting enzyme inhibitors or angiotensin-receptor blockers in patients who are already using them at home, and assessment should be made on the basis of individual patient condition [128,129]. Furthermore, those who have torsades de pointes risk and are treated with drugs for QTc prolongation should be monitored by telemetry, and an electrocardiogram should be performed [130]. Above all, in order to minimize the viral transmission risk, the utility of diagnostic modalities (endomyocardial biopsies, invasive hemodynamic assessments, and cardiac imaging) should be considered carefully [131,132]. The preferred approach for most patients with ST-segment elevation MI is primary percutaneous coronary intervention. Furthermore, fibrinolytic therapy in specific patients should be considered if personal protective supplies are unavailable [133–135].

Table 7. Summary of research studies reporting cardiovascular complications in COVID-19 patients.

Author Name, Year, Ref	Country	Type of Study	Demographic	Complication	Incidence	Mortality
Huang et.al., 2020 [104]	China	Prospective Cross-Sectional	N = 41, Male: 30 (73%) Median Age: 49 years (IQR: 41.0–58.0)	Acute cardiac injury	12%	15% 17% still admitted to hospital
Dawei Wang et al., 2020 [136]	China	Retrospective Case Series	N = 138, Male: 75 (54.3%) Median Age: 56 years (IQR: 42–68)	Arrhythmia Acute cardiac injury	16.7% 7.2%	4.3%
Hong et al., 2020 [137]	South Korea	Retrospective Cross-Sectional	N = 98, Female: 60 (61.2%) Mean Age: 55.4 years (SD: 17.1)	Acute cardiac injury	11.2%	5.1% 58.2% still admitted to hospital
Tao Guo et al., 2020 [103]	China	Retrospective Case Series	N = 187, Male: 91 (48.7%) Mean Age: 58.50 years (SD: 14.66)	Ventricular tachycardia/ventricular fibrillation Coagulopathy	5.9% 34.4%	23%
Shaobo Shi et al., 2020 [109]	China	Retrospective Cohort	N = 416, Female: 211 (50.7%) Mean Age: 64 years (Range: 21–95)	Myocardial injury	19.7%	13.7% 76.7% still admitted to hospital
Zhou et al., 2020 [86]	China	Retrospective Cohort	N = 191, Male: 119 (62%) Median Age: 56.0 years (IQR: 46.0–67.0)	Heart failure Coagulopathy Acute cardiac injury	23% 19% 17%	28.27%
Songping Cui et al., 2020 [138]	China	Retrospective Cross-Sectional	N = 81, Female: 44 (54%) Mean Age: 59.9 years (Range 32–91),	Venous thromboembolism	25%	9.87% (All were VTE patients) Overall 11% patients remained in hospital
Chen et al., 2020 [87]	China	Retrospective Case Series	N = 274, Male: 171 (62%), Median Age: 62.0 years (IQR: 44.0–70.0)	Acute cardiac injury Heart failure	44% 24%	77% (Among acute cardiac injury patients) 49% (Among heart failure patients)
Yu Y et al., 2020 [139]	China	Prospective Cross-Sectional	N = 226, Male 139 (61.5%) Age: 64 (IQR: 57–70)	Cardiac injury Arrhythmia	27% 9.3%	38.5% 6.7% of overall patients were still admitted to hospital
Victoria L. Cammann et al., 2020 [140]	Italy, Spain, and Switzerland	Retrospective Cohort	N = 45, Male: 37 (82.2%), Mean Age: 69.7 years (SD: 11.1)	Acute coronary syndromes	0.96%	27.3% (Among COVID-19-positive acute coronary syndrome patients)
Zhou et al., 2020 [141]	China	Retrospective Cross-Sectional	N = 254, Male: 115 (45.28%) Mean Age: 50.6 years (Range: 15–87)	Acute heart failure Arrthymias	2.4% 6.3%	6.3%
Tang et al., 2020 [142]	China	Retrospective Cohort	N = 183, Male 98 (54%) Mean Age: 54.1 years (Range: 14–94)	Disseminated intravascular coagulation	71.4% (Among non-survivors)	11.5%

Table 7. *Cont.*

Author Name, Year, Ref	Country	Type of Study	Demographic	Complication	Incidence	Mortality
Ruan et al., 2020 [143]	China	Retrospective Cohort	N = 150, Female 48 (32%) Mean Age: Died = 67 years (15–31), Discharged = 50 years (44–81)	Among death group: Myocardial damage (some with fulminant myocarditis) Respiratory failure + myocardial damage (some with fulminant myocarditis)	7% 33%	45%
Lang Wang et al., 2020 [144]	China	Retrospective Cross-Sectional	N = 339, Female: 173 (51.0%), Median Age: 69 years (Range: 65–76	Acute cardiac injury Arrhythmia Cardiac insufficiency	21% 10.4% 17.4%	19.2%
K. Liu et al., 2020 [145]	China	Retrospective Cross-Sectional	N = 137, Female: 76 (55.47%) Median Age: 57 years (Range: 20–83 years)	Arrhythmia	7.3%	11.7% (Among patients with complications)
Wang et al., 2020 [136]	China	Retrospective Case Series	N = 138, Male: 75 (54.3%) Age Median:56 years (IQR: 42–58)	Arrhythmia Acute cardiac injury	16.7% 7.2%	4.3%
Wei JF et al., 2020 [146]	China	Prospective Cohort	N = 101, Male: 54 (53.5%) Age: 49 (IQR: 34–62)	Acute myocardial injury	15.8%	2.97% (Among acute myocardial injury)
Sripal Bangalore et al., 2020 [147]	USA	Retrospective Case Series	N = 18, Male: 15 (83%) Median Age: 63 years (Range: 54–73)	ST-segment elevation Myocardial infarction Non-coronary myocardial injury	100% 44.44% 55.56%	50% (Among myocardial infarction patients) 90% (Among non-coronary myocardial injury patients)

Table 8. Summary of case studies reporting cardiovascular complications in COVID-19 patients.

Name of Author, Year, Ref	Age, Gender	Type of Complication	Past History	Laboratory Tests	Treatment	Days of Illness before Hospitalization	Hospital Stays	Outcome
Richard, Robinson et al., 2020 [148]	28-year-old female	Fulminant myocarditis	Diabetes mellitus type 1, diabetic gastroparesis, asthma, anxiety, depression	WBCs: 29 × $10^3/\mu L$, Hb: 10.3 g/dL, hematocrit: 31%, creatinine: 4.4 mg/dL, glucose: 1679 mg/dL, potassium: 2.9 mmol/L, lactic acid level: 17.1 mg/dL, CRP: 2.47 mg/dL, LDH: 296 U/L, ferritin: 119 ng/mL, troponin: 0.04 ng/mL	IV methylprednisolone 1 g daily for three days, IV steroids	NA	NA	Patient clinically improved

Table 8. *Cont.*

Name of Author, Year, Ref	Age, Gender	Type of Complication	Past History	Laboratory Tests	Treatment	Days of Illness before Hospitalization	Hospital Stays	Outcome
Zeng et al., 2020 [149]	63-year-old male	Fulminant myocarditis Disseminated intravascular coagulation	Allergic cough Smoking	NT-proBNP 750 pg/mL, IL-6: 7.63 pg/mL. troponin I: 0.10 g/L, Candida, human α-herpesvirus, and β-herpesvirus were also detected	Lopinavir–ritonavir, methylprednisolone, interferon α-1b, piperacillin–tazobactam immunoglobulin	NA	33 days	Died
Fiore et al., 2021 [150]	45-year-old male	Cardiogenic shock Myocarditis	No	Hs-troponin T: normal, lactate: normal, NT-proBNP: 945 pg/dL, CRP: normal, left ventricular ejection fraction: 40–45%	Hydroxychloroquine 200 mg bid, broad-spectrum empirical antibiotic therapy	4 days	Almost a month	Discharged
Hu, Ma et al., 2021 [151]	37-year-old male	Myocarditis	Chest pain, dyspnea, diarrhea	Increased BNP and CK-MB, ECG: ST↑ (III and AVF), no coronary stenosis in CT angiography	Methylprednisolone (200 mg/day, 4 days), immunoglobulin (20 g/day, 4 days), norepinephrine, diuretic (toracemide and furosemide), milrinone, piperacillin sulbactam, pantoprazole	3 days	NA	NA
Hua et al., 2020 [152]	47-year-old female	Myopericarditis complicated by cardiac tamponade	No	Troponin T levels were 225 and 253 ng/L	IV fluid resuscitation, vasopressor support	NA	NA	NA
Dabbagh et al., 2020 [153]	67-year-old female	Isolated hemorrhagic pericardial effusion with tamponade	Nonischemic cardiomyopathy with left ventricular ejection fraction	Hs-troponin I: <18 ng/L, BNP: 54 pg/mL CRP: 15.9 mg/dL, ferritin: 593 ng/mL, D-dimer: 6.52 mg/mL, interleukin-6: 8 pg/mL	Hydroxychloroquine along with colchicine and glucocorticoid	NA	NA	Discharged
Danzi et al., 2020 [154]	75-year-old female	Acute pulmonary embolism	No	Leucocytosis: 11.360/mm^2, CRP: 180 mg/L, troponin I: 3240.4 ng/mL, D-dimer: 21 μg/mL	LMWH, lopinavir/ritonavir, and hydroxychloroquine	10 days	NA	NA
Meyer et al., 2020 [155]	83-year-old female	Takotsubo syndrome	Chronic hypertension	Cardiac troponin T: 1142 ng/L	Conventional heart failure medication	3 days	10 days	Discharged
Minhas et al., 2020 [156]	58-year-old women	Takotsubo syndrome	Diabetes mellitus type 2, hypertension, and dyslipidemia	Troponin I level: 11.02 ng/mL, lymphocyte count: 1.04 K/mm^3	Hydroxychloroquine, dobutamine	5 days	NA	Not cured completely but discharged

Table 8. *Cont.*

Name of Author, Year, Ref	Age, Gender	Type of Complication	Past History	Laboratory Tests	Treatment	Days of Illness before Hospitalization	Hospital Stays	Outcome
Jud et al., 2021 [157]	24-year-old women	Vascular reactivity and Arterial stiffness	No	Flow-mediated dilation: 0.0%, nitroglycerin-mediated dilation: 17.24%, aortic pulse-wave analysis: 5.6 m/s, ultrasonography revealed augmentation index: 13%, and carotid intima–media thickness of 0.4 mm	NA	NA	NA	NA
Xu et al., 2020 [122]	50-year-old male	Cardiac arrest	No	WBCs: 6.28 $\times 10^9$/L, Hb: 134.00 g/L, latelet count: 205.00 $\times 10^9$/L, Creatininse: 67 µmol/L Pressure of oxygen in arterial blood: 28 mmHg, PT: 14.9 s	Interferon alfa-2b, lopinavir plus ritonavir as antiviral therapy, and moxifloxacin, methylprednisolone (80 mg twice daily, intravenously)	8 days	6 days	Died

Abbreviations: BNP, B-type natriuretic peptide; CRP, C-reactive protein; LDH, lactate dehydrogenase; Hb, hemoglobin; WBCs, white blood cells; NT-proBNP, N-terminal prohormone of brain natriuretic peptide; CK-MB, creatine kinase–myoglobin binding; PT, prothrombin time; hs-troponin T, high-sensitivity troponin T; ECG, electrocardiogram; ST, sinus tachycardia; AVF, arteriovenous fistula.

5. Limitations and Strengths

There are several limitations in this review that must be taken into account. First, we did not perform a meta-analysis due to the large heterogeneity and variations in data collection and study designs. Secondly, a quality assessment of the studies was not performed. Thirdly, it might be possible that a confirmed diagnosis of these complications is lacking in primary studies. Lastly, due to the large body of available literature, complications related to only four major organ systems were covered in the current review. There are certain strengths of the present review that cannot be neglected. Firstly, according to our knowledge, this is the first review that points out the unusual complications in key organ systems after COVID-19. Secondly, the compilation of a large amount of evidence in a single article provides information on the range of incidences of atypical complications caused by the COVID-19 virus and their impact on hospitalization and mortality rates. Thirdly, the findings of the current review highlight the importance of the consideration of other organ systems during the management of COVID-19 infection.

6. Future Prospects

Since the commencement of the SARS-CoV-2 pandemic, an exceeding number of evidence has concentrated on the quick diagnosis, evolution, and divergence of new therapies. Nevertheless, it has been found in various studies, including the current review, that SARS-CoV-2 is not just a respiratory disease. Elevated levels of endogenous chemical substances generated in reaction to inflammation developed by the virus have the potential to generate disturbances and alterations in target tissues all over the human body, which even surpass the protective barriers of innate tissue immunity. Moreover, the cytokine storm developed during sepsis, which also has pleiotropic capabilities, interacts with respective high-density receptors, vasculature, and immune cells. In addition, the overexpression of angiotensin-converting enzyme II receptors (hACE2-R) in numerous tissues permits the virus to proliferate to the vascular system and extend into the entire human body. A vicious cycle develops, which entails the generation of chemical mediators, a decrease in the density of the hACE2-R receptors, and elevated levels of angiotensin II, producing both inflammatory and vascular effects. Moreover, this mechanism prompts the generation of additional hACE2-R via positive feedback. These frequently stimulated cycles multiply the proliferation of infection and consequent expansion in angiotensin II, which widely contribute to the pathophysiological mechanisms of SARS-CoV-2 and generate increased inflammation, vasoconstriction, and fibrosis. This necessitates the focus of healthcare practitioners on not only the respiratory syndrome caused by this virus but also on monitoring for atypical complications in all major body systems and following up on patients for post-COVID and long-COVID health issues, which at times are entirely asymptomatic in nature. Hence, there is a need for a multidisciplinary approach. Moreover, further research is required to identify actual differences as there is a wide variability across studies. Also, the impact of novel variants on long-COVID development and which individuals will be at the most risk will need future study and research.

7. Conclusions

This article reviewed four major organ systems to determine the burden of atypical complications. Major gastric complications found in research studies are bowel ischemia/infarction, GI bleeding, and hepatic ischemia/injury/infarct due to thromboembolism of the portal system. Major neurological complications included acute ischemic stroke, cerebral venous sinus thrombosis, cerebral hemorrhage, anosmia, and dysgeusia. Major renal complications included acute kidney injury (AKI) and acute renal failure. Major cardiovascular complications included acute cardiac injury/non-coronary myocardial injury, arrhythmia/ventricular tachycardia/ventricular fibrillation, coagulopathy/venous thromboembolism, and myocardial infarction/heart failure. The major complications found in these organ systems in case reports were bowel ischemia/hepatic ischemia, acute pancreatitis, bowel perforation, encephalopathy/encephalitis, Guillain–Barré Syndrome, epileptogenicity/focal seizures with impaired awareness, renal/splenic/cerebral infarct or aortic thrombosis, fulminant myocarditis, and Takotsubo syndrome. Hence, it is important for healthcare practitioners, researchers, and policy-makers to opt for early management practices and long-term follow-up of COVID-19 patients, consider evidence-based research practices, and compel effective policy-making, which would help drive the global community toward the successful management of the after-effects of the COVID-19 pandemic.

Author Contributions: Conceptualization, T.H.M., M.H.B. and Y.H.K.; methodology, T.H.M., A.S., M.H.B. and M.S.; software, A.S. and S.N.; validation, M.S., Z.U.M., F.U.K. and Y.H.K.; resources, T.H.M. and M.H.B.; data curation, T.H.M., A.S., M.H.B. and S.N.; writing—original draft preparation, T.H.M., A.S., M.H.B., S.N., Z.U.M. and M.S.; writing—review and editing, T.H.M., M.S., F.U.K. and Y.H.K.; visualization, M.H.B.; supervision, T.H.M. and M.H.B.; project administration, T.H.M., M.H.B. and Y.H.K. All authors have read and agreed to the published version of the manuscript.

Funding: This research received no external funding.

Institutional Review Board Statement: Not applicable.

Informed Consent Statement: Not applicable.

Data Availability Statement: Not applicable.

Conflicts of Interest: The authors declare no conflicts of interest.

References

1. Misbah, S.; Ahmad, A.; Butt, M.H.; Khan, Y.H.; Alotaibi, N.H.; Mallhi, T.H. A systematic analysis of studies on corona virus disease 19 (COVID-19) from viral emergence to treatment. *J. Coll. Physicians Surg. Pak.* **2020**, *30*, 9–18. [PubMed]
2. Cascella, M.; Rajnik, M.; Aleem, A.; Dulebohn, S.C.; Di Napoli, R. *Features, Evaluation, and Treatment of Coronavirus (COVID-19)*; Statpearls: Treasure Island, FL, USA, 2022.
3. World Health Organization. Coronavirus Disease (COVID-19) Pandemic. 2023. Available online: https://www.who.int/europe/emergencies/situations/covid-19 (accessed on 15 September 2023).
4. Jiang, S.; Hillyer, C.; Du, L. Neutralizing Antibodies against SARS-CoV-2 and Other Human Coronaviruses. *Trends Immunol.* **2020**, *41*, 355–359. [CrossRef] [PubMed]
5. Song, W.; Gui, M.; Wang, X.; Xiang, Y. Cryo-EM structure of the SARS coronavirus spike glycoprotein in complex with its host cell receptor ACE2. *PLoS Pathog.* **2018**, *14*, e1007236. [CrossRef] [PubMed]
6. Hoffmann, M.; Kleine-Weber, H.; Schroeder, S.; Krüger, N.; Herrler, T.; Erichsen, S.; Schiergens, T.S.; Herrler, G.; Wu, N.H.; Nitsche, A.; et al. SARS-CoV-2 Cell Entry Depends on ACE2 and TMPRSS2 and Is Blocked by a Clinically Proven Protease Inhibitor. *Cell* **2020**, *181*, 271–280.e8. [CrossRef] [PubMed]
7. Xu, H.; Zhong, L.; Deng, J.; Peng, J.; Dan, H.; Zeng, X.; Li, T.; Chen, Q. High expression of ACE2 receptor of 2019-nCoV on the epithelial cells of oral mucosa. *Int. J. Oral Sci.* **2020**, *12*, 8. [CrossRef] [PubMed]
8. Gupta, A.; Madhavan, M.V.; Sehgal, K.; Nair, N.; Mahajan, S.; Sehrawat, T.S.; Bikdeli, B.; Ahluwalia, N.; Ausiello, J.C.; Wan, E.Y. Extrapulmonary manifestations of COVID-19. *Nat. Med.* **2020**, *26*, 1017–1032. [CrossRef] [PubMed]
9. Coopersmith, C.M.; Antonelli, M.; Bauer, S.R.; Deutschman, C.S.; Evans, L.E.; Ferrer, R.; Hellman, J.; Jog, S.; Kesecioglu, J.; Kissoon, N.; et al. The Surviving Sepsis Campaign: Research Priorities for Coronavirus Disease 2019 in Critical Illness. *Crit. Care Med.* **2021**, *49*, 598–622. [CrossRef]
10. Sarkesh, A.; Sorkhabi, A.D.; Sheykhsaran, E.; Alinezhad, F.; Mohammadzadeh, N.; Hemmat, N.; Baghi, H.B. Extrapulmonary clinical manifestations in COVID-19 patients. *Am. J. Trop. Med. Hyg.* **2020**, *103*, 1783. [CrossRef]
11. Behzad, S.; Aghaghazvini, L.; Radmard, A.R.; Gholamrezanezhad, A. Extrapulmonary manifestations of COVID-19: Radiologic and clinical overview. *Clin. Imaging* **2020**, *66*, 35–41. [CrossRef]
12. Elrobaa, I.H.; New, K.J. COVID-19: Pulmonary and extra pulmonary manifestations. *Front. Public Health* **2021**, *9*, 711616. [CrossRef]
13. Johnson, K.D.; Harris, C.; Cain, J.K.; Hummer, C.; Goyal, H.; Perisetti, A. Pulmonary and extra-pulmonary clinical manifestations of COVID-19. *Front. Med.* **2020**, *7*, 526. [CrossRef] [PubMed]
14. Mallhi, T.H.; Khan, Y.H.; Alzarea, A.I.; Khan, F.U.; Alotaibi, N.H.; Alanazi, A.S.; Butt, M.H.; Alatawi, A.D.; Salman, M.; Alzarea, S.I. Incidence, risk factors and outcomes of acute kidney injury among COVID-19 patients: A systematic review of systematic reviews. *Front. Med.* **2022**, *9*, 973030. [CrossRef] [PubMed]
15. Kaafarani, H.M.; El Moheb, M.; Hwabejire, J.O.; Naar, L.; Christensen, M.A.; Breen, K.; Gaitanidis, A.; Alser, O.; Mashbari, H.; Bankhead-Kendall, B. Gastrointestinal complications in critically ill patients with COVID-19. *Ann. Surg.* **2020**, *272*, e61. [CrossRef] [PubMed]
16. Sheraton, M.; Deo, N.; Kashyap, R.; Surani, S. A review of neurological complications of COVID-19. *Cureus* **2020**, *12*, e8192. [CrossRef]

17. Filatov, A.; Sharma, P.; Hindi, F.; Espinosa, P.S. Neurological complications of coronavirus disease (COVID-19): Encephalopathy. *Cureus* **2020**, *12*, e7352. [CrossRef]
18. Kunutsor, S.K.; Laukkanen, J.A. Renal complications in COVID-19: A systematic review and meta-analysis. *Ann. Med.* **2020**, *52*, 345–353. [CrossRef]
19. Farshidfar, F.; Koleini, N.; Ardehali, H. Cardiovascular complications of COVID-19. *J. Clin. Investig.* **2021**, *6*, e148980. [CrossRef]
20. Carod-Artal, F.J. Neurological complications associated with dengue virus infection. *Rev. Neurol.* **2019**, *69*, 113–122.
21. Prabhat, N.; Ray, S.; Chakravarty, K.; Kathuria, H.; Saravana, S.; Singh, D.; Rebello, A.; Lakhanpal, V.; Goyal, M.K.; Lal, V. Atypical neurological manifestations of dengue fever: A case series and mini review. *Postgrad. Med. J.* **2020**, *96*, 759–765. [CrossRef]
22. Mishra, A.; Saini, R.; Kallani, M. Acute pancreatitis associated with dengue fever: An interesting and rare complication of dengue virus. *Indian J. Case Rep.* **2019**, *5*, 29–32.
23. Kamath, N.; Acharya, V.; Nandakrishna, B.; Sukumaran, C.A.; Siddharth, G.; Varaprasad, B. Atypical Manifestation of Dengue Fever: A Tale of 2 Cases. *J. Indian Acad. Clin. Med.* **2022**, *23*, 151.
24. Platanaki, C.; Leonidou, L.; Siagkris, D.; Giannopoulou, I.; Paliogianni, F.; Velissaris, D. Varicella-zoster virus aseptic meningitis: An atypical presentation in an immunocompetent male patient. *Oxf. Med. Case Rep.* **2021**, *2021*, omab035. [CrossRef] [PubMed]
25. Gnann, J.W., Jr. Varicella-zoster virus: Atypical presentations and unusual complications. *J. Infect. Dis.* **2002**, *186* (Suppl. S1), S91–S98. [CrossRef] [PubMed]
26. Wölfel, R.; Corman, V.M.; Guggemos, W.; Seilmaier, M.; Zange, S.; Müller, M.A.; Niemeyer, D.; Jones, T.C.; Vollmar, P.; Rothe, C. Virological assessment of hospitalized patients with COVID-2019. *Nature* **2020**, *581*, 465–469. [CrossRef]
27. Xiao, F.; Tang, M.; Zheng, X.; Liu, Y.; Li, X.; Shan, H. Evidence for gastrointestinal infection of SARS-CoV-2. *Gastroenterology* **2020**, *158*, 1831–1833.e3. [CrossRef]
28. Zhang, H.; Kang, Z.; Gong, H.; Xu, D.; Wang, J.; Li, Z.; Li, Z.; Cui, X.; Xiao, J.; Zhan, J. Digestive system is a potential route of COVID-19: An analysis of single-cell coexpression pattern of key proteins in viral entry process. *Gut* **2020**, *69*, 1010–1018. [CrossRef]
29. Lamers, M.M.; Beumer, J.; Van Der Vaart, J.; Knoops, K.; Puschhof, J.; Breugem, T.I.; Ravelli, R.B.; Paul van Schayck, J.; Mykytyn, A.Z.; Duimel, H.Q. SARS-CoV-2 productively infects human gut enterocytes. *Science* **2020**, *369*, 50–54. [CrossRef] [PubMed]
30. Varga, Z.; Flammer, A.J.; Steiger, P.; Haberecker, M.; Andermatt, R.; Zinkernagel, A.S.; Mehra, M.R.; Schuepbach, R.A.; Ruschitzka, F.; Moch, H. Endothelial cell infection and endotheliitis in COVID-19. *Lancet* **2020**, *395*, 1417–1418. [CrossRef]
31. Mak, J.W.; Chan, F.K.; Ng, S.C. Probiotics and COVID-19: One size does not fit all. *Lancet Gastroenterol. Hepatol.* **2020**, *5*, 644–645. [CrossRef]
32. Mao, R.; Qiu, Y.; He, J.-S.; Tan, J.-Y.; Li, X.-H.; Liang, J.; Shen, J.; Zhu, L.-R.; Chen, Y.; Iacucci, M. Manifestations and prognosis of gastrointestinal and liver involvement in patients with COVID-19: A systematic review and meta-analysis. *Lancet Gastroenterol. Hepatol.* **2020**, *5*, 667–678. [CrossRef]
33. Nobel, Y.; Phipps, M.; Zucker, J.; Lebwohl, B.; Wang, T.C.; Sobieszczyk, M.E.; Freedberg, D.E. Gastrointestinal symptoms and COVID-19: Case–control study from the United States. *Gastroenterology* **2020**, *159*, 373–375.e2. [CrossRef]
34. Lui, R.N.; Wong, S.H.; Sánchez-Luna, S.A.; Pellino, G.; Bollipo, S.; Wong, M.Y.; Chiu, P.W.; Sung, J.J. Overview of guidance for endoscopy during the coronavirus disease 2019 pandemic. *J. Gastroenterol. Hepatol.* **2020**, *35*, 749–759. [CrossRef] [PubMed]
35. Sultan, S.; Lim, J.K.; Altayar, O.; Davitkov, P.; Feuerstein, J.D.; Siddique, S.M.; Falck-Ytter, Y.; El-Serag, H.B. AGA rapid recommendations for gastrointestinal procedures during the COVID-19 pandemic. *Gastroenterology* **2020**, *159*, 739–758.e4. [CrossRef] [PubMed]
36. Fix, O.K.; Hameed, B.; Fontana, R.J.; Kwok, R.M.; McGuire, B.M.; Mulligan, D.C.; Pratt, D.S.; Russo, M.W.; Schilsky, M.L.; Verna, E.C. Clinical best practice advice for hepatology and liver transplant providers during the COVID-19 pandemic: AASLD expert panel consensus statement. *Hepatology* **2020**, *72*, 287–304. [CrossRef] [PubMed]
37. El Moheb, M.; Naar, L.; Christensen, M.A.; Kapoen, C.; Maurer, L.R.; Farhat, M.; Kaafarani, H.M. Gastrointestinal complications in critically ill patients with and without COVID-19. *JAMA* **2020**, *324*, 1899–1901. [CrossRef]
38. Mauro, A.; De Grazia, F.; Lenti, M.V.; Penagini, R.; Frego, R.; Ardizzone, S.; Savarino, E.; Radaelli, F.; Bosani, M.; Orlando, S. Upper gastrointestinal bleeding in COVID-19 inpatients: Incidence and management in a multicenter experience from Northern Italy. *Clin. Res. Hepatol. Gastroenterol.* **2021**, *45*, 101521. [CrossRef] [PubMed]
39. Drake, T.M.; Riad, A.M.; Fairfield, C.J.; Egan, C.; Knight, S.R.; Pius, R.; Hardwick, H.E.; Norman, L.; Shaw, C.A.; McLean, K.A. Characterisation of in-hospital complications associated with COVID-19 using the ISARIC WHO Clinical Characterisation Protocol UK: A prospective, multicentre cohort study. *Lancet* **2021**, *398*, 223–237. [CrossRef]
40. Qayed, E.; Deshpande, A.R.; Elmunzer, B.J. Low Incidence of Severe Gastrointestinal Complications in COVID-19 Patients Admitted to the Intensive Care Unit: A Large, Multicenter Study. *Gastroenterology* **2021**, *160*, 1403–1405. [CrossRef]
41. Bhayana, R.; Som, A.; Li, M.D.; Carey, D.E.; Anderson, M.A.; Blake, M.A.; Catalano, O.; Gee, M.S.; Hahn, P.F.; Harisinghani, M. Abdominal imaging findings in COVID-19: Preliminary observations. *Radiology* **2020**, *297*, E207–E215. [CrossRef]
42. Dane, B.; Brusca-Augello, G.; Kim, D.; Katz, D.S. Unexpected findings of coronavirus disease (COVID-19) at the lung bases on abdominopelvic CT. *Am. J. Roentgenol.* **2020**, *215*, 603–606. [CrossRef]
43. De Nardi, P.; Parolini, D.C.; Ripa, M.; Racca, S.; Rosati, R. Bowel perforation in a Covid-19 patient: Case report. *Int. J. Color. Dis.* **2020**, *35*, 1797–1800. [CrossRef]

44. Del Hoyo, J.; López-Muñoz, P.; Fernández-de la Varga, M.; Garrido-Marín, A.; Valero-Pérez, E.; Prieto, M.; Aguilera, V. Hepatobiliary and Pancreatic: A fatal case of extensive splanchnic vein thrombosis in a patient with COVID-19. *J. Gastroenterol. Hepatol.* **2020**, *35*, 1853. [CrossRef] [PubMed]
45. Karna, S.T.; Panda, R.; Maurya, A.P.; Kumari, S. Superior mesenteric artery thrombosis in COVID-19 pneumonia: An underestimated diagnosis—First case report in Asia. *Indian J. Surg.* **2020**, *82*, 1235–1237. [CrossRef] [PubMed]
46. Carll, W.C.; Rady, M.Y.; Salomao, M.A.; Patel, B.; Singh, V.P.; Sen, A. Cytomegalovirus haemorrhagic enterocolitis associated with severe infection with COVID-19. *BMJ Open Gastroenterol.* **2021**, *8*, e000556. [CrossRef]
47. De Barry, O.; Mekki, A.; Diffre, C.; Seror, M.; El Hajjam, M.; Carlier, R.-Y. Arterial and venous abdominal thrombosis in a 79-year-old woman with COVID-19 pneumonia. *Radiol. Case Rep.* **2020**, *15*, 1054–1057. [CrossRef] [PubMed]
48. Chan, K.H.; Lim, S.L.; Damati, A.; Maruboyina, S.P.; Bondili, L.; Hanoud, A.A.; Slim, J. Coronavirus disease 2019 (COVID-19) and ischemic colitis: An under-recognized complication. *Am. J. Emerg. Med.* **2020**, *38*, 2758.e1–2758.e4. [CrossRef]
49. Corrêa Neto, I.J.F.; Viana, K.F.; Silva, M.B.S.d.; Silva, L.M.d.; Oliveira, G.d.; Cecchini, A.R.d.S.; Rolim, A.S.; Robles, L. Perforated acute abdomen in a patient with COVID-19: An atypical manifestation of the disease. *J. Coloproctol.* **2020**, *40*, 269–272. [CrossRef]
50. Hadi, A.; Werge, M.; Kristiansen, K.T.; Pedersen, U.G.; Karstensen, J.G.; Novovic, S.; Gluud, L.L. Coronavirus disease-19 (COVID-19) associated with severe acute pancreatitis: Case report on three family members. *Pancreatology* **2020**, *20*, 665–667. [CrossRef]
51. Marchi, G.; Vianello, A.; Crisafulli, E.; Maroccia, A.; Crinò, S.F.; Pecori, S.; Zamboni, G.A.; Mazzaferri, F.; Tacconelli, E.; Girelli, D. Cytomegalovirus-induced gastrointestinal bleeding and pancreatitis complicating severe COVID-19 pneumonia: A paradigmatic case. *Mediterr. J. Hematol. Infect. Dis.* **2020**, *12*, e2020060. [CrossRef]
52. Kangas-Dick, A.; Prien, C.; Rojas, K.; Pu, Q.; Hamshow, M.; Wan, E.; Chawla, K.; Wiesel, O. Gastrointestinal perforation in a critically ill patient with COVID-19 pneumonia. *SAGE Open Med. Case Rep.* **2020**, *8*, 1–4. [CrossRef]
53. Farina, D.; Rondi, P.; Botturi, E.; Renzulli, M.; Borghesi, A.; Guelfi, D.; Ravanelli, M. Gastrointestinal: Bowel ischemia in a suspected coronavirus disease (COVID-19) patient. *J. Gastroenterol. Hepatol.* **2020**, *36*, 41. [CrossRef] [PubMed]
54. Moazzam, Z.; Salim, A.; Ashraf, A.; Jehan, F.; Arshad, M. Intussusception in an infant as a manifestation of COVID-19. *J. Pediatr. Surg. Case Rep.* **2020**, *59*, 101533. [CrossRef] [PubMed]
55. Paul, T.; Joy, A.R.; Alsoub, H.A.R.S.; Parambil, J.V. Case report: Ischemic colitis in severe COVID-19 pneumonia: An unforeseen gastrointestinal complication. *Am. J. Trop. Med. Hyg.* **2021**, *104*, 63. [CrossRef] [PubMed]
56. Ibrahim, Y.S.; Karuppasamy, G.; Parambil, J.V.; Alsoub, H.; Al-Shokri, S.D. Case report: Paralytic ileus: A potential extrapulmonary manifestation of severe COVID-19. *Am. J. Trop. Med. Hyg.* **2020**, *103*, 1600. [CrossRef] [PubMed]
57. Sungnak, W.; Huang, N.; Bécavin, C.; Berg, M.; Queen, R.; Litvinukova, M.; Talavera-López, C.; Maatz, H.; Reichart, D.; Sampaziotis, F. SARS-CoV-2 entry factors are highly expressed in nasal epithelial cells together with innate immune genes. *Nat. Med.* **2020**, *26*, 681–687. [CrossRef] [PubMed]
58. Ziegler, C.G.; Allon, S.J.; Nyquist, S.K.; Mbano, I.M.; Miao, V.N.; Tzouanas, C.N.; Cao, Y.; Yousif, A.S.; Bals, J.; Hauser, B.M. SARS-CoV-2 receptor ACE2 is an interferon-stimulated gene in human airway epithelial cells and is detected in specific cell subsets across tissues. *Cell* **2020**, *181*, 1016–1035.e19. [CrossRef]
59. Lechien, J.R.; Chiesa-Estomba, C.M.; De Siati, D.R.; Horoi, M.; Le Bon, S.D.; Rodriguez, A.; Dequanter, D.; Blecic, S.; El Afia, F.; Distinguin, L. Olfactory and gustatory dysfunctions as a clinical presentation of mild-to-moderate forms of the coronavirus disease (COVID-19): A multicenter European study. *Eur. Arch. Oto-Rhino-Laryngol.* **2020**, *277*, 2251–2261. [CrossRef]
60. Spinato, G.; Fabbris, C.; Polesel, J.; Cazzador, D.; Borsetto, D.; Hopkins, C.; Boscolo-Rizzo, P. Alterations in smell or taste in mildly symptomatic outpatients with SARS-CoV-2 infection. *JAMA* **2020**, *323*, 2089–2090. [CrossRef]
61. Vaira, L.A.; Deiana, G.; Fois, A.G.; Pirina, P.; Madeddu, G.; De Vito, A.; Babudieri, S.; Petrocelli, M.; Serra, A.; Bussu, F. Objective evaluation of anosmia and ageusia in COVID-19 patients: Single-center experience on 72 cases. *Head Neck* **2020**, *42*, 1252–1258. [CrossRef]
62. Mehta, P.; McAuley, D.F.; Brown, M.; Sanchez, E.; Tattersall, R.S.; Manson, J.J. COVID-19: Consider cytokine storm syndromes and immunosuppression. *Lancet* **2020**, *395*, 1033–1034. [CrossRef]
63. Leadership, A.A.S.C. Temporary emergency guidance to US stroke centers during the coronavirus disease 2019 (COVID-19) pandemic: On behalf of the American Heart Association/American Stroke Association Stroke Council Leadership. *Stroke* **2020**, *51*, 1910–1912.
64. Faigle, R.; Butler, J.; Carhuapoma, J.R.; Johnson, B.; Zink, E.K.; Shakes, T.; Rosenblum, M.; Saheed, M.; Urrutia, V.C. Safety trial of low-intensity monitoring after thrombolysis: Optimal Post Tpa-Iv Monitoring in Ischemic STroke (OPTIMIST). *Neurohospitalist* **2020**, *10*, 11–15. [CrossRef] [PubMed]
65. Hartung, H.-P.; Aktas, O. COVID-19 and management of neuroimmunological disorders. *Nat. Rev. Neurol.* **2020**, *16*, 347–348. [CrossRef] [PubMed]
66. Klopfenstein, T.; Kadiane-Oussou, N.; Toko, L.; Royer, P.-Y.; Lepiller, Q.; Gendrin, V.; Zayet, S. Features of anosmia in COVID-19. *Med. Mal. Infect.* **2020**, *50*, 436–439. [CrossRef] [PubMed]
67. Bagheri, S.H.; Asghari, A.; Farhadi, M.; Shamshiri, A.R.; Kabir, A.; Kamrava, S.K.; Jalessi, M.; Mohebbi, A.; Alizadeh, R.; Honarmand, A.A. Coincidence of COVID-19 epidemic and olfactory dysfunction outbreak in Iran. *Med. J. Islam. Repub. Iran* **2020**, *34*, 62. [CrossRef] [PubMed]

68. Giacomelli, A.; Pezzati, L.; Conti, F.; Bernacchia, D.; Siano, M.; Oreni, L.; Rusconi, S.; Gervasoni, C.; Ridolfo, A.L.; Rizzardini, G Self-reported olfactory and taste disorders in patients with severe acute respiratory coronavirus 2 infection: A cross-sectional study. *Clin. Infect. Dis.* **2020**, *71*, 889–890. [CrossRef] [PubMed]
69. Li, Y.; Li, M.; Wang, M.; Zhou, Y.; Chang, J.; Xian, Y.; Wang, D.; Mao, L.; Jin, H.; Hu, B. Acute cerebrovascular disease following COVID-19: A single center, retrospective, observational study. *Stroke Vasc. Neurol.* **2020**, *5*, 279–284. [CrossRef]
70. Lu, L.; Xiong, W.; Liu, D.; Liu, J.; Yang, D.; Li, N.; Mu, J.; Guo, J.; Li, W.; Wang, G. New onset acute symptomatic seizure and risk factors in coronavirus disease 2019: A retrospective multicenter study. *Epilepsia* **2020**, *61*, e49–e53. [CrossRef]
71. Mao, L.; Jin, H.; Wang, M.; Hu, Y.; Chen, S.; He, Q.; Chang, J.; Hong, C.; Zhou, Y.; Wang, D. Neurologic manifestations of hospitalized patients with coronavirus disease 2019 in Wuhan, China. *JAMA Neurol.* **2020**, *77*, 683–690. [CrossRef]
72. Lodigiani, C.; Iapichino, G.; Carenzo, L.; Cecconi, M.; Ferrazzi, P.; Sebastian, T.; Kucher, N.; Studt, J.-D.; Sacco, C.; Bertuzzi, A. Venous and arterial thromboembolic complications in COVID-19 patients admitted to an academic hospital in Milan, Italy. *Thromb. Res.* **2020**, *191*, 9–14. [CrossRef]
73. Flores-Silva, F.D.; Garcia-Grimshaw, M.; Valdes-Ferrer, S.I.; Vigueras-Hernandez, A.P.; Dominguez-Moreno, R.; Tristan-Samaniego, D.P.; Michel-Chavez, A.; Gonzalez-Duarte, A.; Vega-Boada, F.A.; Reyes-Melo, I. Neurologic manifestations in hospitalized patients with COVID-19 in Mexico City. *PLoS ONE* **2021**, *16*, e0247433. [CrossRef] [PubMed]
74. Romero-Sánchez, C.M.; Díaz-Maroto, I.; Fernández-Díaz, E.; Sánchez-Larsen, Á.; Layos-Romero, A.; García-García, J.; González, E.; Redondo-Peñas, I.; Perona-Moratalla, A.B.; Del Valle-Pérez, J.A. Neurologic manifestations in hospitalized patients with COVID-19: The ALBACOVID registry. *Neurology* **2020**, *95*, e1060–e1070. [CrossRef] [PubMed]
75. Karadaş, Ö.; Öztürk, B.; Sonkaya, A.R. A prospective clinical study of detailed neurological manifestations in patients with COVID-19. *Neurol. Sci.* **2020**, *41*, 1991–1995. [CrossRef] [PubMed]
76. Luigetti, M.; Iorio, R.; Bentivoglio, A.R.; Tricoli, L.; Riso, V.; Marotta, J.; Piano, C.; Primiano, G.; Zileri Del Verme, L.; Lo Monaco, M.R. Assessment of neurological manifestations in hospitalized patients with COVID-19. *Eur. J. Neurol.* **2020**, *27*, 2322–2328. [CrossRef]
77. Moriguchi, T.; Harii, N.; Goto, J.; Harada, D.; Sugawara, H.; Takamino, J.; Ueno, M.; Sakata, H.; Kondo, K.; Myose, N. A first case of meningitis/encephalitis associated with SARS-Coronavirus-2. *Int. J. Infect. Dis.* **2020**, *94*, 55–58. [CrossRef] [PubMed]
78. Poyiadji, N.; Shahin, G.; Noujaim, D.; Stone, M.; Patel, S.; Griffith, B. COVID-19–associated acute hemorrhagic necrotizing encephalopathy: Imaging features. *Radiology* **2020**, *296*, E119–E120. [CrossRef] [PubMed]
79. Gutiérrez-Ortiz, C.; Méndez-Guerrero, A.; Rodrigo-Rey, S.; San Pedro-Murillo, E.; Bermejo-Guerrero, L.; Gordo-Mañas, R.; de Aragón-Gómez, F.; Benito-León, J. Miller Fisher syndrome and polyneuritis cranialis in COVID-19. *Neurology* **2020**, *95*, e601–e605. [CrossRef]
80. Sharifi-Razavi, A.; Karimi, N.; Rouhani, N. COVID-19 and intracerebral haemorrhage: Causative or coincidental? *New Microbes New Infect.* **2020**, *35*, 100669. [CrossRef]
81. Paybast, S.; Gorji, R.; Mavandadi, S. Guillain-Barré syndrome as a neurological complication of novel COVID-19 infection: A case report and review of the literature. *Neurologist* **2020**, *25*, 101–103. [CrossRef]
82. Bozzali, M.; Grassini, A.; Morana, G.; Zotta, M.; Cabras, S.; Romagnolo, A.; Artusi, C.A.; Montalenti, E.; Rizzone, M.G.; Garbossa, D. Focal seizures with impaired awareness as long-term neurological complication of COVID-19: A case report. *Neurol. Sci.* **2021**, *42*, 2619–2623. [CrossRef]
83. Zhao, H.; Shen, D.; Zhou, H.; Liu, J.; Chen, S. Guillain-Barré syndrome associated with SARS-CoV-2 infection: Causality or coincidence? *Lancet Neurol.* **2020**, *19*, 383–384. [CrossRef] [PubMed]
84. Zhao, K.; Huang, J.; Dai, D.; Feng, Y.; Liu, L.; Nie, S. Acute myelitis after SARS-CoV-2 infection: A case report. *MedRxiv* **2020**. [CrossRef]
85. Sedaghat, Z.; Karimi, N. Guillain Barre syndrome associated with COVID-19 infection: A case report. *J. Clin. Neurosci.* **2020**, *76*, 233–235. [CrossRef] [PubMed]
86. Zhou, F.; Yu, T.; Du, R.; Fan, G.; Liu, Y.; Liu, Z.; Xiang, J.; Wang, Y.; Song, B.; Gu, X.; et al. Clinical course and risk factors for mortality of adult inpatients with COVID-19 in Wuhan, China: A retrospective cohort study. *Lancet* **2020**, *395*, 1054–1062. [CrossRef]
87. Chen, T.; Wu, D.; Chen, H.; Yan, W.; Yang, D.; Chen, G.; Ma, K.; Xu, D.; Yu, H.; Wang, H. Clinical characteristics of 113 deceased patients with coronavirus disease 2019: Retrospective study. *BMJ* **2020**, *368*, m1091. [CrossRef]
88. Su, H.; Yang, M.; Wan, C.; Yi, L.-X.; Tang, F.; Zhu, H.-Y.; Yi, F.; Yang, H.-C.; Fogo, A.B.; Nie, X. Renal histopathological analysis of 26 postmortem findings of patients with COVID-19 in China. *Kidney Int.* **2020**, *98*, 219–227. [CrossRef]
89. Pan, X.-w.; Xu, D.; Zhang, H.; Zhou, W.; Wang, L.-h.; Cui, X.-g. Identification of a potential mechanism of acute kidney injury during the COVID-19 outbreak: A study based on single-cell transcriptome analysis. *Intensive Care Med.* **2020**, *46*, 1114–1116. [CrossRef] [PubMed]
90. Hamming, I.; Timens, W.; Bulthuis, M.; Lely, A.; Navis, G.v.; van Goor, H. Tissue distribution of ACE2 protein, the functional receptor for SARS coronavirus. A first step in understanding SARS pathogenesis. *J. Pathol. A J. Pathol. Soc. Great Br. Irel.* **2004**, *203*, 631–637. [CrossRef]
91. Iwasaki, A.; Pillai, P.S. Innate immunity to influenza virus infection. *Nat. Rev. Immunol.* **2014**, *14*, 315–328. [CrossRef]
92. Peerapornratana, S.; Manrique-Caballero, C.L.; Gómez, H.; Kellum, J.A. Acute kidney injury from sepsis: Current concepts, epidemiology, pathophysiology, prevention and treatment. *Kidney Int.* **2019**, *96*, 1083–1099. [CrossRef]

93. Cheng, Y.; Luo, R.; Wang, K.; Zhang, M.; Wang, Z.; Dong, L.; Li, J.; Yao, Y.; Ge, S.; Xu, G. Kidney disease is associated with in-hospital death of patients with COVID-19. *Kidney Int.* **2020**, *97*, 829–838. [CrossRef] [PubMed]
94. Pei, G.; Zhang, Z.; Peng, J.; Liu, L.; Zhang, C.; Yu, C.; Ma, Z.; Huang, Y.; Liu, W.; Yao, Y. Renal involvement and early prognosis in patients with COVID-19 pneumonia. *J. Am. Soc. Nephrol.* **2020**, *31*, 1157–1165. [CrossRef] [PubMed]
95. Ronco, C.; Reis, T.; Husain-Syed, F. Management of acute kidney injury in patients with COVID-19. *Lancet Respir. Med.* **2020**, *8*, 738–742. [CrossRef] [PubMed]
96. Gupta, S.; Coca, S.G.; Chan, L.; Melamed, M.L.; Brenner, S.K.; Hayek, S.S.; Sutherland, A.; Puri, S.; Srivastava, A.; Leonberg-Yoo, A. AKI treated with renal replacement therapy in critically ill patients with COVID-19. *J. Am. Soc. Nephrol.* **2021**, *32*, 161–176. [CrossRef] [PubMed]
97. Hirsch, J.S.; Ng, J.H.; Ross, D.W.; Sharma, P.; Shah, H.H.; Barnett, R.L.; Hazzan, A.D.; Fishbane, S.; Jhaveri, K.D.; Abate, M. Acute kidney injury in patients hospitalized with COVID-19. *Kidney Int.* **2020**, *98*, 209–218. [CrossRef]
98. Guan, W.-j.; Ni, Z.-y.; Hu, Y.; Liang, W.-h.; Ou, C.-q.; He, J.-x.; Liu, L.; Shan, H.; Lei, C.-l.; Hui, D.S. Clinical characteristics of coronavirus disease 2019 in China. *N. Engl. J. Med.* **2020**, *382*, 1708–1720. [CrossRef] [PubMed]
99. Yan, Q.; Zuo, P.; Cheng, L.; Li, Y.; Song, K.; Chen, Y.; Dai, Y.; Yang, Y.; Zhou, L.; Yu, W. Acute kidney injury is associated with in-hospital mortality in older patients with COVID-19. *J. Gerontol. Ser. A* **2021**, *76*, 456–462. [CrossRef] [PubMed]
100. Abramovitz, B.W.; Oguntuwase, E.; Abo-Zed, A.; DeSilva, R. Hypertriglyceridemia as a Cause of Continuous Renal Replacement Therapy Circuit Clotting: A Case Series. *Blood Purif.* **2023**, *52*, 352–358. [CrossRef]
101. Aggarwal, S.; Garcia-Telles, N.; Aggarwal, G.; Lavie, C.; Lippi, G.; Henry, B.M. Clinical features, laboratory characteristics, and outcomes of patients hospitalized with coronavirus disease 2019 (COVID-19): Early report from the United States. *Diagnosis* **2020**, *7*, 91–96. [CrossRef]
102. Arentz, M.; Yim, E.; Klaff, L.; Lokhandwala, S.; Riedo, F.X.; Chong, M.; Lee, M. Characteristics and outcomes of 21 critically ill patients with COVID-19 in Washington State. *JAMA* **2020**, *323*, 1612–1614. [CrossRef]
103. Guo, T.; Fan, Y.; Chen, M.; Wu, X.; Zhang, L.; He, T.; Wang, H.; Wan, J.; Wang, X.; Lu, Z. Cardiovascular implications of fatal outcomes of patients with coronavirus disease 2019 (COVID-19). *JAMA Cardiol.* **2020**, *5*, 811–818. [CrossRef] [PubMed]
104. Huang, C.; Wang, Y.; Li, X.; Ren, L.; Zhao, J.; Hu, Y.; Zhang, L.; Fan, G.; Xu, J.; Gu, X. Clinical features of patients infected with 2019 novel coronavirus in Wuhan, China. *Lancet* **2020**, *395*, 497–506. [CrossRef] [PubMed]
105. Richardson, S.; Hirsch, J.S.; Narasimhan, M.; Crawford, J.M.; McGinn, T.; Davidson, K.W.; Barnaby, D.P.; Becker, L.B.; Chelico, J.D.; Cohen, S.L. Presenting characteristics, comorbidities, and outcomes among 5700 patients hospitalized with COVID-19 in the New York City area. *JAMA* **2020**, *323*, 2052–2059. [CrossRef]
106. Chan, L.; Chaudhary, K.; Saha, A.; Chauhan, K.; Vaid, A.; Zhao, S.; Paranjpe, I.; Somani, S.; Richter, F.; Miotto, R. AKI in hospitalized patients with COVID-19. *J. Am. Soc. Nephrol.* **2021**, *32*, 151–160. [CrossRef] [PubMed]
107. Mohamed, M.M.; Lukitsch, I.; Torres-Ortiz, A.E.; Walker, J.B.; Varghese, V.; Hernandez-Arroyo, C.F.; Alqudsi, M.; LeDoux, J.R.; Velez, J.C.Q. Acute kidney injury associated with coronavirus disease 2019 in urban New Orleans. *Kidney360* **2020**, *1*, 614. [CrossRef]
108. Argenziano, M.G.; Bruce, S.L.; Slater, C.L.; Tiao, J.R.; Baldwin, M.R.; Barr, R.G.; Chang, B.P.; Chau, K.H.; Choi, J.J.; Gavin, N. Characterization and clinical course of 1000 patients with coronavirus disease 2019 in New York: Retrospective case series. *BMJ* **2020**, *369*, m1996. [CrossRef]
109. Shi, S.; Qin, M.; Shen, B.; Cai, Y.; Liu, T.; Yang, F.; Gong, W.; Liu, X.; Liang, J.; Zhao, Q. Association of cardiac injury with mortality in hospitalized patients with COVID-19 in Wuhan, China. *JAMA Cardiol.* **2020**, *5*, 802–810. [CrossRef]
110. Moeinzadeh, F.; Dezfouli, M.; Naimi, A.; Shahidi, S.; Moradi, H. Newly diagnosed glomerulonephritis during COVID-19 infection undergoing immunosuppression therapy, a case report. *Iran. J. Kidney Dis.* **2020**, *14*, 239–242.
111. Haque, T.S.U.; Jahan, I.; Rahim, M.A.; Chowdhury, T.A.; Ananna, M.A.; Iqbal, S. A tale of an unfortunate outcome in COVID-era. *BIRDEM Med. J.* **2020**, *10*, 115–119. [CrossRef]
112. Mavraganis, G.; Ioannou, S.; Kallianos, A.; Rentziou, G.; Trakada, G. A COVID-19 patient with simultaneous renal infarct, splenic infarct and aortic thrombosis during the severe disease. *Healthcare* **2022**, *10*, 150. [CrossRef]
113. Göre, B.; Yenigün, E.C.; Cevher, Ş.K.; Cankaya, E.; Aydın, N.; Dede, F. IGA nephropathy and spinal epidural abscess after COVID-19 infection: A case report. *Future Virol.* **2022**, *17*, 611–615. [CrossRef] [PubMed]
114. Rigual, R.; Ruiz-Ares, G.; Rodriguez-Pardo, J.; Fernández-Prieto, A.; Navia, P.; Novo, J.R.; de Leciñana, M.A.; Alonso-Singer, P.; Fuentes, B.; Díez-Tejedor, E. Concurrent cerebral, splenic, and renal infarction in a patient with COVID-19 infection. *Neurologist* **2022**, *27*, 143. [CrossRef] [PubMed]
115. Brem, F.L.; Al Tayef, T.A.; Rasras, H.; El Mahi, O.; El Ouafi, N.; Zakaria, B. Concomitant renal and splenic infarctions in a COVID-19-patient with a catastrophic thrombotic syndrome. *Radiol. Case Rep.* **2022**, *17*, 4030–4033. [CrossRef] [PubMed]
116. Gjonbalaj, N.; Uka, S.; Olluri, E.; Sulovari, A.; Vishaj, M.; Kamberi, L.; Berisha, H.; Gjonbalaj, E. Renal artery thrombosis as a long-term complication of COVID-19. *Radiol. Case Rep.* **2023**, *18*, 260–265. [CrossRef] [PubMed]
117. Gallagher, P.E.; Ferrario, C.M.; Tallant, E.A. Regulation of ACE2 in cardiac myocytes and fibroblasts. *Am. J. Physiol.-Heart Circ. Physiol.* **2008**, *295*, H2373–H2379. [CrossRef] [PubMed]
118. Puelles, V.G.; Lütgehetmann, M.; Lindenmeyer, M.T.; Sperhake, J.P.; Wong, M.N.; Allweiss, L.; Chilla, S.; Heinemann, A.; Wanner, N.; Liu, S. Multiorgan and renal tropism of SARS-CoV-2. *N. Engl. J. Med.* **2020**, *383*, 590–592. [CrossRef] [PubMed]

119. Tavazzi, G.; Pellegrini, C.; Maurelli, M.; Belliato, M.; Sciutti, F.; Bottazzi, A.; Sepe, P.A.; Resasco, T.; Camporotondo, R.; Bruno, R. Myocardial localization of coronavirus in COVID-19 cardiogenic shock. *Eur. J. Heart Fail.* **2020**, *22*, 911–915. [CrossRef]
120. Wichmann, D.; Sperhake, J.; Lütgehetmann, M.; Steurer, S.; Edler, C.; Heinemann, A.; Heinrich, F.; Mushumba, H.; Kniep, I.; Schröder, A.S.; et al. Autopsy findings and venous thromboembolism in patients with COVID-19: A prospective cohort study. *Ann. Intern. Med.* **2020**, *10*, M20-2003. [CrossRef]
121. Sala, S.; Peretto, G.; Gramegna, M.; Palmisano, A.; Villatore, A.; Vignale, D.; De Cobelli, F.; Tresoldi, M.; Cappelletti, A.M.; Basso, C. Acute myocarditis presenting as a reverse Tako-Tsubo syndrome in a patient with SARS-CoV-2 respiratory infection. *Eur. Heart J.* **2020**, *41*, 1861–1862. [CrossRef]
122. Xu, Z.; Shi, L.; Wang, Y.; Zhang, J.; Huang, L.; Zhang, C.; Liu, S.; Zhao, P.; Liu, H.; Zhu, L. Pathological findings of COVID-19 associated with acute respiratory distress syndrome. *Lancet Respir. Med.* **2020**, *8*, 420–422. [CrossRef]
123. Li, H.; Liu, L.; Zhang, D.; Xu, J.; Dai, H.; Tang, N.; Su, X.; Cao, B. SARS-CoV-2 and viral sepsis: Observations and hypotheses. *Lancet* **2020**, *395*, 1517–1520. [CrossRef] [PubMed]
124. Kwong, J.C.; Schwartz, K.L.; Campitelli, M.A.; Chung, H.; Crowcroft, N.S.; Karnauchow, T.; Katz, K.; Ko, D.T.; McGeer, A.J.; McNally, D. Acute myocardial infarction after laboratory-confirmed influenza infection. *N. Engl. J. Med.* **2018**, *378*, 345–353. [CrossRef] [PubMed]
125. Ullah, W.; Saeed, R.; Sarwar, U.; Patel, R.; Fischman, D.L. COVID-19 complicated by acute pulmonary embolism and right-sided heart failure. *Case Rep.* **2020**, *2*, 1379–1382. [CrossRef] [PubMed]
126. Creel-Bulos, C.; Hockstein, M.; Amin, N.; Melhem, S.; Truong, A.; Sharifpour, M. Acute cor pulmonale in critically ill patients with COVID-19. *N. Engl. J. Med.* **2020**, *382*, e70. [CrossRef] [PubMed]
127. Repesse, X.; Vieillard-Baron, A. Right heart function during acute respiratory distress syndrome. *Ann. Transl. Med.* **2017**, *5*, 295. [CrossRef] [PubMed]
128. De Simone, G. Position statement of the ESC council on hypertension on ACE-inhibitors and angiotensin receptor blockers. *Eur. Soc. Cardiol.* **2020**, *13*.
129. Bozkurt, B.; Kovacs, R.; Harrington, B. Joint HFSA/ACC/AHA statement addresses concerns re: Using RAAS antagonists in COVID-19. *J. Card. Fail.* **2020**, *26*, 370. [CrossRef]
130. Anca, D.; Reyes, O.; Mitra, R.L.; Epstein, L.M.; Shore-Lesserson, L. Electrophysiology practice during COVID-19 pandemic: A New York tertiary hospital experience. *J. Cardiothorac. Vasc. Anesth.* **2021**, *35*, 1281–1285. [CrossRef]
131. Kirkpatrick, J.N.; Mitchell, C.; Taub, C.; Kort, S.; Hung, J.; Swaminathan, M. ASE statement on protection of patients and echocardiography service providers during the 2019 novel coronavirus outbreak: Endorsed by the American College of Cardiology. *J. Am. Coll. Cardiol.* **2020**, *75*, 3078–3084. [CrossRef]
132. Al Zaghrini, E.; Emmanuel, N.; Zibara, V.; Terro, W.D.; Hanna, S. COVID-19 myocarditis clinical presentation, diagnosis and management: A narrative review. *Int. J. Clin. Res.* **2020**, *1*, 135–150. [CrossRef]
133. Welt, F.G.; Shah, P.B.; Aronow, H.D.; Bortnick, A.E.; Henry, T.D.; Sherwood, M.W.; Young, M.N.; Davidson, L.J.; Kadavath, S.; Mahmud, E. Catheterization laboratory considerations during the coronavirus (COVID-19) pandemic: From the ACC's Interventional Council and SCAI. *J. Am. Coll. Cardiol.* **2020**, *75*, 2372–2375. [CrossRef] [PubMed]
134. Szerlip, M.; Anwaruddin, S.; Aronow, H.D.; Cohen, M.G.; Daniels, M.J.; Dehghani, P.; Drachman, D.E.; Elmariah, S.; Feldman, D.N.; Garcia, S. Considerations for cardiac catheterization laboratory procedures during the COVID-19 pandemic perspectives from the Society for Cardiovascular Angiography and Interventions Emerging Leader Mentorship (SCAI ELM) Members and Graduates. *Catheter. Cardiovasc. Interv.* **2020**, *96*, 586–597. [CrossRef]
135. Ranard, L.S.; Ahmad, Y.; Masoumi, A.; Chuich, T.; Romney, M.-L.S.; Gavin, N.; Sayan, O.R.; Kirtane, A.J.; Rabbani, L.E. Clinical pathway for management of suspected or positive novel coronavirus-19 patients with ST-segment elevation myocardial infarction. *Crit. Pathw. Cardiol.* **2020**, *19*, 49–54. [CrossRef] [PubMed]
136. Wang, D.; Hu, B.; Hu, C.; Zhu, F.; Liu, X.; Zhang, J.; Wang, B.; Xiang, H.; Cheng, Z.; Xiong, Y. Clinical characteristics of 138 hospitalized patients with 2019 novel coronavirus–infected pneumonia in Wuhan, China. *JAMA* **2020**, *323*, 1061–1069. [CrossRef] [PubMed]
137. Hong, K.S.; Lee, K.H.; Chung, J.H.; Shin, K.C.; Choi, E.Y.; Jin, H.J.; Jang, J.G.; Lee, W.; Ahn, J.H. Clinical Features and Outcomes of 98 Patients Hospitalized with SARS-CoV-2 Infection in Daegu, South Korea: A Brief Descriptive Study. *Yonsei Med. J.* **2020**, *61*, 431–437. [CrossRef] [PubMed]
138. Cui, S.; Chen, S.; Li, X.; Liu, S.; Wang, F. Prevalence of venous thromboembolism in patients with severe novel coronavirus pneumonia. *J. Thromb. Haemost.* **2020**, *18*, 1421–1424. [CrossRef] [PubMed]
139. Yu, Y.; Xu, D.; Fu, S.; Zhang, J.; Yang, X.; Xu, L.; Xu, J.; Wu, Y.; Huang, C.; Ouyang, Y.; et al. Patients with COVID-19 in 19 ICUs in Wuhan, China: A cross-sectional study. *Crit. Care* **2020**, *24*, 219. [CrossRef]
140. Cammann, V.L.; Szawan, K.A.; D'Ascenzo, F.; Gili, S.; Dreiding, S.; Würdinger, M.; Manka, R.; Stähli, B.E.; Holy, E.W.; Siegrist, P. Outcomes of acute coronary syndromes in coronavirus disease 2019. *Clin. Res. Cardiol.* **2020**, *109*, 1601–1604. [CrossRef]
141. Zhou, Z.; Zhao, N.; Shu, Y.; Han, S.; Chen, B.; Shu, X. Effect of gastrointestinal symptoms in patients with COVID-19. *Gastroenterology* **2020**, *158*, 2294. [CrossRef]
142. Tang, N.; Li, D.; Wang, X.; Sun, Z. Abnormal coagulation parameters are associated with poor prognosis in patients with novel coronavirus pneumonia. *J. Thromb. Haemost.* **2020**, *18*, 844–847. [CrossRef]

143. Ruan, Q.; Yang, K.; Wang, W.; Jiang, L.; Song, J. Clinical predictors of mortality due to COVID-19 based on an analysis of data of 150 patients from Wuhan, China. *Intensive Care Med.* **2020**, *46*, 846–848. [CrossRef] [PubMed]
144. Wang, L.; He, W.; Yu, X.; Hu, D.; Bao, M.; Liu, H.; Zhou, J.; Jiang, H. Coronavirus disease 2019 in elderly patients: Characteristics and prognostic factors based on 4-week follow-up. *J. Infect.* **2020**, *80*, 639–645. [CrossRef] [PubMed]
145. Liu, K.; Fang, Y.-Y.; Deng, Y.; Liu, W.; Wang, M.-F.; Ma, J.-P.; Xiao, W.; Wang, Y.-N.; Zhong, M.-H.; Li, C.-H. Clinical characteristics of novel coronavirus cases in tertiary hospitals in Hubei Province. *Chin. Med. J.* **2020**, *133*, 1025–1031. [CrossRef] [PubMed]
146. Wei, J.F.; Huang, F.Y.; Xiong, T.Y.; Liu, Q.; Chen, H.; Wang, H.; Huang, H.; Luo, Y.C.; Zhou, X.; Liu, Z.Y.; et al. Acute myocardial injury is common in patients with COVID-19 and impairs their prognosis. *Heart* **2020**, *106*, 1154–1159. [CrossRef]
147. Bangalore, S.; Sharma, A.; Slotwiner, A.; Yatskar, L.; Harari, R.; Shah, B.; Ibrahim, H.; Friedman, G.H.; Thompson, C.; Alviar, C.L. ST-segment elevation in patients with Covid-19—A case series. *N. Engl. J. Med.* **2020**, *382*, 2478–2480. [CrossRef] [PubMed]
148. Richard, I.; Robinson, B.; Dawson, A.; Aya, A.; Ali, R. An atypical presentation of fulminant myocarditis secondary to COVID-19 infection. *Cureus* **2020**, *12*, e9179. [CrossRef] [PubMed]
149. Zeng, J.-H.; Liu, Y.-X.; Yuan, J.; Wang, F.-X.; Wu, W.-B.; Li, J.-X.; Wang, L.-F.; Gao, H.; Wang, Y.; Dong, C.-F.; et al. First case of COVID-19 complicated with fulminant myocarditis: A case report and insights. *Infection* **2020**, *48*, 773–777. [CrossRef]
150. Fiore, G.; Sanvito, F.; Fragasso, G.; Spoladore, R. Case report of cardiogenic shock in COVID-19 myocarditis: Peculiarities on diagnosis, histology, and treatment. *Eur. Heart J.-Case Rep.* **2021**, *5*, ytab357. [CrossRef]
151. Hu, H.; Ma, F.; Wei, X.; Fang, Y. Coronavirus fulminant myocarditis treated with glucocorticoid and human immunoglobulin. *Eur. Heart J.* **2021**, *42*, 206. [CrossRef]
152. Hua, A.; O'Gallagher, K.; Sado, D.; Byrne, J. Life-threatening cardiac tamponade complicating myo-pericarditis in COVID-19. *Eur. Heart J.* **2020**, *41*, 2130. [CrossRef]
153. Dabbagh, M.F.; Aurora, L.; D'Souza, P.; Weinmann, A.J.; Bhargava, P.; Basir, M.B. Cardiac tamponade secondary to COVID-19. *Case Rep.* **2020**, *2*, 1326–1330. [CrossRef] [PubMed]
154. Danzi, G.B.; Loffi, M.; Galeazzi, G.; Gherbesi, E. Acute pulmonary embolism and COVID-19 pneumonia: A random association? *Eur. Heart J.* **2020**, *41*, 1858. [CrossRef] [PubMed]
155. Meyer, P.; Degrauwe, S.; Van Delden, C.; Ghadri, J.-R.; Templin, C. Typical takotsubo syndrome triggered by SARS-CoV-2 infection. *Eur. Heart J.* **2020**, *41*, 1860. [CrossRef] [PubMed]
156. Minhas, A.S.; Scheel, P.; Garibaldi, B.; Liu, G.; Horton, M.; Jennings, M.; Jones, S.R.; Michos, E.D.; Hays, A.G. Takotsubo syndrome in the setting of COVID-19. *Case Rep.* **2020**, *2*, 1321–1325. [CrossRef]
157. Jud, P.; Kessler, H.H.; Brodmann, M. Case report: Changes of vascular reactivity and arterial stiffness in a patient with COVID-19 infection. *Front. Cardiovasc. Med.* **2021**, *8*, 671669. [CrossRef]

medicina

MDPI

Article

Trends in Group A *Streptococcus* Pharyngitis and Co-Infection with Severe Acute Respiratory Syndrome Coronavirus 2: A Retrospective Observational Study

Hidenori Takahashi [1,2,*], Yugo Satake [1], Saori Shimizu [2], Satomi Fujihara [2], Syunsuke Takano [2], Suzuko Fukasawa [2], Kaeyong Park [2], Naoya Toba [1,2], Takahiko Yano [2], Hiroki Nagamatsu [1], Ryutaro Hirose [1], Mio Toyama-Kousaka [1], Shinichiro Ota [1,2], Miwa Morikawa [1] and Masaharu Shinkai [1]

1 Department of Respiratory Medicine, Tokyo Shinagawa Hospital, Tokyo 140-8522, Japan; ntoba634@gmail.com (N.T.); shin.ohta0915@gmail.com (S.O.)

2 Department of Infection Control, Tokyo Shinagawa Hospital, Tokyo 140-8522, Japan; saokawachi@gmail.com (S.S.); fukasawa@tokyo-shinagawa.jp (S.F.); kansen@tokyo-shinagawa.jp (K.P.)

* Correspondence: hidenori.tsh@gmail.com; Tel.: +81-337640511

Abstract: *Background and Objectives*: Group A *Streptococcus* (GAS) is a leading cause of acute pharyngitis with seasonal outbreaks. The coronavirus disease 2019 (COVID-19) pandemic significantly altered respiratory infection trends; however, its impact on GAS pharyngitis (GAS-P) incidence remains unclear. Additionally, data on co-infections with GAS and severe acute respiratory syndrome coronavirus 2 (SARS-CoV-2) are limited. In this study, temporal trends in GAS-P incidence and characteristics of GAS–SARS-CoV-2 co-infections in Japan were examined. *Materials and Methods*: In this observational study, data from patients who visited the Tokyo Shinagawa Hospital between January 2019 and December 2024 were retrospectively analyzed. Data on GAS and SARS-CoV-2 test results and patient demographics were extracted from medical records. The study period was categorized based on COVID-19-related public health measures as follows: pre-COVID-19 social period (January 2019–April 2020), restricted social period (May 2020–April 2023), and post-restriction period (May 2023–December 2024). GAS incidence stratified by sex, age, and period was calculated. Clinical characteristics of patients co-infected with GAS and SARS-CoV-2 were analyzed. *Results*: Among 4837 GAS tests, 463 (9.6%) were positive. GAS positivity rates varied significantly: 11.4% (pre-COVID-19), 7.1% (restricted social period), and 12.6% (post-restriction period; $p < 0.001$). The proportion of pediatric cases decreased significantly during the restricted social period (24.8–5.3%) before rising sharply in the post-restriction period (47.1%, $p < 0.001$). Among 151 patients tested for GAS and SARS-CoV-2, 14 (9.3%) had co-infections, which were identified exclusively after July 2022. Most patients exhibited mild symptoms, primarily fever and sore throat, with decreased lymphocyte counts despite normal white blood cell counts. *Conclusions*: In our cohort, the incidence of GAS pharyngitis temporarily declined during COVID-19-related public health measures and subsequently increased, particularly among children, after restrictions were lifted. Limited testing may contribute to the underdiagnosis of GAS–SARS-CoV-2 co-infections. Further large-scale studies are warranted to assess microbial interactions, disease severity, and long-term outcomes.

Keywords: group A *Streptococcus*; GAS pharyngitis; SARS-CoV-2; co-infection; rapid antigen test

1. Introduction

Group A *Streptococcus* (GAS) is a Gram-positive, non-motile bacterium and a common cause of acute pharyngitis, which affects approximately 5–15% of adults and 20–30% of children worldwide [1]. In Japan, GAS pharyngitis (GAS-P) has seasonal outbreaks, which occur from winter to spring and during summer. GAS-P typically presents with sudden fever and sore throat and is often associated with recent contact with infected individuals. In some cases, GAS-P can lead to severe complications, such as pneumonia or bacteremia [1,2]. Additionally, GAS infections can trigger immune-mediated complications, including post-streptococcal glomerulonephritis and rheumatic fever, affecting the kidneys, heart, joints, and other organs [1]. The first-line antimicrobial treatment for GAS-P and the prevention of complications is penicillin-based antibiotics, and macrolides are alternative options [1].

After early 2020, reports from Japan and elsewhere showed a marked decline in GAS-P during widespread non-pharmaceutical interventions (NPI) [3–6], followed by a resurgence from mid-2022 to 2023 [2,7,8]. However, there are no Japanese studies where adults and children were followed through the entire pre-pandemic, NPI, and post-restriction timeline, leaving it unclear whether the age-specific trends reported nationally are mirrored within a single cohort. Only two single-case reports of GAS-P with concomitant severe acute respiratory syndrome coronavirus 2 (SARS-CoV-2) infection have been published—one during the early (Wuhan/Alpha) wave and one in the Delta wave [9,10]—and we found no peer-reviewed reports describing such co-infections in the Omicron era. The pathophysiology of co-infection and potential microbial interactions between GAS and SARS-CoV-2 remains unclear, partly because of the limited number of reported cases.

Here, we used 6 years of single-center data to examine age-stratified trends in GAS-P and to characterize contemporary GAS–SARS-CoV-2 co-infection.

2. Materials and Methods

In this single-center observational study, data from patients who visited Tokyo Shinagawa Hospital (Tokyo, Japan) between 1 January 2019 and 31 December 2024 were retrospectively analyzed. Data on patient age, sex, and GAS and SARS-CoV-2 test results were retrospectively collected from medical records. GAS testing was performed by internal medicine physicians, otolaryngologists, and pediatricians in the outpatient fever clinic and emergency outpatient departments for patients clinically suspected of having pharyngitis. Oropharyngeal swabs were collected by specialized nurses. GAS antigens were detected using Capilia Strep A (TAUNS Laboratories, Inc., Izunokuni, Shizuoka, Japan), which has a sensitivity of 93.1% and a specificity of 100% [11].

We defined two points marking changes in GAS transmission dynamics: May 2020 (when the state of emergency was first declared in Japan) and May 2023 (the time of relaxation of mask mandates, the conclusion of the World Health Organization Public Health Emergency of International Concern, and reclassification of coronavirus disease 2019 (COVID-19) from a Category II-equivalent status to Category V in Japan), based on findings from previous Japanese studies [2,6].

To analyze epidemiological changes, we divided the study period into three phases based on COVID-19-related public health measures: pre-COVID-19 social period (January 2019–April 2020), restricted social period (May 2020–April 2023), and post-restriction period (May 2023–December 2024). We compared patient demographics and clinical characteristics across these periods to evaluate the impact of pandemic-related interventions on GAS transmission and incidence trends.

For statistical analysis, we used the Kruskal–Wallis test to compare age distributions among the three periods, while Fisher's exact test was applied to compare GAS positivity rates, the sex distribution, and the proportion of pediatric cases. Pairwise comparisons between two periods were subsequently performed using *t*-tests for age and Fisher's exact test for categorical variables.

All statistical analyses were conducted using R version 4.0.3 (R Core Development Team, Vienna, Austria). Two-sided *p*-values < 0.05 were considered statistically significant. The number of GAS tests performed and positivity rates in our cohort were compared with the incidence of GAS-P reported through the Tokyo Notifiable Disease Surveillance system [6]. Data on the demographic characteristics, symptoms, and clinical characteristics of patients who tested positive for GAS and SARS-CoV-2 simultaneously were collected and processed (Table 1). SARS-CoV-2 was detected using the following methods:

7 May 2020–8 November 2022: in-house polymerase chain reaction (PCR) test;

27 May 2020–31 December 2020: Antigen testing using QuickNavi-COVID-19 Ag (Denka Co., Ltd., Chuo-ku, Tokyo, Japan);

28 December 2020–20 February 2023: ID NOW COVID-19 test (Abbott Laboratories, Abbott Park, IL, USA);

9 November 2022–31 December 2024: GeneXpert SARS-CoV-2 test (Cepheid, Sunnyvale, CA, USA). The criteria for positive results followed contemporary COVID-19 treatment guidelines [12].

Table 1. Comparison of GAS-P incidence across different periods.

Variable	Overall	① Pre-COVID-19 Social Period (January 2019–April 2020)	② Restricted Social Period (May 2020–April 2023)	③ Post-Restriction Period (May 2023–December 2024)	*p*-Value (① vs. ②, ② vs. ③, ① vs. ③)
Positivity rate (%)	463/4837 (9.6)	137/1197 (11.4)	169/2398 (7.0)	157/1242 (12.6)	<0.001 (0.000015, <0.001, 0.459)
Age (mean ± SD, years)	28.0 ± 17.2	27.8 ± 16.5	33.1 ± 14.3	22.6 ± 18.9	<0.001(0.0029, <0.001, 0.013)
Male (%)	278 (60.0)	81 (59.1)	107 (63.3)	90 (57.3)	0.52 (0.48, 0.31, 0.81)
Children aged <15 years (%)	117 (25.3)	34 (24.8)	9 (5.3)	74 (47.1)	<0.001 (<0.001, <0.001, 0.00010)

This table presents the positivity rate, age distribution, and demographic characteristics of patients who were positive for GAS across three distinct study periods: the pre-COVID-19 social period (January 2019–April 2020), the restricted social period (May 2020–April 2023), and the post-restriction period (May 2023–December 2024). GAS, group A *Streptococcus*; GAS-P, group A *Streptococcus* pharyngitis; COVID-19, coronavirus disease; SD, standard deviation.

This study was approved by the Ethics Committee of Tokyo Shinagawa Hospital (approval number: 22-A-14) on 25 January 2023. Consent was obtained using the "opt-out method", thereby allowing patients to decline participation. Therefore, the research ethics committee waived the requirement for written informed consent. Additionally, the graphical abstract and symptom-related icons were generated with the assistance of ChatGPT-4o (OpenAI, May 2024 version), a generative AI tool, and were edited accordingly for presentation purposes.

3. Results

During the study period, a total of 4837 rapid antigen tests were performed to detect GAS antigens, and 463 (9.6%) were positive for GAS. The number of tests conducted ranged from 22–117 per month, except in January and July 2022. The monthly trends in GAS test results are summarized in Figure 1, while the age and sex distributions of positive cases are presented in Table S1. Among the patients who were GAS-positive, 278 (60.0%) were male, and the overall mean age ± standard deviation (SD) was 28.0 ± 17.2 years (Table 1). In total, 346 (74.7%) of those who were positive for GAS were aged ≥15 years, and 117 (25.3%) were children aged <15 years.

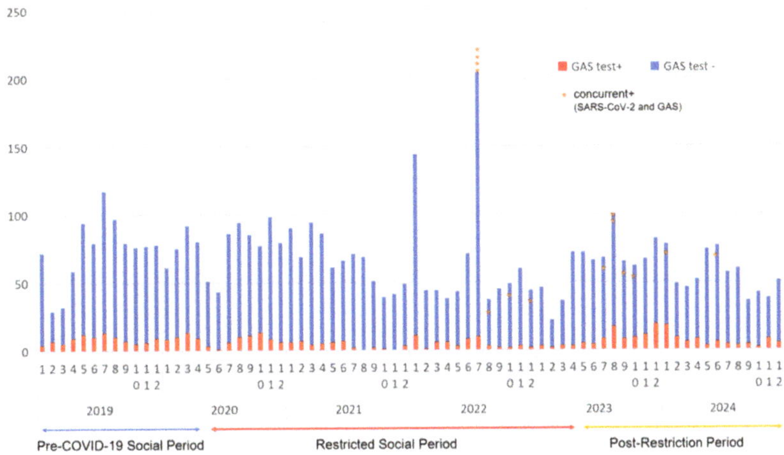

Figure 1. Trends in GAS-P incidence before and after the COVID-19 pandemic. Monthly trends in GAS-P cases between January 2019 and December 2024. Asterisks (*) indicate (number of) cases of concurrent GAS and SARS-CoV-2 infections. GAS-P, group A *Streptococcus* pharyngitis; COVID-19, coronavirus disease 2019; SARS-CoV-2, severe acute respiratory syndrome coronavirus 2.

The positivity rate was 11.4% (137/1197) in the pre-COVID-19 social period, significantly decreasing to 7.1% (169/2398, p = 0.000015 vs. pre-COVID-19) during the restricted social period, and then increasing to 12.6% (157/1242, p < 0.001 vs. restricted, p = 0.459 vs. pre-COVID-19) in the post-restriction period. The proportion of children aged <15 years was 24.8% (34/137) in the pre-COVID-19 social period, which significantly decreased to 5.3% (9/169, p < 0.001 vs. pre-COVID-19) during the restricted period, then markedly increased to 47.1% (74/157, p < 0.001 vs. restricted, p = 0.00010 vs. pre-COVID-19) in the post-restriction period.

These findings indicate a significant reduction in GAS positivity rates and pediatric cases during the restricted social period, followed by a sharp resurgence in the post-restriction period, particularly among younger age groups.

Among the 151 patients who tested positive for GAS and underwent simultaneous SARS-CoV-2 testing throughout the study period, 14 were diagnosed with co-infection (Table 2). Their clinical characteristics are shown in Table 3. These co-infection cases spanned a wide age range and included both sexes, with one case occurring in a pediatric patient. All co-infections occurred after July 2022, when the Omicron variant and subsequent lineages predominated.

Table 2. Yearly distribution of GAS positivity and SARS-CoV-2 co-infection among patients.

Category	2019	2020	2021	2022	2023	2024
GAS-positive cases (pediatric cases)	97 (23)	98 (13)	43 (3)	57 (1)	92 (42)	76 (35)
SARS-CoV-2 testing among GAS-positive cases (pediatric cases tested)	0 (0)	21 (0)	5 (0)	42 (1)	43 (3)	40 (5)
Co-infection cases: GAS and SARS-CoV-2 (pediatric co-infections)	0 (0)	0 (0)	0 (0)	7 (0)	6 (1)	1 (0)

This table shows a summary of the yearly counts of patients with GAS-positive results, those tested for SARS-CoV-2, and confirmed co-infections, with pediatric cases shown in parentheses. Co-infection cases were observed only after 2022. GAS, group A *Streptococcus*; SARS-CoV-2, severe acute respiratory syndrome coronavirus 2.

Table 3. Clinical characteristics of patients with GAS–SARS-CoV-2 co-infection.

Characteristics	
Total patients	14
Age (mean ± SD)	34.4 ± 17.7
Sex (male/female)	7/7
History of COVID-19	2
Immunodeficiency	0
Number of COVID-19 vaccine doses	
≥2	10
None	4
Days from onset (mean ± SD, [range])	1.5 ± 1.2 [0–4]
Symptoms	
Fever	14 (100%)
Sore throat	12 (85.7%)
Cough	7 (50%)
Headache	6 (42.9%)
Malaise	6 (42.9%)
Arthralgia	4 (28.6%)
Nasal discharge	3 (21.4%)
Muscle pain	2 (14.3%)
Nasal congestion	2 (14.3%)
Chills	2 (14.3%)
Nausea	2 (14.3%)
Vital signs	
Body temperature (mean ± SD, [range])	38.4 ± 1.2 °C [37.1–40.0]
Pulse oximetry oxygen saturation (mean ± SD, [range])	98.0 ± 1.0% [97–99]
Systolic blood pressure (mean ± SD, [range])	122.5 ± 16.9 [90–149]
Heart rate (mean ± SD, [range])	97.1 ± 15.5 [72–120]
Laboratory and imaging data	
White blood cell count (/μL)	5812.5 ± 660.0 [4400–6600]
Neutrophil count (/μL)	4342 ± 911 [3089–5316]
Lymphocyte count (/μL)	954 ± 542 [180–1401]
C-reactive protein (mg/dL)	2.0 ± 1.5 [0.6–4.0]
SARS-CoV-2 PCR (C_t values)	20.2 ± 4.3 [15.2–29.4]
Pneumonia findings on chest imaging/patients who underwent imaging (%)	1/5 (20%)
Clinical course and treatment	
Hospitalized/outpatient cases	3/11
Treatment	Regimen Details (Number of Patients)
Antibiotics only (nine patients)	AMPC/CVA (5), CAM (2), ABPC/SBT (1), CFPN-PI (1)
Antibiotics + antiviral agents (five patients)	CCL + ensitrelvir (2), AMPC/CVA + molnupiravir (1), ABPC/SBT + CAM + remdesivir (1), ABPC/SBT + nirmatrelvir (1)
Outcomes	Recovery: 14/14 (100%)

This table shows a summary of the demographic data, symptoms, laboratory findings, and treatment details of 14 patients diagnosed with GAS-P and SARS-CoV-2 infection. ABPC/SBT, ampicillin/sulbactam; AMPC/CVA, amoxicillin/clavulanic acid; CAM, clarithromycin; CCL, cefaclor; CFPN-PI, cefcapene pivoxil; COVID-19, coronavirus disease 2019; GAS, group A *Streptococcus*; GAS-P, group A *Streptococcus* pharyngitis; PCR, polymerase chain reaction; SARS-CoV-2, severe acute respiratory syndrome coronavirus 2; SD, standard deviation.

Despite the co-infection, the clinical course was mild in most cases. Fever was observed in all patients (100%), followed by sore throat (85.7%), cough (50.0%), headache (42.9%), and malaise (42.9%) as the most frequently reported symptoms. None of the patients developed hypoxemia or hypotension, and only three of them required hospitalization because of a severe sore throat, limiting oral intake.

Laboratory findings showed that white blood cell and neutrophil counts remained within normal ranges or were mildly elevated, whereas lymphopenia was common, consistent with known hematologic features of SARS-CoV-2 infections. Pneumonia was detected in only one of the five patients who underwent chest imaging.

All patients responded well to antimicrobial therapy. Penicillin-based antibiotics were most commonly used, followed by macrolides and cephalosporins; approximately one-third of the patients also received antiviral agents. No cases progressed to post-streptococcal complications or long COVID-19.

4. Discussion

Our study provides the first contiguous 6-year view of laboratory-confirmed GAS-P in Japan, spanning the pre-COVID-19 era, successive NPI phases, and the post-restriction period. We demonstrated that GAS-P incidence fell sharply after the first state of emergency in May 2020, lost its typical winter–spring and summer peaks, and then rebounded above the pre-pandemic baseline from May 2023—an increase driven predominantly in children.

These phases have been separately addressed in previous studies. The National Institute of Infectious Diseases documented a pandemic-associated collapse of pediatric GAS-P notifications, while an ecological time-series analysis showed a broader decline in communicable diseases during NPIs [13,14].

More recently, surveillance data highlighted a post-2023 surge in GAS-P and streptococcal toxic shock syndrome after public health restrictions were relaxed [15,16]. Using a retrospective enumeration of laboratory-confirmed cases in our center from 2019 to 2024, we linked these separate national observations: our data corroborate the NPI-related suppression of GAS-P, show the documentation of the loss and return of its seasonality and the size quantification of the post-restriction rebound. The initial decrease in the incidence of GAS-P is consistent with observations that stringent NPIs decreased the incidence of other infectious diseases [2,6]. In Japan, the reported incidence of *Streptococcus pyogenes* infections decreased by 32.1% (95% confidence interval: 0.06–0.589) after nationwide mandates on masking, hand hygiene, school closures, and social distancing [2,5,17–19]. Because GAS-P peaks are driven largely by child-to-child transmission [19], prolonged masking probably curtailed exposure and delayed immunity accrual [20]. Once mandates were relaxed (13 March 2023 for masks; 8 May 2023 for legal reclassification [21]), incidence rebounded, mirroring the post-restriction surges reported in Europe [22–24]. In Japan, the increase lagged until NPIs were lifted despite earlier respiratory syncytial virus and influenza waves [25–27], underscoring the dominant effect of behavioral measures on GAS transmission.

A similar study from Italy, in which 2230 swabs were analyzed over a 6-year period (2018–2023) using antigen testing, reported epidemiological trends comparable to those observed in Europe. Despite being a single-center study, a temporary decline in GAS-P cases was documented, followed by a resurgence, aligning with our findings [7].

Nonetheless, in the Italian study, co-infections with viral pathogens were not examined. In our cohort, 14 (9.3%) patients were co-infected with GAS and SARS-CoV-2.

GAS-P symptoms include fever and pharyngodynia, whereas headache, malaise, and cough are COVID-19 symptoms [1,28]. Laboratory findings showed that total leukocyte and neutrophil counts were normal to mildly elevated, although absolute lymphopenia was common (mean lymphocyte count: $0.95 \times 10^3/\mu L$). In contrast, a previous study showed that the prevalence of absolute leukocytosis and relative lymphopenia in GAS-P cases was 78.9% and 56%, respectively; in turn, the prevalence of absolute lymphopenia was less than 10% based on the results of throat cultures [29]. Thus, lymphocyte depletion in our cohort may reflect the additive effect of SARS-CoV-2, which decreases lymphocyte counts even in mild cases [30]. All our patients recovered uneventfully. Nonetheless, the potential for post-streptococcal or post-COVID-19 complications remains unknown and warrants prospective follow-up.

In our cohort, every GAS–SARS-CoV-2 co-infection case was documented after July 2022, a period dominated by Omicron sub-lineages. Notably, these cases emerged while influenza circulation in Japan was minimal, indicating that influenza-related confounding is unlikely. The temporal clustering, therefore, raises the possibility of a positive interaction between the Omicron variant and *S. pyogenes* in the upper airway [27,31]. Since Omicron preferentially replicates in the oropharynx, unlike pre-Omicron strains that infect the lower respiratory tract [32–34], two non-mutually exclusive mechanisms are plausible. First, Omicron-mediated epithelial damage may enhance streptococcal adherence and invasion [35–38]. Second, SARS-CoV-2-induced lymphopenia could impair mucosal immunity; a phenomenon also linked to enhanced *Candida* colonization [39]. Nonetheless, strong evidence for such virus–bacterium synergy is lacking; in our cohort, the high co-infection rate supports this hypothesis but cannot establish causality. Thus, integrated virologic, bacteriologic, and immunologic studies that analyze pathogen loads and mucosal immune profiling are needed to assess whether Omicron facilitates GAS colonization or whether the association reflects the high circulation of both pathogens in community settings.

This study has some limitations. First, SARS-CoV-2 testing among patients who were GAS-positive was not routinely performed, particularly in children, for whom obtaining swab samples poses practical challenges. In addition, the limited testing infrastructure during the early stages of the pandemic may have resulted in the underdetection of co-infections, especially before the Omicron wave, when testing resources were more constrained and diagnostic focus was narrower. Second, no multiplex diagnostic tests capable of detecting *S. pyogenes* and SARS-CoV-2 in a single assay were available in Japan during the study period. Therefore, clinicians ceased testing once one pathogen was identified, potentially missing additional infections [10]. Third, the use of multiple SARS-CoV-2 diagnostic platforms over time, each with varying sensitivities and specificities, may have decreased the accuracy of detection of co-infections. Fourth, the single-center nature of this study may limit the generalizability of the findings. However, the sentinel surveillance of acute respiratory infections nationwide since April 2025, including simultaneous monitoring for GAS and SARS-CoV-2, may help address these knowledge gaps [40,41].

Considering these diagnostic challenges, a substantial number of co-infections with SARS-CoV-2 may have been undetected. Moreover, it is unknown whether these co-infections can be effectively treated with antibiotic monotherapy versus combination therapy with antiviral agents. Thus, SARS-CoV-2 testing should be considered in patients who are GAS-positive with symptoms suggestive of COVID-19, such as cough or lymphopenia.

5. Conclusions

During the COVID-19 pandemic, the incidence of GAS-P significantly declined across all age groups, likely because of the widespread implementation of NPIs, which also disrupted the seasonal pattern of GAS-P. The incidence of GAS-P increased after the relaxation of COVID-19 restrictions, particularly among children. Co-infections with GAS and SARS-CoV-2 may be underrecognized owing to limited testing. Moreover, all co-infection cases in our cohort were mild; nevertheless, the potential impact of viral–bacterial interactions on disease severity and long-term complications remains unclear. Thus, larger prospective studies are warranted to elucidate these associations.

Supplementary Materials: The following supporting information can be downloaded at https://www.mdpi.com/article/10.3390/medicina61050937/s1: Table S1A: Number of positive cases of group A *Streptococcus* pharyngitis in 2019 and 2020, stratified by sex and age group; Table S1B: Number of positive cases of group A *Streptococcus* pharyngitis in 2021 and 2022, stratified by sex and age group; Table S1C: Number of positive cases of group A *Streptococcus* pharyngitis in 2023 and 2024, stratified by sex and age group.

Author Contributions: Conceptualization, H.T.; methodology, H.T., S.S., S.F. (Satomi Fujihara), and S.F. (Suzuko Fukasawa); formal analysis, H.T.; investigation, H.T., S.S., S.F. (Satomi Fujihara), and S.F. (Suzuko Fukasawa); resources, S.S., S.F. (Satomi Fujihara), and S.F. (Suzuko Fukasawa); data curation, H.T.; writing—original draft preparation, H.T.; writing—review and editing, Y.S., S.S., S.F. (Satomi Fujihara) S.T., S.F. (Suzuko Fukasawa), K.P., N.T., T.Y., H.N., R.H., M.T.-K., S.O., M.M., and M.S.; visualization, H.T., Y.S., and S.S.; supervision, S.F. (Suzuko Fukasawa); project administration, M.S. All authors have read and agreed to the published version of the manuscript.

Funding: This research received no external funding.

Institutional Review Board Statement: This study was approved by the Ethics Committee of Tokyo Shinagawa Hospital (Approval No. 22-A-14 approved on 25 January 2023).

Informed Consent Statement: Consent was obtained using the "opt-out method", thereby allowing patients to decline participation. Therefore, the research ethics committee waived the requirement for written informed consent.

Data Availability Statement: The data that support the findings of this study are available from the corresponding author upon reasonable request.

Acknowledgments: The authors acknowledge using ChatGPT-4o (OpenAI, May 2024 version) to create the illustrative symptom-related icons included in the graphical abstract. The content of this manuscript was solely developed and approved by the authors.

Conflicts of Interest: The authors declare no conflicts of interest.

Abbreviations

The following abbreviations are used in this manuscript:

COVID-19	coronavirus disease 2019
GAS	group A *Streptococcus*
GAS-P	group A *Streptococcus* pharyngitis
NPIs	non-pharmaceutical interventions
PCR	polymerase chain reaction
RSV	respiratory syncytial virus
SARS-CoV-2	severe acute respiratory syndrome coronavirus 2
SD	standard deviation

References

1. Ashurst, J.V.; Weiss, E.; Tristram, D.; Edgerley-Gibb, L. Streptococcal pharyngitis. In *StatPearls*; StatPearls Publishing: Treasure Island, FL, USA, 2025. Available online: https://www.ncbi.nlm.nih.gov/books/NBK525997/ (accessed on 24 April 2025).
2. Kakimoto, M.; Miyamori, D.; Omori, K.; Kobayashi, T.; Ikeda, K.; Kashiyama, S.; Ohge, H.; Ito, M. Impact of the early phase of COVID-19 on the trends of isolated bacteria in the national database of Japan: An interrupted time-series analysis. *J. Infect.* **2023**, *86*, 147–153. [CrossRef] [PubMed]
3. McBride, J.A.; Eickhoff, J.; Wald, E.R. Impact of COVID-19 quarantine and school cancelation on other common infectious diseases. *Pediatr. Infect. Dis. J.* **2020**, *39*, e449–e452. [CrossRef] [PubMed]
4. Li, A.; Zhang, L. Reduced incidence of acute pharyngitis and increased incidence of chornic pharyngitis under COVID-19 control strategy in Beijing. *J. Infect.* **2022**, *85*, 174–211. [CrossRef] [PubMed]
5. Boyanton, B.L., Jr.; Snowden, J.N.; Frenner, R.A.; Rosenbaum, E.R.; Young, H.L.; Kennedy, J.L. SARS-CoV-2 infection mitigation strategies concomitantly reduce group a streptococcus pharyngitis. *Clin. Pediatr.* **2023**, *62*, 683–687. [CrossRef]
6. Tokyo Metropolitan Infectious Disease Surveilance Center. Available online: https://idsc.tmiph.metro.tokyo.lg.jp/diseases/group-a/group-a/ (accessed on 22 May 2023).
7. Massese, M.; La Sorda, M.; De Maio, F.; Gatto, A.; Rosato, R.; Pansini, V.; Caroselli, A.; Fiori, B.; Sanguinetti, M.; Chiaretti, A.; et al. Epidemiology of group A streptococcal infection: Are we ready for a new scenario? *Lancet Microbe* **2024**, *5*, 620–621. [CrossRef]

8. Lassoued, Y.; Assad, Z.; Ouldali, N.; Caseris, M.; Mariani, P.; Birgy, A.; Bonacorsi, S.; Bidet, P.; Faye, A. Unexpected increase in invasive Group A streptococcal infections in children after respiratory viruses outbreak in France: A 15-year time-series analysis. *Open Forum Infect. Dis.* **2023**, *10*, ofad188. [CrossRef]
9. Chan, K.H.; Veeraballi, S.; Ahmed, E.; Yakobi, R.; Slim, J. A case of co-occurrence of COVID-19 and group A streptococcal pharyngitis. *Cureus* **2021**, *13*, e14729. [CrossRef]
10. Khaddour, K.; Sikora, A.; Tahir, N.; Nepomuceno, D.; Huang, T. Case report: The importance of novel coronavirus disease (COVID-19) and coinfection with other respiratory pathogens in the current pandemic. *Am. J. Trop. Med. Hyg.* **2020**, *102*, 1208–1209. [CrossRef]
11. Capilia™ Strep A. Available online: https://www.tauns.co.jp/en/wp-content/uploads/2021/08/capilia_strep_a_Brochure_2007A.pdf (accessed on 22 May 2023).
12. Ministry of Health, Labour and Welfare. Clinical Management of Patients with COVID-19. Available online: https://www.niph.go.jp/h-crisis/wp-content/uploads/2020/07/20200706103735_content_000646531.pdf (accessed on 17 November 2023).
13. Ghaznavi, C.; Sakamoto, H.; Kawashima, T.; Horiuchi, S.; Ishikane, M.; Abe, S.K.; Yoneoka, D.; Eguchi, A.; Tanoue, Y.; Hashizume, M.; et al. Decreased incidence followed by comeback of pediatric infections during the COVID-19 pandemic in Japan. *World J. Pediatr.* **2022**, *18*, 564–567. [CrossRef]
14. Hirae, K.; Hoshina, T.; Koga, H. Impact of the COVID-19 pandemic on the epidemiology of other communicable diseases in Japan. *Int. J. Infect. Dis.* **2023**, *128*, 265–271. [CrossRef]
15. Ujiie, M. Emerging trends in streptococcal toxic shock syndrome, Japan. *Emerg. Infect. Dis.* **2025**, *31*, 847–849. [CrossRef] [PubMed]
16. Fukushima, S.; Saito, T.; Iwamoto, Y.; Takehara, Y.; Yamada, H.; Fujita, K.; Yoshida, M.; Nakano, Y.; Hagiya, H. Trends in the growing impact of group A Streptococcus infection on public health after COVID-19 pandemic: A multicentral observational study in Okayama, Japan. *Eur. J. Clin. Microbiol. Infect. Dis.* **2025**, *44*, 383–391. [CrossRef] [PubMed]
17. Nakamoto, D.; Nojiri, S.; Taguchi, C.; Kawakami, Y.; Miyazawa, S.; Kuroki, M.; Nishizaki, Y. The impact of declaring the state of emergency on human mobility during COVID-19 pandemic in Japan. *Clin. Epidemiol. Glob. Health* **2022**, *17*, 101149. [CrossRef]
18. Mettias, B.; Jenkins, D.; Rea, P. Ten-year prevalence of acute hospital ENT infections and the impact of COVID: A large population study. *Clin. Otolaryngol.* **2023**, *48*, 10–16. [CrossRef]
19. Kennis, M.; Tagawa, A.; Kung, V.M.; Montalbano, G.; Narvaez, I.; Franco-Paredes, C.; Vargas Barahona, L.; Madinger, N.; Shapiro, L.; Chastain, D.B.; et al. Seasonal variations and risk factors of *Streptococcus pyogenes* infection: A multicenter research network study. *Ther. Adv. Infect. Dis.* **2022**, *9*, 20499361221132101. [CrossRef]
20. Frenck, R.W., Jr.; Laudat, F.; Liang, J.; Giordano-Schmidt, D.; Jansen, K.U.; Gruber, W.; Anderson, A.S.; Scully, I.L. A longitudinal study of Group A streptococcal colonization and pharyngitis in US children. *Pediatr. Infect. Dis. J.* **2023**, *42*, 1045–1050. [CrossRef]
21. Japan Relaxes Mask Guidelines in COVID Milestone. Available online: https://asia.nikkei.com/Spotlight/Coronavirus/Japan-relaxes-mask-guidelines-in-COVID-milestone (accessed on 22 May 2023).
22. de Gier, B.; Marchal, N.; de Beer-Schuurman, I.; Te Wierik, M.; Hooiveld, M.; de Melker, H.E.; van Sorge, N.M.; Stuart, J.C.; Melles, D.C.; Van Dijk, K.; et al. Increase in invasive group A streptococcal (*Streptococcus pyogenes*) infections (iGAS) in young children in the Netherlands, 2022. *Euro Surveill.* **2023**, *28*, 2200941. [CrossRef]
23. Cobo-Vázquez, E.; Aguilera-Alonso, D.; Carrasco-Colom, J.; Calvo, C.; Saavedra-Lozano, J.; PedGAS-Net Working Group. Increasing incidence and severity of invasive Group A streptococcal disease in Spanish children in 2019–2022. *Lancet Reg. Health Eur.* **2023**, *27*, 100597. [CrossRef]
24. Jain, N.; Lansiaux, E.; Reinis, A. Group A streptococcal (GAS) infections amongst children in Europe: Taming the rising tide. *New Microbes New Infect.* **2023**, *51*, 101071. [CrossRef]
25. Ujiie, M.; Tsuzuki, S.; Nakamoto, T.; Iwamoto, N. Resurgence of respiratory syncytial virus infections during COVID-19 pandemic, Tokyo, Japan. *Emerg. Infect. Dis.* **2021**, *27*, 2969–2970. [CrossRef]
26. Ohnishi, T.; Kang, Y.; Kawano, Y.; Kunikata, T.; Ichihashi, K. An atypical surge in RSV infections among children in Saitama, Japan in 2021. *IJID Reg.* **2023**, *7*, 124–126. [CrossRef]
27. Takahashi, H.; Nagamatsu, H.; Yamada, Y.; Toba, N.; Toyama-Kousaka, M.; Ota, S.; Morikawa, M.; Shinoda, M.; Takano, S.; Fukasawa, S.; et al. Surveillance of seasonal influenza viruses during the COVID-19 pandemic in Tokyo, Japan, 2018–2023, a single-center study. *Influ. Other Respir. Viruses* **2024**, *18*, e13248. [CrossRef]
28. Akaishi, T.; Kushimoto, S.; Katori, Y.; Sugawara, N.; Egusa, H.; Igarashi, K.; Fujita, M.; Kure, S.; Takayama, S.; Abe, M.; et al. COVID-19-related symptoms during the SARS-CoV-2 Omicron (B.1.1.529) variant surge in Japan. *Tohoku J. Exp. Med.* **2022**, *258*, 103–110. [CrossRef]
29. Herbinger, K.H.; Hanus, I.; Beissner, M.; Berens-Riha, N.; Kroidl, I.; von Sonnenburg, F.; Löscher, T.; Hoelscher, M.; Nothdurft, H.D.; Schunk, M. Lymphocytosis and lymphopenia induced by imported infectious diseases: A controlled cross-sectional study of 17,229 diseased German travelers returning from the tropics and subtropics. *Am. J. Trop. Med. Hyg.* **2016**, *94*, 1385–1391. [CrossRef]

30. Tan, L.; Wang, Q.; Zhang, D.; Ding, J.; Huang, Q.; Tang, Y.Q.; Wang, Q.; Miao, H. Lymphopenia predicts disease severity of COVID-19: A descriptive and predictive study. *Signal Transduct. Target. Ther.* **2020**, *5*, 33. [CrossRef]
31. Matsumura, Y.; Yamamoto, M.; Tsuda, Y.; Shinohara, K.; Tsuchido, Y.; Yukawa, S.; Noguchi, T.; Takayama, K.; Nagao, M. Epidemiology of respiratory viruses according to age group, 2023–2024 winter season, Kyoto, Japan. *Sci. Rep.* **2025**, *15*, 924. [CrossRef] [PubMed]
32. Sreenath, K.; Batra, P.; Vinayaraj, E.V.; Bhatia, R.; SaiKiran, K.; Singh, V.; Singh, S.; Verma, N.; Singh, U.B.; Mohan, A.; et al. Coinfections with other respiratory pathogens among patients with COVID-19. *Microbiol. Spectr.* **2021**, *9*, e0016321. [CrossRef]
33. Kawaguchi, A.; Nagaoka, K.; Kawasuji, H.; Kawagishi, T.; Fuchigami, T.; Ikeda, K.; Kanatani, J.I.; Doi, T.; Oishi, K.; Yamamoto, Y. COVID-19 complicated with severe $M1_{UK}$-lineage *Streptococcus pyogenes* infection in elderly patients: A report of two cases. *Int. J. Infect. Dis.* **2024**, *148*, 107246. [CrossRef]
34. Takahashi, H.; Morikawa, M.; Satake, Y.; Nagamatsu, H.; Hirose, R.; Yamada, Y.; Toba, N.; Toyama-Kousaka, M.; Ota, S.; Shinoda, M.; et al. Diagnostic utility of pharyngeal follicular structures in COVID-19: A large-scale cross-sectional study. *Int. J. Infect. Dis.* **2024**, *149*, 107244. [CrossRef]
35. Herrera, A.L.; Huber, V.C.; Chaussee, M.S. The association between invasive group a streptococcal diseases and viral respiratory tract infections. *Front. Microbiol.* **2016**, *7*, 342. [CrossRef]
36. Okamoto, S.; Nagase, S. Pathogenic mechanisms of invasive group A Streptococcus infections by influenza virus–group A Streptococcus superinfection. *Microbiol. Immunol.* **2018**, *62*, 141–149. [CrossRef] [PubMed]
37. Fan, Y.; Li, X.; Zhang, L.; Wan, S.; Zhang, L.; Zhou, F. SARS-CoV-2 Omicron variant: Recent progress and future perspectives. *Signal Transduct. Target. Ther.* **2022**, *7*, 141. [CrossRef] [PubMed]
38. Piersiala, K.; Kakabas, L.; Bruckova, A.; Starkhammar, M.; Cardell, L.O. Acute odynophagia: A new symptom of COVID-19 during the SARS-CoV-2 Omicron variant wave in Sweden. *J. Intern. Med.* **2022**, *292*, 154–161. [CrossRef] [PubMed]
39. Boia, E.R.; Huț, A.R.; Roi, A.; Luca, R.E.; Munteanu, I.R.; Roi, C.I.; Riviș, M.; Boia, S.; Duse, A.O.; Vulcănescu, D.D.; et al. Associated bacterial coinfections in COVID-19-positive patients. *Medicina* **2023**, *59*, 1858. [CrossRef]
40. Ministry of Health, Labour and Welfare. Acute Respiratory Infection: ARI. Available online: https://www.mhlw.go.jp/stf/seisakunitsuite/bunya/kenkou/kekkaku-kansenshou19/ari.html (accessed on 24 April 2025).
41. The Japan Times. Japan Begins Monitoring Acute Respiratory Infections. Available online: https://www.japantimes.co.jp/news/2025/04/08/japan/science-health/japan-respiratory-infections-monitor/ (accessed on 24 April 2025).

medicina

MDPI

Article

The Efficacy and Tolerability of Colistin Versus Non-Colistin Antimicrobial Regimens Among Hospitalized COVID-19 Patients with Multidrug-Resistant Bacterial Superinfection: An Observational Multicenter Study

Alzahraa M. Fahmy [1], Marwa O. Elgendy [2,3,*], Alaa Aboud Mohamed [4], Mohamed S. Imam [5,*], Abdullah Nasser Alharbi [6], Muhammad Husayn Al-Anezi [6], Omar Mana Aldhafeeri [6], Saif Mamdouh Aldhafeeri [6], Jawaher A. Ajeebi [7], Marwa Kamal [8] and Hasnaa Osama [9]

1 Tropical Medicine and Infectious Diseases Department, Faculty of Medicine, Beni-Suef University, Beni-Suef 62511, Egypt; alzhraamohamed@med.bsu.edu.eg
2 Department of Clinical Pharmacy, Beni-Suef University Hospitals, Faculty of Medicine, Beni-Suef University, Beni-Suef 62511, Egypt
3 Department of Clinical Pharmacy, Faculty of Pharmacy, Nahda University (NUB), Beni-Suef 62511, Egypt
4 Department of Tropical Medicine, Faculty of Medicine, Beni-Suef University, Beni-Suef 62511, Egypt; dralaaboud2005@yahoo.com
5 Department of Clinical Pharmacy, National Cancer Institute, Cairo University, Fom El Khalig Square, Kasr Al-Aini Street, Cairo 11796, Egypt
6 College of Pharmacy, Hafr Al Batin University, Hafr Al-Batin 31991, Saudi Arabia; abdullah.aldugaim@outlook.sa (A.N.A.); omarmani029@gmail.com (O.M.A.); callofnow@gmail.com (S.M.A.)
7 College of Pharmacy, Jazan University, Jazan 82912, Saudi Arabia; jawaher.ajeebi@gmail.com
8 Department of Clinical Pharmacy, Faculty of Pharmacy, Fayoum University, Fayoum 63514, Egypt; marwa.tolba@yahoo.com
9 Clinical Pharmacy Department, Faculty of Pharmacy, Beni-Suef University, Beni-Suef 62511, Egypt; hasnaa_osama2010@yahoo.com
* Correspondence: marwa.elgendy@nub.edu.eg or marwaosamaelgendy@yahoo.com (M.O.E.); imammohamed311@gmail.com (M.S.I.)

Abstract: *Background and Objectives*: Bacterial infections amongst COVID-19 patients could be associated with worsened outcomes. This study aimed to investigate the efficacy of colistin antibiotic in multidrug-resistant (MDR) Gram-negative (-ve) secondary bacterial infections among hospitalized COVID-19 patients. *Materials and Methods*: In this multi-centered retrospective study, we analyzed data from the medical records of 116 patients diagnosed with COVID-19 infection and secondary Gram-negative MDR bacterial respiratory infections. *Results*: We compared those assigned to colistin versus non-colistin-based antimicrobial therapy. The two arms of the study were similar in baseline clinical features, demographics, and Gram-negative pathogens' distribution. Acinetobacter baumannii (51.7%) was the major pathogen, followed by Klebsiella pneumonia (26.7%). Patients who received colistin-based antimicrobial regimen showed a non-significant difference compared to non-colistin antimicrobial (NCA) therapy ($p > 0.05$) in the main outcomes. Nephrotoxicity was significantly higher in the IV colistin group, compared to the control (34.1% and 15.3%, $p = 0.018$). There were substantial differences observed in the levels of serum creatinine and urea among the study arms ($p = 0.029$ and <0.001, respectively). *Conclusions*: The combination of colistin with other antimicrobial agents showed comparable results to that of NCA regimens in hospitalized COVID-19 patients with superinfections with multidrug-resistant bacterial isolates; however, there was a notably elevated incidence of nephrotoxicity with colistin antimicrobial therapy. Further randomized controlled trials are needed to assess the therapeutic benefits and tolerability of colistin antimicrobial therapy.

Medicina **2025**, *61*, 884 https://doi.org/10.3390/medicina61050884

Keywords: colistin; COVID-19; Gram-negative bacteria; secondary infection

1. Introduction

Since the emergence of the COVID-19 outbreak, the majority of efforts has been directed to the management of the virus [1–3]. Several emerging variants have been isolated with substantial variability in disease severity, evasion of the immune system, and response to therapeutics [4–6]. According to the World Health Organization (WHO), five variants of SARS-CoV-2 are designated as variants of concern with higher rates of transmission and relatively severe illnesses [7,8], and they warrant close monitoring [9,10].

Many studies reported respiratory bacterial superinfection among patients with COVID-19, with variable prevalence across the globe, especially among hospitalized patients. Severe cases of COVID-19 infections have much lower CD4 and CD8 T cells, which is conducive to higher vulnerability to bacterial coinfection and, consequently, higher fatality [11,12].

Bacterial infection transmission occurs within hospitals [13], either directly or indirectly, among hospitalized patients through contact with workers in healthcare settings and hospital equipment, such as ventilators and catheters [14]. Several isolates are well linked with nosocomial infections, such as Acinetobacter species, Klebsiella, Pseudomonas, and Staphylococcus species [15,16].

There is evidence indicating that the presence of bacterial pathogens as secondary infections can exacerbate the clinical prognosis of individuals with COVID-19 [17,18]. Bacterial infections acquired during a hospital stay are likely resistant to multiple antimicrobial drugs, resulting in a considerable challenge in managing COVID-19 patients [19,20].

Colistin is an antibacterial agent that has been used for several decades [21,22]. However, it was withdrawn due to safety concerns, including its neurotoxicity and nephrotoxicity [23,24]. Recently, because of the global concern about widespread nosocomial infections with carbapenem-resistant bacterial isolates, colistin has re-emerged [25,26].

The emergence of antibiotic resistance through the COVID-19 outbreak is significantly linked to the prevalence of Klebsiella pneumoniae, particularly carbapenemase-producing strains. The prior report indicated that the incidence of carbapenem-resistant K. pneumoniae (CRKP) escalated during the initial wave of the pandemic [27]. Numerous studies have indicated that the incidence of CRKP infections escalated during the pandemic. Currently, colistin in combination with other antimicrobial agents, such as meropenem or tigecycline, has been considered the cornerstone therapy for Gram-negative resistant isolates despite its considerable adverse effects [22,28]. Although colistin use has considerably increased in clinical practice, no standardized consensus has been developed for the optimum dose or route of administration.

Therefore, the main purpose of this study was to evaluate the tolerance and effectiveness of colistin-based treatment regimens for MDR Gram-negative bacterial superinfection in hospitalized patients with COVID-19.

2. Results

2.1. Baseline Study Population Characteristics

In total, 116 COVID-19-confirmed patients using PCR met the inclusion criteria and were included in the analysis. Out of the total, 44 (37.9%) patients received IV colistin-based regimen, and 72 (62.1%) received NCA regimen. Figure 1 summarizes the study's flowchart.

The demographics, clinical characteristics, and other therapeutic regimens of antimicrobials or specific drugs for COVID-19 of patients are illustrated in Table 1. The mean ± SD age was 57.9 ± 8.7 years and ranged between 46 and 79 years. Males made up 49.1% of the overall study population. The difference in baseline demographic data and comorbidities upon admission of patients in the study groups was statistically non-significant. In the two arms of the study, the combination with antimicrobial therapy was non-significantly different. Carbapenem antibiotics were commonly prescribed in both colistin (47.7%) and non-colistin (40.3%) groups.

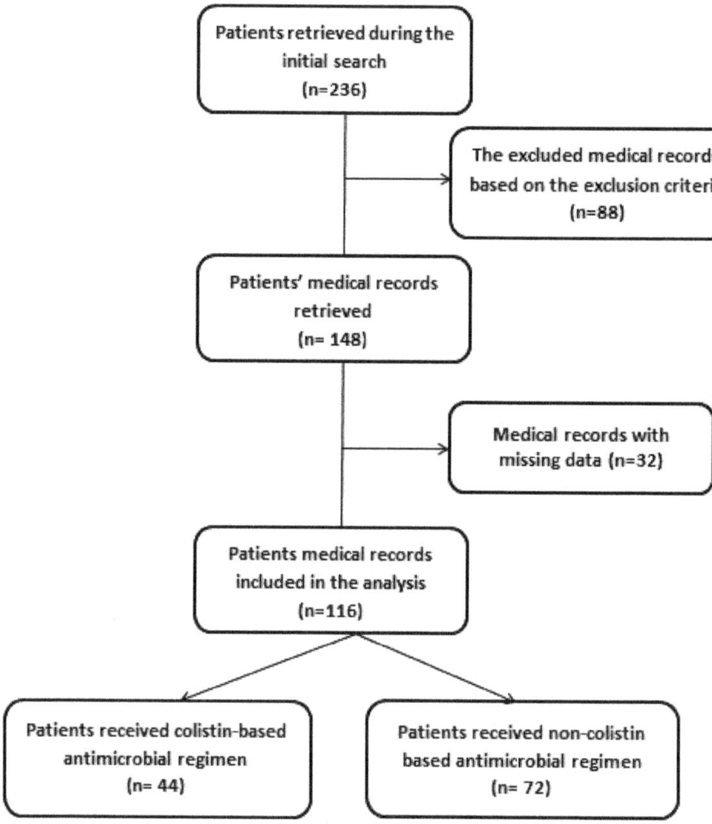

Figure 1. Flowchart of the study.

Table 1. Baseline demographic and clinical characteristics in the study groups.

Parameter	Intravenous Colistin Group (n = 44)	Non-Colistin (Control Group) (n = 72)	*p*-Value
Age	58.9 ± 9.6	57.3 ± 8.2	0.316
Gender (male, %)	18 (40.9%)	39 (54.2)	0.166
Co-administered antibiotic therapy (n, %)			
Carbapenem	21 (47.7)	29 (40.3)	0.432
Piperacillin–tazobactam	12 (27.3)	16 (22.2)	0.537
Macrolides	10 (22.7)	18 (25)	0.781
Cephalosporins	4 (9.1)	11 (15.3)	0.335
Fluoroquinolones	3 (6.8)	7 (9.7)	0.589
Comorbidities (n, %)			
Obesity	12 (27.3)	15 (20.8)	0.426

Table 1. *Cont.*

Parameter	Intravenous Colistin Group (n = 44)	Non-Colistin (Control Group) (n = 72)	*p*-Value
Chronic respiratory diseases	3 (6.8)	2 (2.8)	0.298
Diabetes mellitus	16 (36.4)	23 (31.9)	0.625
Hypertension	10 (22.7)	13 (18.1)	0.540
Laboratory findings (mean ± SD)			
Hemoglobin (g/dL)	12.6 ± 1.37	12.4 ± 1.34	0.310
Platelet (cells/mm^3)	349.6 ± 49.7	331.8 ± 69.8	0.132
Lymphocytes (%)	19.3 ± 6.2	18.9 ± 6.7	0.716
Serum urea (mg/dL)	34.3 ± 7.9	36.2 ± 8.1	0.217
Serum creatinine (mg/dL)	0.86 ± 0.16	0.91 ± 0.17	0.071
CRP (mg/L)	91.6 ± 28.4	94.5 ± 31.4	0.616
D-dimer (ng/mL)	683 ± 541.1	882 ± 598.3	0.232
AST (U/L)	48.7 ± 16.5	50.9 ± 19.7	0.532
ALT (U/L)	42.6 ± 18.4	46.1 ± 17.1	0.298
Pathogen causing super-infection (n, %)			
Acinetobacter spp.	23 (52.3)	37 (51.4)	0.926
Pseudomonas aeruginosa	7 (15.9)	15 (20.8)	0.512
Klebsiella	12 (27.3)	19 (26.4)	0.917
Poly-microbial infections	2 (4.5)	1 (1.4)	0.299
Smoking status (yes, n %)	23 (52.3)	30 (41.7)	0.266
Special therapy for COVID-19 treatment (n, %)			
Steroids	29 (65.9)	38 (52.8)	0.165
Lopinavir/ritonavir	6 (13.6)	9 (12.5)	0.860
Remdesivir	8 (18.2)	21 (29.2)	0.185
Tocilizumab	6 (13.6)	17 (23.6)	0.191

CRP, C-reactive protein; AST, aspartate aminotransferase; ALT, Alanine aminotransferase.

Of all included patients, co-infections with Klebsiella pneumonia, Acinetobacter baumannii, and Pseudomonas aeruginosa infections were the most common bacterial isolates, with a non-significant difference in the distribution of microbial isolates between the study groups ($p > 0.05$) (Figure 2).

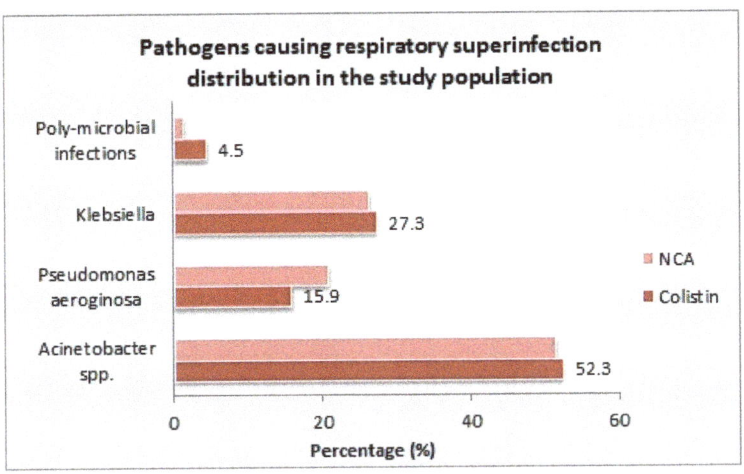

Figure 2. Microbial distribution in the study population. NCA, non-colistin antimicrobial regimen.

2.2. Assessment of Efficacy

The use of the colistin-based regimen was linked with a reduced length of hospitalization, with a mean ± SD of 11.3 ± 3.8 days, compared to the non-colistin group (12.8 ± 4.7); however, the difference was non-significant (p = 0.073). The number of patients assigned for mechanical ventilation did not differ significantly between the study groups: 22.7% and and 23.6%, p-value = 0.913, for colistin and non-colistin based regimens, respectively. The outcomes of the study groups are presented in Table 2. In the same context, a non-significant difference was observed in the other outcomes: the need for admission to the ICU, the duration of the ICU stay, and the all-cause mortality at 30 days between the two study arms. The colistin group showed a higher microbiological eradication rate (n = 35, 79.5%) than that observed with non-colistin-based antibiotic regimen (n = 52, 72.2%); however, the difference did not reach significance (p = 0.377).

Table 2. Outcomes of subjects in the two arms of the study.

Outcome	Colistin Group (n = 44)	Non-Colistin (Control Group) (n = 72)	p-Value
Hospitalization duration (days) mean	11.3 ± 3.8	12.8 ± 4.7	0.073
Admission for ICU (yes, %)	14 (31.8)	31 (43.1)	0.228
Duration of ICU stay (days)	9.3 ± 3.1	10.4 ± 3.8	0.108
Mechanical ventilation (yes, %)	10 (22.7)	17 (23.6)	0.913
All-cause-mortality at 30 days (n, %)	14 (31.8)	17 (23.6)	0.332
Microbiological eradication rate (n, %)	35 (79.5)	52 (72.2)	0.377

2.3. Assessment of Systemic Toxicity

Of the overall included patients, 13 (11.2%) showed elevations in ALT and AST serum levels with treatment. Of them, eight (18.2%) were receiving IV colistin-based regimens, and the other five (6.9%) patients were in the NCA group. However, no significant difference was observed between the study groups (p = 0.063).

Nephrotoxicity incidence was higher in the colistin group compared to the NCA group (34.1% vs. 15.3%, p = 0.018). Among the 44 patients who received IV colistin, risk and injury KDIGO categories occurred in 8 (18.2%) and 5 (11.4%), respectively, and failure was observed in 2 (4.5%) patients who required discontinuation of treatment. Eleven (15.3%) patients in the control group had nephrotoxicity in the risk category of KDIGO.

At baseline, the difference in creatinine levels between the study population was non-significant (p = 0.071), with an overall mean ± SD of 0.89 ± 0.16 mg/dL. After treatment, the overall difference in serum creatinine levels between the study arms was significant (p = 0.048), with a high increase in SCr levels observed with colistin-based regimens and a mean difference (MD) of 0.28 [95%CI; 0.2, 0.39; p-value < 0.001], while the control group showed lower change in creatinine levels [MD: 0.04; 95% CI; −0.01, 0.09; p = 0.109] (Figure 3A).

The difference in urea levels between the study populations at baseline was non-significant (p = 0.217), with an overall mean ± SD of 35.5 ± 8.01 mg/dL. Following the completion of therapy, urea levels increased from baseline with intravenous colistin [MD: 4.1, 95% CI: 2.04 to 6.22, p < 0.001]. Furthermore, there was a significant difference between the two arms of the study (p = 0.002) (Figure 3B).

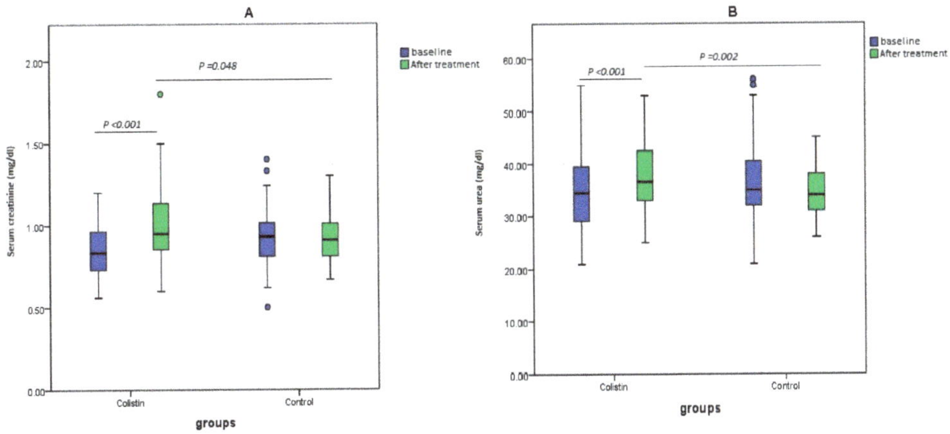

Figure 3. The changes in (**A**) serum creatinine (mg/dL) and (**B**) serum urea (mg/dL) levels in the study groups.

To determine the risk factors associated with nephrotoxicity as defined by KDIGO criteria in both colistin- and NCA-treated cohort arms, logistic regression analyses were performed. The outcomes showed that patients receiving colistin experienced significantly higher nephrotoxicity (OR: 2.86; 95%CI: 1.17 to 7.02, $p = 0.021$). In other words, the incidence of AKI in the colistin group was 2.86 times higher than that experienced in non-colistin based regimens. Other factors significantly associated with nephrotoxicity were age older than 60 years (OR: 1.08; 95%CI: 1.012 to 1.13; p value = 0.017), diabetes mellitus (OR: 2.65; 95% CI, 1.07 to 6.51, $p = 0.034$), remdesivir use (OR: 2.93; 95%CI: 1.15 to 7.463, $p = 0.024$), and tocilizumab use (OR: 2.57; 95% CI, 1.02 to 6.46; $p = 0.045$) (Supplementary Table S1).

Multivariate logistic regression analysis showed a significant association between chronic respiratory diseases, nephrotoxicity, and the incidence of mortality at 30 days, with odds ratios (ORs) of 1.9 [95% CI; 1.02, 3.9] and [OR: 2.6, 95% CI: 1.1, 6.2], respectively (Table 3).

Table 3. Logistic regression of the independent predictors associated with the all-cause mortality at 30 days.

Parameter	Odds Ratio	95% Confidence Interval (CI)
Age (>60)	1.3	0.74–2.5
Chronic respiratory diseases	1.9	1.02–3.9
Colistin use	1.5	0.7–3.5
Nephrotoxicity	2.6	1.1–6.2
Main pathogen		
Acinetobacter baumannii	0.76	0.48–1.2
Pseudomonas aeruginosa	1.4	0.49–3.7
Klebsiella pneumonia	1.7	0.96–3.1

3. Discussion

The primary objective of this study was to examine the clinical outcomes and tolerability of using a colistin-based regimen of antimicrobial therapy in the treatment of hospitalized patients with COVID-19 who have developed MDR bacterial superinfection. The main finding of this study is that the colistin-based antimicrobial regimen did not show superiority compared to the other antimicrobial regimens. Moreover, nephrotoxicity was significantly higher with colistin-based antimicrobial therapy among COVID-19 patients with MDR Gram-negative respiratory superinfection.

The significance of secondary bacterial infection, especially with Gram-negative pathogens, is well recognized by many researchers [29,30]. Many studies investigated the prevalence of microbiological pathogens in the respiratory tract specimens of adult COVID-19 cases admitted to hospitals [31]. Most of these studies reported that K. pneumoniae, A. baumannii, and Pseudomonas species were the most commonly isolated Gram-negative agents from patients' specimens [32], as were S. aureus for Gram-positive bacteria [33,34]. In this study, Acinetobacter baumannii (51.7%) was found to be the most common Gram-negative microorganism, followed by K. pneumonia (26.7%) and P. aeruginosa (18.97%).

Colistin, a polymyxin E antibiotic, gradually restored its popularity because of its potential efficacy against infections that result from multidrug-resistant (MDR) pathogens [35,36]. However, only limited examinations of its efficacy and tolerability are available for COVID-19 patients with secondary MDR bacterial infections [37,38].

Lim et al. assessed the effects of different combinations against MDR Gram-negative bacterial infections and observed non-significant differences in mortality rates among cases treated with colistin and NCA arms (35.5% and 38.5%, respectively, $p = 0.80$) [39]. The same was also reported by Balkan et al., thus conforming to our findings. In a prospective trial, including patients assigned to colistin versus comparators, including meropenem or imipenem or ampicillin–sulbactam, the administration of beta-lactams antimicrobial therapy was found to be linked with lower overall mortality [40]. The same was observed in our results, where higher mortality was associated with colistin-based regimens; however, the effect did not reach significance.

A previous study reported that four bacterial species were predominantly found in COVID-19 patients: Klebsiella pneumoniae, Acinetobacter baumannii, Pseudomonas aeruginosa, and *Escherichia coli*. Among these, *K. pneumoniae** and *A. baumannii* showed the highest rates of co-infection with SARS-CoV-2, which was associated with increased mortality in this study. The colistin showed highly efficacy against Pseudomonas aeruginosa and Klebsiella pneumonia [41,42].

The regression analysis of our results revealed nephrotoxicity and chronic pulmonary disease as the two important factors highly linked with mortality among our study population. Indeed, these results are consistent with several studies which identified acute kidney injury and pulmonary diseases as predictors of in-hospital mortality [43,44]. The administration of colistin-based antimicrobial therapy showed a higher microbiological eradication rate than that observed with the non-colistin-based antibiotic regimen, with non-significant difference between groups (79.5% vs. 72.2%, $p = 0.377$).

It is noteworthy that several factors have been identified in the clinical response to colistin therapy, including IV colistin loading dose, sepsis, nephrotoxicity, gender, and the score of Acute Physiology and Chronic Health Evaluation II [45]. Considering the limited sample size, considerable variation in clinical and demographic attributes within our study cohort, and comorbidity with COVID-19, it might be challenging to detect significant predictive factors for response to colistin therapy.

The infection of COVID-19 mainly affects the lungs; however, the incidence of acute kidney injury (AKI), shown as a notable increase in serum creatinine and urea levels, is also well documented [46]. Replicated studies reported an incidence rate of AKI ranging from 5% to 23% among hospitalized COVID-19 patients and reaching over 60% in severe cases [47,48]. Since colistin is associated with the possibility of nephrotoxicity, the potential synergistic effect of the harmful effects of COVID-19 on the kidney would be a subject of concern. In the current study, the incidence rate of nephrotoxicity appeared to be significantly higher with colistin-based regimens (34.1% vs. 15.3%, $p = 0.018$).

Furthermore, the conducted multivariable regression analyses to assess the robustness of our main findings revealed that colistin-based regimens increased the risk of nephrotoxicity by 2.86 times that of NCA (95%CI: 1.17 to 7.02, $p = 0.021$). Old age (>60 years) and diabetes mellitus comorbidity were consistently associated with nephrotoxicity. Remdesivir and tocilizumab were also identified as risk factors for the incidence of AKI I in the study cohorts. Hence, based on our findings, the risk of nephrotoxicity among COVID-19 patients seems to be multifactorial. These findings are in accordance with those reported by Rocco et al.'s (2013) study, which identified older age and sepsis as strongly associated risk factors for the incidence of AKI with receiving a high dose of colistin methanesulfonate intravenously, either alone or in combination with other potentially nephrotoxic antibiotics [49]. Similarly, numerous studies reported a significant association of remdesivir, tocilizumab, and lopinavir/ritonavir with an increased odds of AKI among COVID-19 patients [50,51].

It is worth noting that we could not observe significant hepatotoxicity with colistin-based regimens; however, a relative elevation in liver enzymes with the IV colistin regimen compared to NCA regimens [8 (18.2%) vs. 5 (6.9%), $p = 0.063$] was detected. These findings were consistent with previous studies [35,52].

Therefore, polymyxin-based antimicrobial regimens might be an adequate alternative option for MDR Gram-negative bacterial respiratory infection, especially in conditions where resistance for β-lactam–β-lactamase inhibitors is present [53]. However, kidney function should be cautiously monitored in such cases. In addition, the inhalation route of colistin can be a less toxic alternative according to several recent studies [36,54,55].

The retrospective design is the major limitation of our investigation. Other limitations encompass the relatively small sample size; the presence of other antimicrobial therapies; and the absence of follow-up for long-term, recurrence, or emergence of resistance assessment. In addition, we could not assess the neurotoxic effects of colistin. Additional randomized controlled studies that use genomic and artificial intelligence techniques like WGCNA and LIME may be able to pinpoint the important genes affecting the toxicity and efficacy of colistin in COVID-19 patients. Examining hub genes, like PGLYRP4 and HEPHL1, that have been connected to COVID-19 may shed light on how colistin affects the immune system. Colistin may improve results and lessen nephrotoxicity when used in conjunction with FDA-approved medications that target certain genes [56].

4. Materials and Methods

4.1. Ethical Approval

Before proceeding with the trial, the protocol underwent a comprehensive evaluation and received approval from the research ethics committee of Faculty of pharmacy, Beni-Suef University.

4.2. Study Design and Target Population

This cohort study was conducted retrospectively at many Egyptian healthcare centers between March 2021 and August 2021. In this study, we compared the tolerability and effectiveness of IV colistin in comparison to non-colistin antimicrobial (NCA) regimens in COVID-19 patients with MDR-secondary Gram-negative bacterial infection. Patients who were treated with colistin or NCA regimens for ≥72 h were identified from medical records. Severe, non-critically ill COVID-19 adult patients aged > 18 years and who had pneumonia and with confirmed MDR Gram-negative bacterial superinfection were eligible for the study. The determination of the severity of the COVID-19 infection was made in accordance with the definitions provided by the World Health Organization (WHO) [57]. The included patients were identified as positive COVID-19 cases using the reverse transcription–polymerase chain reaction (RT-PCR) test. Pneumonia diagnosis in patients was defined either by chest imaging and at least 2 clinical features of pneumonia [58,59].

A bacterial infection was confirmed using microbiological cultures. MDR bacteria were defined as microbial pathogens exhibiting resistance to a minimum of one antibiotic in three or more distinct antibiotic groups [11,60].

The exclusion criteria included patients younger than 18 years old; pregnancy; immunocompromised patients with malignancy or HIV infection; and patients with renal impairment, such as chronic kidney disease (CKD), or assignment to renal-replacement therapy (RRT). Patients' records that fulfilled the predetermined inclusion criteria were included in the analysis.

We divided the whole cohort into two groups as follows: the intravenous colistin-based antimicrobial regimen (9 million international units (MIU) of colistin in divided doses for 10 days, adjusted according to the renal function), and the control group, which included patients who received systemic antibiotic regimens without colistin. The Sanford guide on antimicrobial therapy was used to determine the adequate dose of antimicrobial therapy for each patient.

4.3. *Study Outcomes*

The following data were extracted from the medical records of the included patients: demographics, medical history, hospital settings, dosage of colistin used, and the co-administered antibiotics. The main outcomes included microbiological eradication rate, defined as the absence of Gram-negative isolates with respiratory cultures at the end of antibiotic therapy, hospital duration of stay, admission to intensive care unit (ICU), ventilation needs, and survival rate of the participants. Laboratory test outcomes such as alanine aminotransferase (ALT), aspartate aminotransferase (AST), D-dimer hemoglobin, platelet count, and C-reactive protein (CRP) were also collected. Serum creatinine (SCr) and urea levels at baseline and post-intervention were recorded to detect antibiotic-associated nephrotoxicity, in accordance with the Kidney Disease Outcomes Quality Initiative (KDOQI) guidelines [61].

Drug-sensitivity tests and sputum cultures were performed according to hospital laboratory standards using the disk diffusion method. The microbiological-susceptibility testing was performed on the causative pathogen to common antibiotics, including carbapenem, amino-glycosides, cephalosporins, piperacillin/tazobactam, fluoroquinolones, colistin, and tigecycline. The breakpoints identified by the Clinical and Laboratory Standards Institute (CLSI) were applied in the susceptibility testing. Susceptibility to colistin was defined as in vitro minimum inhibitory concentration (MIC) < 2 mg/L.

4.4. *Statistical Analysis*

IBM SPSS Statistics version 16 software, created by Install Shield Corporation, Inc., Chicago, IL, USA, was used to perform the descriptive analysis. The Kolmogorov–Smirnov test was performed to determine the normality of the data, and the continuous variables were represented by the mean $\pm$ standard deviation (SD). The categorical data were represented in the form of frequencies and percentages. A pairwise comparison utilizing a paired Student's *t*-test for normally distributed data was employed to evaluate the differences between the research groups. Wilcoxon signed rank was used for paired comparisons with values that were not normally distributed, and the Mann–Whitney U test was used for comparisons between two independent groups. Categorical variables were compared using the Chi-square test. A logistic regression analysis was conducted to investigate the variables that are correlated with death at the 30-day outcome and the independent predictors associated with acute kidney injury in the study population.

5. Conclusions

The presence of multidrug-resistant respiratory infections in severe cases of COVID-19 infections is considerably challenging for healthcare professionals. The effectiveness of colistin combined with other antimicrobial therapies showed comparable results to that of non-colistin-based regimens among hospitalized COVID-19 patients with secondary infections with multidrug-resistant bacterial isolates; however, there was a substantial change in the occurrence of nephrotoxicity between the groups with and without colistin antimicrobial therapy. Further robustly designed randomized controlled studies with a larger cohort are necessary to assess the therapeutic benefits of colistin, its safety, and its potential antiviral activity against COVID-19.

Supplementary Materials: The following supporting information can be downloaded at: https://www.mdpi.com/article/10.3390/medicina61050884/s1, Table S1: Logistic regression analysis of the independent predictors associated with acute kidney injury in the study population.

Author Contributions: Conception and design, H.O. and M.O.E.; methodology, A.M.F., A.A.M. and M.K.; software, H.O.; validation and investigation, M.O.E. and M.K.; original draft preparation, H.O., A.M.F., M.O.E., M.S.I., A.N.A. and O.M.A.; resources, M.S.I., A.N.A., O.M.A., S.M.A. and J.A.A.; data curation, M.O.E., H.O. and M.K.; funding acquisition, A.N.A., M.S.I., O.M.A., S.M.A., J.A.A. and M.H.A.-A.; writing review and editing, M.K., A.M.F., M.O.E., M.S.I., S.M.A., J.A.A. and H.O.; visualization, H.O.; supervision, H.O. and M.O.E. All authors have read and agreed to the published version of the manuscript.

Funding: This research received no external funding.

Institutional Review Board Statement: The study was conducted in accordance with the Declaration of Helsinki and approved by the Ethics Committee of the Faculty of Pharmacy at Beni-Suef University (Rec-H-phBsu 23055, 5 May 2023).

Informed Consent Statement: Not applicable.

Data Availability Statement: The datasets generated and/or analyzed during the current study are available from the corresponding author upon reasonable request.

Conflicts of Interest: The authors have no relevant affiliations or financial involvement with any organization or entity with a financial interest in or financial conflict with the subject matter or materials discussed in the manuscript.

References

1. Bazaid, A.S.; Barnawi, H.; Qanash, H.; Alsaif, G.; Aldarhami, A.; Gattan, H.; Alharbi, B.; Alrashidi, A.; Al-Soud, W.A.; Moussa, S. Bacterial coinfection and antibiotic resistance profiles among hospitalised COVID-19 patients. *Microorganisms* **2022**, *10*, 495. [CrossRef] [PubMed]
2. Khalaf, A.M.; Elgendy, M.O.; Fahmy, A.M.; El Gendy, S.O.; El-Gendy, A.O.; Abdelrahman, M.A.; El-Bahrawy, A.H.; Elsisi, A.M.M.; Shafiq, S.N. Relation between ABO and RhD and prevalence and severity of COVID-19 disease. *Int. J. Clin. Med. Res.* **2024**, *2*, 78–86. [CrossRef]
3. Zawbaa, H.M.; El-Gendy, A.; Saeed, H.; Osama, H.; Ali, A.M.; Gomaa, D.; Abdelrahman, M.; Harb, H.S.; Madney, Y.M.; Abdelrahim, M.E. A study of the possible factors affecting COVID-19 spread, severity and mortality and the effect of social distancing on these factors: Machine learning forecasting model. *Int. J. Clin. Pract.* **2021**, *75*, e14116. [CrossRef]
4. AbdelHalim, M.M.; El Sherbini, S.A.; Ahmed, E.S.S.; Gharib, H.A.A.; Elgendy, M.O.; Ibrahim, A.R.; Abdel Aziz, H.S. Management of Ventilator-Associated Pneumonia Caused by Pseudomonas and Acinetobacter Organisms in a Pediatric Center: A Randomized Controlled Study. *Medicina* **2024**, *60*, 2098. [CrossRef]

5. Aziz, H.S.A.; Ismail, D.K.; Mohammed, N.S.A.; Elgendy, M.O.; Bassiouny, D.M. Distribution and antifungal susceptibility profiles of Candida species isolated from candidemia patients admitted to Egyptian tertiary hospitals: A cross-sectional study. *BMC Infect. Dis.* **2024**, *24*, 1177. [CrossRef]
6. Yuki, K.; Fujiogi, M.; Koutsogiannaki, S. COVID-19 pathophysiology: A review. *Clin. Immunol.* **2020**, *215*, 108427. [CrossRef]
7. Abdelgawad, M.A.; Bakr, R.B.; El-Gendy, A.O.; Kamel, G.M.; Azouz, A.A.; Bukhari, S.N.A. Discovery of a COX-2 selective inhibitor hit with anti-inflammatory activity and gastric ulcer protective effect. *Future Med. Chem.* **2017**, *9*, 1899–1912. [CrossRef] [PubMed]
8. Abo-Elela, M.M.; ElKasabgy, N.A. COVID-19 a global crisis: Features, complications and suggested treatments. *Int. J. Clin. Med. Res.* **2023**, *1*, 43–55. [CrossRef]
9. Chavda, V.P.; Patel, A.B.; Vaghasiya, D.D. SARS-CoV-2 variants and vulnerability at the global level. *J. Med. Virol.* **2022**, *94*, 2986–3005. [CrossRef]
10. Carabelli, A.M.; Peacock, T.P.; Thorne, L.G.; Harvey, W.T.; Hughes, J.; Peacock, S.J.; Barclay, W.S.; De Silva, T.I.; Towers, G.J.; Robertson, D.L. SARS-CoV-2 variant biology: Immune escape, transmission and fitness. *Nat. Rev. Microbiol.* **2023**, *21*, 162–177. [CrossRef]
11. Khalifa, R.; Ismail, B.; Al-Jahdali, H.; Alghamdi, H.; Joharjy, H.; Eibani, K.; Sabour, R.; Almalki, F.; Alfarhan, S.; Alatram, M. Secondary multidrug resistant bacterial pneumonia among adult COVID-19 patients: A molecular study. *Microbes Infect. Dis.* **2023**, *4*, 11–26. [CrossRef]
12. Mutua, J.M.; Njeru, J.M.; Musyoki, A.M. Multidrug resistant bacterial infections in severely ill COVID-19 patients admitted in a national referral and teaching hospital, Kenya. *BMC Infect. Dis.* **2022**, *22*, 877. [CrossRef] [PubMed]
13. Naguib, M.M.; El-Gendy, A.O.; Khairalla, A.S. Microbial diversity of mer operon genes and their potential rules in mercury bioremediation and resistance. *Open Biotechnol. J.* **2018**, *12*, 56–77. [CrossRef]
14. Sayed, A.M.; Alhadrami, H.A.; El-Gendy, A.O.; Shamikh, Y.I.; Belbahri, L.; Hassan, H.M.; Abdelmohsen, U.R.; Rateb, M.E. Microbial natural products as potential inhibitors of SARS-CoV-2 main protease (Mpro). *Microorganisms* **2020**, *8*, 970. [CrossRef]
15. Garcia-Vidal, C.; Sanjuan, G.; Moreno-García, E.; Puerta-Alcalde, P.; Garcia-Pouton, N.; Chumbita, M.; Fernandez-Pittol, M.; Pitart, C.; Inciarte, A.; Bodro, M.; et al. Incidence of co-infections and superinfections in hospitalized patients with COVID-19: A retrospective cohort study. *Clin. Microbiol. Infect.* **2021**, *27*, 83–88. [CrossRef] [PubMed]
16. Ahmed, E.; El-Gendy, A.O.; Hamblin, M.R.; Mohamed, T. The effect of femtosecond laser irradiation on the growth kinetics of Staphylococcus aureus: An in vitro study. *J. Photochem. Photobiol. B Biol.* **2021**, *221*, 112240. [CrossRef]
17. Behera, B.; Tripathy, S.; Venkateshan, M.; Mahapatra, A.; Mohanty, S.; Gupta, K.; Mishra, B.; Rao, P.B.; Mitra, J.K.; Mohapatra, P.R.; et al. Spectrum of Bacterial Pathogens in Critical COVID-19 Patients Admitted in Intensive Care Units of a Tertiary Care Hospital During the First and Second Wave of the Pandemic. *J. Assoc. Physicians India* **2022**, *70*, 11–12.
18. El-Gendy, A.O.; Saeed, H.; Ali, A.M.; Zawbaa, H.M.; Gomaa, D.; Harb, H.S.; Madney, Y.M.; Osama, H.; Abdelrahman, M.A.; Abdelrahim, M.E. Bacillus Calmette–Guérin vaccine, antimalarial, age and gender relation to COVID-19 spread and mortality. *Vaccine* **2020**, *38*, 5564–5568. [CrossRef]
19. Wang, L.; Zhou, K.-H.; Chen, W.; Yu, Y.; Feng, S.-F. Epidemiology and risk factors for nosocomial infection in the respiratory intensive care unit of a teaching hospital in China: A prospective surveillance during 2013 and 2015. *BMC Infect. Dis.* **2019**, *19*, 145. [CrossRef]
20. Sayed, A.M.; Sherif, N.H.; El-Gendy, A.O.; Shamikh, Y.I.; Ali, A.T.; Attia, E.Z.; El-Katatny, M.H.; Khalifa, B.A.; Hassan, H.M.; Abdelmohsen, U.R. Metabolomic profiling and antioxidant potential of three fungal endophytes derived from Artemisia annua and Medicago sativa. *Nat. Prod. Res.* **2022**, *36*, 2404–2408. [CrossRef]
21. Abdelrahman, M.A.; Zaki, A.; Salem, S.A.; Salem, H.F.; Ibrahim, A.R.; Hassan, A.; Elgendy, M.O. The Impact of Cefepime and Ampicillin/Sulbactam on Preventing Post-Cesarean Surgical Site Infections, Randomized Controlled Trail. *Antibiotics* **2023**, *12*, 1666. [CrossRef] [PubMed]
22. El-Gendy, A.; Essam, T.; Amin, M.; Ahmed, S.; Nes, I. Clinical screening for bacteriocinogenic *Enterococcus faecalis* isolated from intensive care unit inpatient in Egypt. *J. Microb. Biochem. Technol.* **2013**, *4*, 161–167. [CrossRef]
23. Babar, Z.U.; Dodani, S.K.; Nasim, A. Treatment outcome and adverse effects of colistin in adult patients with carbapenem-resistant gram-negative bacteremia from Pakistan. *Int. J. Infect. Dis.* **2021**, *106*, 171–175. [CrossRef]
24. Alessio, B. COVID-19's effects on undergraduate medical education. *Int. J. Clin. Med. Res.* **2024**, *2*, 60–61. [CrossRef]
25. Audrick, J. Immediate and long-term effects of COVID-19's on the pharmaceutical industry. *Int. J. Clin. Med. Res.* **2024**, *2*, 209–213. [CrossRef]
26. Mahmoud Farhan, S.; Mahmoud Abd El-Baky, R.; Abdalla, M.; Osama El-Gendy, A.; Farag Azmy, A. Efficacy of Amikacin and Imipenem Against Multi-Drug Resistant Gram-Negative Bacteria Isolated from Wound Infections, Egypt. *Iran. J. Med. Microbiol.* **2023**, *17*, 218–229. [CrossRef]
27. Farhan, S.M.; Raafat, M.; Abourehab, M.A.; Abd El-Baky, R.M.; Abdalla, S.; El-Gendy, A.O.; Azmy, A.F. Effect of imipenem and amikacin combination against multi-drug resistant Pseudomonas aeruginosa. *Antibiotics* **2021**, *10*, 1429. [CrossRef]

28. Kengkla, K.; Kongpakwattana, K.; Saokaew, S.; Apisarnthanarak, A.; Chaiyakunapruk, N. Comparative efficacy and safety of treatment options for MDR and XDR Acinetobacter baumannii infections: A systematic review and network meta-analysis. *J. Antimicrob. Chemother.* **2018**, *73*, 22–32. [CrossRef]
29. Zhou, P.; Liu, Z.; Chen, Y.; Xiao, Y.; Huang, X.; Fan, X.-G. Bacterial and fungal infections in COVID-19 patients: A matter of concern. *Infect. Control Hosp. Epidemiol.* **2020**, *41*, 1124–1125. [CrossRef]
30. Rawson, T.M.; Moore, L.S.; Zhu, N.; Ranganathan, N.; Skolimowska, K.; Gilchrist, M.; Satta, G.; Cooke, G.; Holmes, A. Bacterial and fungal coinfection in individuals with coronavirus: A rapid review to support COVID-19 antimicrobial prescribing. *Clin. Infect. Dis.* **2020**, *71*, 2459–2468. [CrossRef]
31. Salah, H.; Sinan, I.; Alsamani, O.; Abdelghani, L.S.; ElLithy, M.H.; Bukamal, N.; Jawad, H.; Hussein, R.R.S.; Elgendy, M.O.; Rabie, A.S.I.; et al. COVID-19 booster doses: A multi-center study reflecting healthcare providers' perceptions. *Vaccines* **2023**, *11*, 1061. [CrossRef] [PubMed]
32. Haggag, Y.A.E.G.; Saafan, A.E.; El-Gendy, A.O.; Hefzy, E.M.; AbdelGhani, S. Molecular Characterization of Quinolone Resistant Urinary Isolates of *Escherichia coli*. *J. Pure Appl. Microbiol.* **2020**, *14*, 1269–1278. [CrossRef]
33. Lee, S.H.; Ruan, S.-Y.; Pan, S.-C.; Lee, T.-F.; Chien, J.-Y.; Hsueh, P.-R. Performance of a multiplex PCR pneumonia panel for the identification of respiratory pathogens and the main determinants of resistance from the lower respiratory tract specimens of adult patients in intensive care units. *J. Microbiol. Immunol. Infect.* **2019**, *52*, 920–928. [CrossRef]
34. Molham, F.; Khairalla, A.S.; Azmy, A.F.; El-Gebaly, E.; El-Gendy, A.O.; AbdelGhani, S. Anti-proliferative and anti-biofilm potentials of bacteriocins produced by non-pathogenic *Enterococcus* sp. *Probiotics Antimicrob. Proteins* **2021**, *13*, 571–585. [CrossRef]
35. Gu, W.-J.; Wang, F.; Tang, L.; Bakker, J.; Liu, J.-C. Colistin for the treatment of ventilator-associated pneumonia caused by multidrug-resistant Gram-negative bacteria: A systematic review and meta-analysis. *Int. J. Antimicrob. Agents* **2014**, *44*, 477–485. [CrossRef] [PubMed]
36. Almangour, T.A.; Alruwaili, A.; Almutairi, R.; Alrasheed, A.; Alhifany, A.A.; Eljaaly, K.; Alkofide, H.; Alhammad, A.M.; Ghonem, L.; Alsharidi, A. Aerosolized plus intravenous colistin vs intravenous colistin alone for the treatment of nosocomial pneumonia due to multidrug-resistant Gram-negative bacteria: A retrospective cohort study. *Int. J. Infect. Dis.* **2021**, *108*, 406–412. [CrossRef] [PubMed]
37. Khalil, E.M.; Madney, Y.M.; Hassan, M.; Fahmy, A.M.; Alshammari, S.O.; Alshammari, Q.A.; Abou-Taleb, H.A.; Taha, A.A.; Elgendy, M.O.; Ali, H.A. Maternal and Fetal Outcome of COVID-19 Infection among Pregnant Women. *Medicina* **2024**, *60*, 1676. [CrossRef]
38. Ismael, M.S.; Elgendy, M.O.; Binsaleh, A.Y.; Saleh, A.; Abdelrahim, M.E.; Osama, H. Impulsivity and Its Association with Depression and Anxiety in the Normal Egyptian Population Post COVID-19 Pandemic. *Medicina* **2024**, *60*, 1367. [CrossRef]
39. Lim, S.-K.; Lee, S.-O.; Choi, S.-H.; Choi, J.-P.; Kim, S.-H.; Jeong, J.-Y.; Choi, S.-H.; Woo, J.H.; Kim, Y.S. The outcomes of using colistin for treating multidrug resistant Acinetobacter species bloodstream infections. *J. Korean Med. Sci.* **2011**, *26*, 325–331. [CrossRef]
40. Balkan, I.I.; Batirel, A.; Karabay, O.; Agalar, C.; Akalin, S.; Alici, O.; Alp, E.; Altay, F.A.; Altin, N.; Arslan, F. Comparison of colistin monotherapy and non-colistin combinations in the treatment of multi-drug resistant *Acinetobacter* spp. bloodstream infections: A Multicenter retrospective analysis. *Indian J. Pharmacol.* **2015**, *47*, 95–100. [CrossRef]
41. Said, K.B.; Alsolami, A.; Moussa, S.; Alfouzan, F.; Bashir, A.I.; Rashidi, M.; Aborans, R.; Taha, T.E.; Almansour, H.; Alazmi, M. COVID-19 clinical profiles and fatality rates in hospitalized patients reveal case aggravation and selective co-infection by limited gram-negative bacteria. *Int. J. Environ. Res. Public Health* **2022**, *19*, 5270. [CrossRef]
42. Abbas, A.M.; Hamed, R.M.R.; Elgendy, M.O.; Abdel Aziz, H.S. Prevalence and Antimicrobial Susceptibility Profile of Gram-negative and Gram-positive Bacteria in a Tertiary Hospital: A Retrospective Study. *Egypt. J. Med. Microbiol.* **2025**, *34*, 89–104. [CrossRef]
43. Cheng, Y.; Luo, R.; Wang, K.; Zhang, M.; Wang, Z.; Dong, L.; Li, J.; Yao, Y.; Ge, S.; Xu, G. Kidney disease is associated with in-hospital death of patients with COVID-19. *Kidney Int.* **2020**, *97*, 829–838. [CrossRef]
44. Branco, C.G.; Duarte, I.; Gameiro, J.; Costa, C.; Marques, F.; Oliveira, J.; Bernardo, J.; Fonseca, J.N.; Carreiro, C.; Braz, S. Presentation and outcomes of chronic kidney disease patients with COVID-19. *Braz. J. Nephrol.* **2021**, *44*, 321–328. [CrossRef] [PubMed]
45. Jung, S.; Chung, E.K.; Jun, M.S.; Son, E.S.; Rhie, S.J. Differences in colistin administration and bacterial and treatment outcomes in critically ill patients. *Sci. Rep.* **2019**, *9*, 8781. [CrossRef] [PubMed]
46. Elgendy, M.O.; Khalaf, A.M.; El-Gendy, A.O.; Abdelrahman, M.A.; El Gendy, S.O.; Hamied, A.M.A.; Essam, O.; Al Amir, K.; Yousry, E.M.; Abdelrahim, M.E. An observational study on the management of COVID-19 patients in limited-resource hospitals. *J. Clin. Nurs. Res.* **2022**, *6*, 43–53. [CrossRef]
47. Yarijani, Z.M.; Najafi, H. Kidney injury in COVID-19 patients, drug development and their renal complications: Review study. *Biomed. Pharmacother.* **2021**, *142*, 111966.

48. Elgendy, M.O.; El-Gendy, A.O.; Elgendy, S.O.; Abdelaty, L.N.; Abdelrahim, M.E.; Abdelrahman, M.A. Perceptions, Knowledge, and Experiences of Using Face Masks among Egyptian Healthcare Workers during the COVID-19 Pandemic: A Cross-Sectional Study. *Healthcare* **2023**, *11*, 838. [CrossRef]
49. Rocco, M.; Montini, L.; Alessandri, E.; Venditti, M.; Laderchi, A.; De Gennaro, P.; Raponi, G.; Vitale, M.; Pietropaoli, P.; Antonelli, M. Risk factors for acute kidney injury in critically ill patients receiving high intravenous doses of colistin methanesulfonate and/or other nephrotoxic antibiotics: A retrospective cohort study. *Crit. Care* **2013**, *17*, R174. [CrossRef]
50. Zhou, Y.; Li, J.; Wang, L.; Zhu, X.; Zhang, M.; Zheng, J. Acute kidney injury and drugs prescribed for COVID-19 in diabetes patients: A real-world disproportionality analysis. *Front. Pharmacol.* **2022**, *13*, 833679. [CrossRef]
51. Binois, Y.; Hachad, H.; Salem, J.-E.; Charpentier, J.; Lebrun-Vignes, B.; Pène, F.; Cariou, A.; Chiche, J.-D.; Mira, J.-P.; Nguyen, L.S. Acute kidney injury associated with lopinavir/ritonavir combined therapy in patients with COVID-19. *Kidney Int. Rep.* **2020**, *5*, 1787–1790. [CrossRef] [PubMed]
52. Kalin, G.; Alp, E.; Demiraslan, H.; Doganay, M.; Coskun, R.; Gündogan, K. Use of high-dose IV and aerosolized colistin for the treatment of multidrug-resistant Acinetobacter baumannii ventilator-associated pneumonia: Do we really need this treatment? *J. Infect. Chemother.* **2012**, *18*, 872–877. [CrossRef]
53. Ahmed, E.; El-Gendy, A.O.; Moniem Radi, N.A.; Mohamed, T. The bactericidal efficacy of femtosecond laser-based therapy on the most common infectious bacterial pathogens in chronic wounds: An in vitro study. *Lasers Med. Sci.* **2021**, *36*, 641–647. [CrossRef]
54. Lu, Q.; Luo, R.; Bodin, L.; Yang, J.; Zahr, N.; Aubry, A.; Golmard, J.-L.; Rouby, J.-J. Efficacy of high-dose nebulized colistin in ventilator-associated pneumonia caused by multidrug-resistant Pseudomonas aeruginosa and Acinetobacter baumannii. *Surv. Anesthesiol.* **2013**, *57*, 222–223. [CrossRef]
55. Boisson, M.; Grégoire, N.; Cormier, M.; Gobin, P.; Marchand, S.; Couet, W.; Mimoz, O. Pharmacokinetics of nebulized colistin methanesulfonate in critically ill patients. *J. Antimicrob. Chemother.* **2017**, *72*, 2607–2612. [CrossRef] [PubMed]
56. Karami, H.; Derakhshani, A.; Ghasemigol, M.; Fereidouni, M.; Miri-Moghaddam, E.; Baradaran, B.; Tabrizi, N.J.; Najafi, S.; Solimando, A.G.; Marsh, L.M.; et al. Weighted gene co-expression network analysis combined with machine learning validation to identify key modules and hub genes associated with SARS-CoV-2 infection. *J. Clin. Med.* **2021**, *10*, 3567. [CrossRef]
57. World Health Organization. *Clinical Care for Severe Acute Respiratory Infection: Toolkit: COVID-19 Adaptation*; World Health Organization: Geneva, Switzerland, 2022.
58. Zaki, A.; Elgendy, M.O.; Abdelrahman, M.A.; Ali, H.; Khalil, E.M.; Hassan, M.; Fahmy, A.M.; Gad, R.A.; Salem, H.F. The efficacy of using different antibiotics to prevent maternal surgical site infections in COVID-19-infected cases. *Eur. Chem. Bull.* **2023**, *6*, 1342–1348.
59. Shaban, M.; Elgendy, M.O.; Fahmy, A.M.; Khalil, D.M.; El-Gendy, A.O.; Mahmoud, T.M.; Abdelrahim, M.E. The Outcomes of COVID-19 Patients with Spontaneous Intracerebral Hemorrhage Comorbidity and the Efficacy of Enoxaparin in Decreasing the Mortality Rate in Them: Single Egyptian Center Report. *J. Pers. Med.* **2022**, *12*, 1822. [CrossRef]
60. Martin-Loeches, I.; Torres, A.; Rinaudo, M.; Terraneo, S.; de Rosa, F.; Ramirez, P.; Diaz, E.; Fernández-Barat, L.; Ferrer, M. Resistance patterns and outcomes in intensive care unit (ICU)-acquired pneumonia. Validation of European Centre for Disease Prevention and Control (ECDC) and the Centers for Disease Control and Prevention (CDC) classification of multidrug resistant organisms. *J. Infect.* **2015**, *70*, 213–222.
61. Kellum, J.A.; Lameire, N.; Group KAGW. Diagnosis, evaluation, and management of acute kidney injury: A KDIGO summary (Part 1). *Crit. Care* **2013**, *17*, 204. [CrossRef]

medicina

MDPI

Article

Assessing the Diagnostic Values of the Neutrophil-to-Lymphocyte Ratio (NLR) and Systematic Immunoinflammatory Index (SII) as Biomarkers in Predicting COVID-19 Severity: A Multicentre Comparative Study

Anwar A. Sayed

Department of Basic Medical Sciences, Taibah University, Madinah 42353, Saudi Arabia; dsayed@taibahu.edu.sa; Tel.: +966-014-861-8888

Abstract: COVID-19 has been notoriously unpredictable in its clinical course. Such unpredictability poses a challenge to clinicians in predicting patients who will develop severe cases and possibly die from the infection. This study aims to assess and compare the diagnostic value of the NLR and SII as biomarkers in predicting COVID-19 severity, represented by mortality, with a multicentre comparative study including 855 patients in Saudi Arabia. Descriptive and analytical statistics were used to compare haematological indices between survivors and non-survivors. The median age of patients included was 41 years old, with an almost equal ratio of men to women. Most participants were Saudis, and the mortality rate in the study cohort was 13.22%. Non-survivors, as compared to survivors, were significantly older, had lower RBC counts, haemoglobin and haematocrit levels, as well as significantly higher WBC and neutrophil counts. Both the NLR and SII were capable of differentiating between survivors and non-survivors, with the latter having significantly higher values. However, the NLR was superior to the SII in such differentiation, as it had a larger area under the curve. This study further confirms the diagnostic values of the NLR and SII as biomarkers in predicting COVID-19 severity and mortality, with the NLR being more sensitive and specific. Clinical guidelines on managing COVID-19 cases should benefit from these findings by harnessing the value of the NLR in COVID-19 management.

Keywords: biomarkers; COVID-19; diagnostics; mortality; multicentre; NLR; Saudi Arabia; SII; systematic immunoinflammatory index

1. Introduction

Four years ago, the world was faced with its first pandemic of the 21st century, with the novel coronavirus disease 2019 (COVID-19) spreading all over the world [1]. In response, countries took unprecedented measures to tackle the spread of the infection, including Saudi Arabia. Saudi Arabia took a series of progressive public measures, including halting public religious activities, travel bans and 24-h curfews [2].

COVID-19, even after 4 years of its first declaration as a pandemic and the end of its pandemic status [3], remains a medical dilemma for physicians. When it was first described, COVID-19 was described as a respiratory virus, affecting mainly the respiratory system [4]. However, subsequent studies found that the infection extends beyond the respiratory system, causing haematological abnormalities, leading to thrombotic abnormalities [5]. Furthermore, the condition was described to lead to hyperactivation of the immune system, leading to subsequent harmful autoimmune reactions damaging other parts of the body, such as the kidneys and the heart [6,7].

Another unsolved issue with COVID-19 is its unpredictable course. The pathophysiology of COVID-19 remains extremely heterogeneous, and, hence, efforts were made to develop tools to predict its course [8]. However, most of these predicting tools depend on clinical presentations and parameters that may differ significantly between countries. Thus, the applicability of these clinical tools remains limited to the geographical location in which these tools were developed.

Several studies proposed novel biomarkers that depend on haematological parameters to predict the course of COVID-19. These include the neutrophil-to-lymphocyte ratio (NLR) [9], systemic immune-inflammatory index (SII) and, more recently, the COMPred indicator [10]. Most of these studies focused on a particular tool, which makes the comparison between these tools difficult as the study cohorts were different. This study aims to address this gap in the literature and compare the NLR and SII in predicting the course of COVID-19 and, more specifically, its associated mortality.

2. Materials and Methods

2.1. Study Design and Setting

This is a multicentre cross-sectional retrospective study that included three tertiary hospitals in Saudi Arabia. This study included 855 patients who were hospital-admitted with a suspicion of COVID-19. The diagnosis of COVID-19 was confirmed using a quantitative polymerase chain reaction (qPCR) test of a nasopharyngeal swab. Patients were admitted to the hospitals between June 2020 and December 2021. Patients were admitted based on the recommendation of the Saudi Ministry of Health (MoH) criteria for COVID-19 patients [11]. In brief, patients with any one of the following symptoms were to be admitted: clinical evidence of pneumonia, age older than 65 years, low oxygen saturation on a pulsometer of less than 94% in room air, acute respiratory distress syndrome, chronic pulmonary or kidney disease and a history of comorbidities or morbid obesity (BMI equal or more than 40). Those who yielded a negative COVID-19 diagnosis or had missing information were not included in this study.

The management of these admitted patients was consistent between the three hospitals as the national COVID-19 management protocol, i.e., the Saudi MoH for Patients Suspected of/Confirmed with COVID-19 [11], was followed throughout the course of their management. Patients who were admitted to the intensive care unit (ICU) were managed according to the Saudi MoH Protocol for Patients Suspected of/Confirmed to have severe COVID-19 [11]. These patients showed clinical signs of pneumonia, e.g., fever, cough, dyspnea and one of the following: respiratory rate more than 30/min, oxygen saturation on pulsometer less than 93% in room air or severe respiratory distress.

All of the included patients had a series of laboratory investigations performed on them, and some were repeated over the course of their hospital stay. To ensure the consistency of the compared parameters, only the first readings of their investigations were included in this study, which were conducted upon admission. Venous blood samples were collected from patients for analysis as a part of their in-hospital management. Venous blood samples were tested for a complete blood count using the Mindray BC-3200. Auto Hematology Analyzer (Shenzhen Mindray Bio-Medical Electronics Co., Ltd., Shenzhen, China). The collected parameters were based on the complete blood count investigation, which includes the red blood cell (RBC), haemoglobin level, mean corpuscular volume (MCV), mean concentration of haemoglobin (MCH), the platelet count, the white blood cell (WBC) count, neutrophil count, lymphocyte count, monocyte count and eosinophil count. The NLR was calculated by dividing the neutrophil count by the lymphocyte count, and the SII was calculated by multiplying the platelet count by the NLR.

2.2. Statistical Analysis

Categorical data, such as gender and nationality, was described using absolute numbers and percentages. Descriptive statistics were used to describe numerical data, such as haemoglobin levels and the NLR, in accordance with their distribution. The Shapiro–Wilk test was used to determine the data distribution in order to determine whether the data follow a normal Gaussian distribution (parametric) or not (nonparametric). Means and standard deviations were used to describe parametric data, whereas medians and interquartile ranges were used for nonparametric data. Analytical statistics were used to compare the different data sets, including the t-test for parametric data and the Mann–Whitney U test to compare nonparametric data.

A receiver operating characteristic (ROC) curve analysis was made, and the area under the curve was calculated to determine the indicator's sensitivity and specificity of both the NLR and the SII. A p-value of less than 0.05 was considered statistically significant. A data analysis was carried out using GraphPad Prism Version 10.1.2 for Windows.

2.3. Ethical Considerations

No personal or sensitive patient information was collected as part of this study. Collected data were stored on a password-protected drive and was backed up on a password-protected server. This study was conducted in accordance with the declaration of Helsinki and ethically approved by the Taibah University College of Medicine Research Ethics Committee no. TU-21-010 on 10 February 2022. Given the retrospective nature of this study, the patients' consent was waived by the approving IRB ethics committee.

3. Results

3.1. Participant Characteristics

The analysis encompassed a total of 855 patients within the clinical cohort. The average age of patients was determined to be 41 years, with an interquartile range spanning from 27 to 57 years, indicating a relatively homogeneous distribution across age groups. Among the patients, 426 were identified as male, while 429 were female, suggesting a nearly equal gender distribution within the cohort. In terms of nationality, 550 patients were Saudi nationals, whereas 305 patients were non-Saudis, including but not limited to other nationalities such as Egyptians and Sudanese Indians.

The examination of admission outcomes revealed notable disparities within the cohort. A total of 742 patients were discharged alive, constituting the majority of the cohort's population. Conversely, 113 patients experienced mortality during their hospital stay, indicating a mortality rate of 13.22% within the cohort. These characteristics are described in Table 1.

Table 1. Patients' Characteristics.

Characteristic (Unit)	Values
Age (years)	41 (27–57) *
Gender	Male: 426 Female: 429
Nationality	Saudi: 550 Non-Saudi: 305
Admission outcome	Alive: 742 Deceased: 113

* Years are expressed as median (interquartile range).

3.2. Patients' Baseline Investigations

The investigation into haematological parameters revealed significant insights into the blood profiles of the study population. Analysis of red blood cell (RBC) count demonstrated a median value of 4.74 (4.35–5.13) $\times 10^6$/mL, which falls within the reference ranges for both genders. Haemoglobin levels' median value was at 13.40 (11.99–14.60) g/dL, similar to the RBC count, falling within the reference range for males and females. Additional parameters such as mean corpuscular volume (MCV), mean corpuscular haemoglobin (MCH), platelet count, white blood cell (WBC) count, and differential leukocyte counts were also assessed and are described in Table 2.

Table 2. Patients' laboratory investigations at baseline.

Investigation (Unit)	Patients' Readings	Reference Levels
RBC count ($\times 10^6$/mL)	4.74 (4.35–5.13)	Male: 4.0–5.9 Female: 3.8–5.2
Haemoglobin (g/dL)	13.40 (11.99–14.60)	Male: 13.8–17.2 Female: 12.1–15.1
Haematocrit (%)	40.70 (37.13–44.10)	Male: 40–54 Female: 36–48
MCV (fl)	86.25 (81.53–89.80)	80–100
MCH (pg)	28.60 (26.80–30)	27–31
Platelet count ($\times 10^6$/mL)	229.5 (182–290.5)	150–450
WBC ($\times 10^3$/mL)	6.24 (4.57–9.29)	4–11
Neutrophil count ($\times 10^3$/mL)	4.28 (2.71–7.49)	2.5–7
Lymphocyte count ($\times 10^3$/mL)	1.07 (0.69–1.59)	1–4.8
Monocyte Count ($\times 10^3$/mL)	0.33 (0.23–0.48)	0.2–0.8
Eosinophil count ($\times 10^3$/mL)	0.04 (0.01–0.08)	0.03–0.35

All values are expressed using the median value (interquartile range).

Interestingly, the median readings of the laboratory investigations of the study participants were within the reference levels.

3.3. Non-Survivors Demonstrate a Different Haematological Profile Compared to Survivors

In examining the characteristics and investigations of survivors (n = 742) compared to non-survivors (n = 113), notable distinctions were observed. Survivors exhibited a significantly younger median age of 38 years (27–52), contrasting starkly with non-survivors, who had a median age of 62 years (49–75.50) ($p < 0.0001$). Gender distribution showed no significant difference between survivors and non-survivors, with 361 males and 381 females among survivors and 65 males and 48 females among non-survivors ($p = 0.08$). While red blood cell (RBC) counts, haemoglobin levels, haematocrit percentages, mean corpuscular volume (MCV), mean corpuscular haemoglobin (MCH) and platelet counts did not display substantial variations between the two groups, white blood cell (WBC) counts, neutrophil counts, lymphocyte counts and eosinophil counts exhibited significant differences ($p < 0.0001$). Survivors demonstrated lower median WBC counts (5.96×10^3/mL) compared to non-survivors (8.33×10^3/mL), along with lower neutrophil and lymphocyte counts, indicating potential immune response variations between the groups. Eosinophil counts also varied significantly ($p = 0.002$), with survivors presenting higher median counts (0.04×10^3/mL) than non-survivors (0.02×10^3/mL). Despite the significant differences in the haematological parameters between survivors and non-survivors, they were still within the reference range of these parameters. These findings underscore the relevance of age and immune response indicators in predicting patient outcomes, providing valuable insights for clinical prognosis and management strategies. These results are summarised in Table 3.

Table 3. Comparison of patients' characteristics and lab investigations between survivors and non-survivors.

Characteristics/Investigation (Unit)	Survivors (n = 742)	Non-Survivors (n = 113)	*p*-Value
Age (years)	**38 (27–52)**	**62 (49–75.50)**	**<0.0001**
Gender	Male: 361 Female: 381	Male: 65 Female: 48	0.08 ^
RBC count ($\times 10^6$/mL)	4.76 (4.37–5.14)	4.60 (4.09–5.08)	0.09
Haemoglobin (g/dL)	**13.50 (12.20–14.70)**	**12.88 (11.60–14.35)**	**0.007**
Haematocrit (%)	**41 (37.30–44.20)**	**39.70 (35.70–43.30)**	**0.046**
MCV (fl)	86.20 (81.70–89.80)	86.70 (80.90–89.90)	0.73
MCH (pg)	28.70 (26.90–30)	28.10 (26.40–29.90)	0.23
Platelet count ($\times 10^6$/mL)	228.5 (185–294)	235 (160.9–285)	0.46

Table 3. *Cont.*

Characteristics/Investigation (Unit)	Survivors (n = 742)	Non-Survivors (n = 113)	*p*-Value
WBC count (×10³/mL)	**5.96 (4.45–8.56)**	**8.33 (5.78–11.60)**	**<0.0001**
Neutrophil count (×10³/mL)	**3.93 (2.57–6.63)**	**6.16 (4.16–9.86)**	**<0.0001**
Lymphocyte count (×10³/mL)	**1.13 (0.74–1.66)**	**0.76 (0.53–1.25)**	**<0.0001**
Monocyte Count (×10³/mL)	0.33 (0.23–0.48)	0.33 (0.20–0.53)	0.32
Eosinophil count (×10³/mL)	**0.04 (0.01–0.08)**	**0.02 (0.00–0.06)**	**0.002**

All values, except for gender, are described as a median (interquartile range). All comparisons, except for gender, were performed using the Mann–Whitney U test, given the nonparametric distribution of the data. Values written in bold denote statistically significant differences between survivors and non-survivors. ^ Chi-square test was used.

3.4. The Value of Using the Neutrophil-to-Lymphocyte Ratio (NLR) and the Systematic Immunoinflammatory Index (SII) to Discriminate between Survivors and Non-Survivors

As the median of all the haematological parameters of both survivors and non-survivors were within the reference range, it was important to develop a tool that could differentiate between survivors and non-survivors. The NLR, which depends on both the neutrophil and lymphocyte counts, can be used for such a purpose. Upon comparing the NLR between survivors and non-survivors, non-survivors had a significantly higher NLR compared to survivors (*p*-value < 0.0001; Figure 1A). The SII depends on both the platelet count and NLR to be calculated. In this study cohort, both survivors and non-survivors had comparable platelet counts (Figure 1B). However, the SII showed a statistically significant difference when compared between survivors and non-survivors, with the latter having a higher SII (*p*-value < 0.001; Figure 1C).

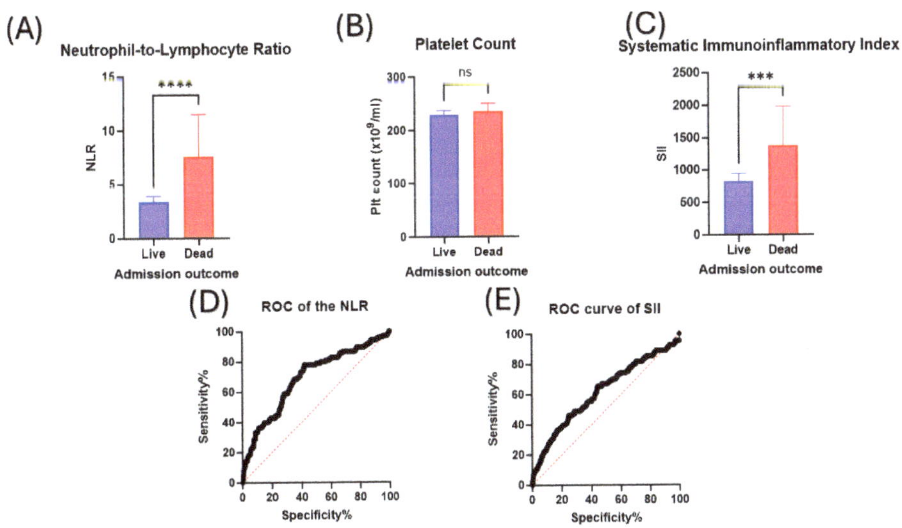

Figure 1. Comparison of key parameters between survivors and non-survivors. (**A**) A comparison between the NLR of patients who survived (blue column) and to those who passed away (red column). (**B**) Comparisons of platelet count and (**C**) the systematic immunoinflammatory index between survivors and non-survivors. The ROC curves of (**D**), the NLR and (**E**) the SII, demonstrating their sensitivity and specificity in differentiating between survivors and non-survivors. NLR: Neutrophil-to-Lymphocyte Ratio, ns: Non-significant, Plt: Platelet, ROC: Receiver Operating Curve, SII: Systematic Immunoinflammatory Index. *** denotes a statistically significant difference at a *p*-value < 0.001. **** denotes a statistically significant difference at a *p*-value < 0.0001.

Next was to evaluate and compare the value of these tools, the NLR and SII, as prognostic tools for COVID-19 mortality. Using the ROC analysis, the NLR demonstrated a larger area under the curve of 0.69 (0.6334 to 0.7510 95% confidence interval; p-value < 0.0001) (Figure 1D) compared to the SII of 0.61 (0.5555 to 0.6809 95% confidence interval; p-value 0.0001) (Figure 1E). The discriminatory cutoff values for the NLR and SII were 5.3 (sensitivity and specificity > 66%) and 1051 (sensitivity and specificity > 58%), such values indicating that the NLR is superior in its sensitivity and specificity in predicting COVID-19 mortality when compared to the SII.

4. Discussion

Clinically, COVID-19 has always been a challenge to manage, especially given its unanticipated clinical course. Hence, the need arose among clinicians to develop predictors of disease severity upon first encounter with patients. However, most of these predictors were based on clinical examination, which may vary across physicians and populations, and some were based on a theoretical basis, such as the presence of comorbidities or in immunocompromised subjects whose immune system may not be capable of mounting a proper immune response.

In this study, age has been identified as a risk factor for mortality among COVID-19 patients. It is not surprising, the find of the low mortality rate of over 13% among the study cohort, given that the majority of survivors were younger than 40 years of age. This rate is significantly lower than in other countries [12] and could be partially attributed to the age of this study cohort. Ageing is associated with a series of biological changes that consequently lead to a reduction in the capability of the immune system to respond properly to infections [13]. As immune competency deteriorates with age, it is no surprise that it is constantly considered a risk factor, especially among subjects older than 45 years old, based on the current literature [14].

COVID-19 is considered a proinflammatory condition, hence, haematological indices are expected to change accordingly. This gives the basis for the use of haematological parameters as a monitoring tool. This study builds on the previous extensive work that validated the use of the NLR in the context of COVID-19. Our previous multicentre study in Saudi Arabia demonstrated the prognostic value of the NLR in detecting severe COVID-19 cases, i.e., admitted to the ICU, compared to both non-severe cases and non-COVID-19 patients [9]. Such a finding was later confirmed and was found to be applicable to other cohorts locally [15,16] and internationally [17–19]. More recently, the works of Regolo et al. demonstrated the value of the NLR as an independent predictor of mortality in separate studies including over 1000 patients with COVID-19 [20,21]. A proper immune response requires a complex interaction between cells of the innate and adaptive immune systems. Hence, the NLR represents both of these systems, neutrophils (innate immune system) and lymphocytes (adaptive immune system). So, the changes in the NLR represented by significantly high levels of the NLR among non-survivors may reflect a sign of deranged interplay between these systems [22]. This could be in the form of hyperactivation of the innate immune system, leading to a significant rise in the neutrophil count. On the other hand, the engagement and consumption of the lymphocytes, both T and B cells, leading to a significant reduction in the lymphocytic count, could be an indicator of COVID-19 severity and, subsequently, mortality. Severe forms of COVID-19 that lead to mortality have been described to be of significantly high viral load and reduced adaptive immune response, namely, T and B cell responses [23]. In this study, the NLR had the capacity to predict mortality on its own and remains an invaluable tool in the management of COVID-19 cases given its wide availability and cost-effectiveness in comparison to other laboratory investigations [24].

Platelets are well known for their role in haemostasis. However, in more recent years platelets were found to play an important role in immunity against viral infections and have the capacity to directly interact with immune cells [25]. In the context of COVID-19, several mechanisms were suggested that could lead to a reduced platelet count as part of the COVID-19 pathophysiology. In some patients, COVID-19 lead to a cytokine storm, a state of hyperinflammatory milieu, which would subsequently reduce the production of platelets [7,26]. Another alternative mechanism of reduced platelet count could be attributed to their increased destruction by autoantibodies as a side effect of SARS-CoV-2 infection [27]. Despite the safety and effectiveness of COVID-19 vaccines [28], several reports have suggested that COVID-19 vaccines could have the adverse reaction of a reduced platelet count [29]. Such an adverse reaction has been attributed to an autoimmune response that is triggered by adeno-vector vaccines such as the AstraZeneca vaccine, leading to a case referred to as vaccine-induced immune thrombotic thrombocytopaenia (VITT) [30]. VITT was explained to be due to an interaction between antiplatelet factor 4 (PF4) antibodies and platelets, leading to their destruction through Fc receptors and opsonisation by phagocytes. Another possible mechanism is that these PF4 antibodies activate platelets causing them to start the thrombotic cascade, and hence their consumption in the process [31].

Given the value of platelets in the immune response against viruses, it was only logical to include it as a predictor of severity and incorporate it with the NLR to develop the SII [32]. In this study, platelet count was not sufficient to differentiate between survivors and non-survivors, in line with the work of Yuan and colleagues [33]. However, the SII was capable of predicting mortality, but with lesser sensitivity and specificity as compared to the NLR. Such findings confirm the previous work of Ghobadi and his team [34], Gutiérrez-Pérez and colleagues [35] and Yılmaz and her team [36], as well as in Turkey [37]. In contrast, previous studies either refuted and excluded the value of the SII in the context of COVID-19 [38] or found it to be exclusively useful and to surpass the limited value of the NLR [32]. Such contradictory findings may be explained by the limited study sample sizes, which were not sufficient to determine the value of the NLR, or the skewed study cohort by including elderly patients only.

The primary objective of this study was to compare the diagnostic value of the NLR and SII in predicting mortality among patients with COVID-19. However, more results came out of this study that provide further insights into the pathophysiology of severe COVID-19. Patients who did not survive due to COVID-19 were significantly older than those who survived, confirming the previous findings that age is an independent risk factor for the severity of COVID-19 cases. This is due to the biological changes associated with the ageing process that lead to the gradual deterioration of the immune system, also known as immunosenescence [13]. These changes include but are not limited to a low lymphocytic repertoire (leading to an immunological response against a limited number of pathogens), shorter telomere length as well as structural changes within immune organs. Given the inverse correlation between age and the fitness of the immune response, many studies have considered it an important predictor of the severity of COVID-19 cases and include it in their COVID-19 mortality prediction tools [10,14].

Another possible side effect of COVID-19 infections is the development of anaemia. Although several mechanisms are proposed for COVID-19-related anaemia, such as via the haemolytic pathway caused as part of the COVID-19 pathophysiology [39,40], it remains a sign of severe COVID-19 infection. The findings of this study further confirm this principle, but not necessarily to the degree of overt anaemia. In this study, non-survivors had significantly lower haemoglobin levels compared to survivors. Nevertheless, the haemoglobin levels in both cohorts, despite the statistically significant difference, were within the normal reference values. Indeed, the results of Bergamaschi and colleagues on 206 COVID-19 patients found that the presence of anaemia is not a direct predictor of severity in COVID-19, but rather an indication of old age and frailty [41]. The study by Mi Oh and colleagues showed that anaemia upon admission increased the odds of all-cause mortality among COVID-19 patients, with anaemia of haemoglobin of less than 11 g/dL considered an independent risk factor [42]. While such a conclusion may oppose the findings of this study, it is important to consider the age factor, as the median age in this study cohort was 41 years old, whereas in Mi Oh's study, it was 65 years old. Hence, anaemia, as defined by haemoglobin below the reference range, could be a predictor of COVID-19-related severity, and possibly mortality, in elderly patients.

Despite the merits of this study of providing new insights to the current scientific literature, this study is not without limitations. Firstly, this study is a retrospective cross-sectional study, which is at risk of sampling bias [43]. Secondly, this study did not consider other influencing factors, such as the presence of comorbidities and smoking status, which may significantly affect the mortality associated with COVID-19. Lastly, this study focused merely on values obtained and derived from an ordinary CBC. However, this does not negate the importance of other haematological markers that have shown their value in predicting COVID-19-related mortality, such as C-reactive protein (CRP) and interleukin (IL)-6 [44,45].

Future studies should aim to further build on the findings of this study and address the limitations of this study. For example, a prospective multicentre study with more comprehensive data should be conducted to assess the sensitivity and specificity of these indicators, the NLR and SII.

5. Conclusions

In conclusion, this study presents both tools, the NLR and SII, as valuable assets that can be used by clinicians to predict COVID-19 severity. These tools are affordable, widely available and rapid, which should facilitate the decision-making process when managing the uncertainties associated with COVID-19 cases. These tools, the NLR more specifically, should be incorporated into medical guidelines on the management of COVID-19.

Funding: This research was funded by the King Salman Center For Disability Research, grant number KSRG-2023-460.

Institutional Review Board Statement: This study was conducted in accordance with the Declaration of Helsinki and approved by the Institutional Review Board (or Ethics Committee) of the Taibah University College of Medicine (protocol code TU-21-010, 10 February 2022).

Informed Consent Statement: Patient consent was waived due to the retrospective nature of this study and as the patients' anonymity was maintained throughout the duration of this study.

Data Availability Statement: The data presented in this study are available on reasonable request from the corresponding author.

Acknowledgments: The author extends his appreciation to the King Salman Center for Disability Research for funding this work through Research Group no KSRG-2023-460. The author wishes to express his gratitude to Barah T. Daghistani for her generous assistance and efforts in the data collection process. Many thanks to the study participants for their time and generous participation.

Conflicts of Interest: The author declares no conflicts of interest. The funders had no role in the design of this study; in the collection, analyses, or interpretation of data; in the writing of the manuscript or in the decision to publish the results.

References

1. Guan, W.; Ni, Z.; Hu, Y.; Liang, W.; Ou, C.; He, J.; Liu, L.; Shan, H.; Lei, C.; Hui, D.S.C.; et al. Clinical Characteristics of Coronavirus Disease 2019 in China. *N. Engl. J. Med.* **2020**, *382*, 1708–1720. [CrossRef] [PubMed]
2. Sayed, A.A. The Progressive Public Measures of Saudi Arabia to Tackle Covid-19 and Limit Its Spread. *Int. J. Environ. Res. Public Health* **2021**, *18*, 783. [CrossRef] [PubMed]
3. Wise, J. Covid-19: WHO declares end of global health emergency. *BMJ* **2023**, *381*, 1041. [CrossRef] [PubMed]
4. Anka, A.U.; Tahir, M.I.; Abubakar, S.D.; Alsabbagh, M.; Zian, Z.; Hamedifar, H.; Sabzevari, A.; Azizi, G. Coronavirus disease 2019 (COVID-19): An overview of the immunopathology, serological diagnosis and management. *Scand. J. Immunol.* **2021**, *93*, e12998. [CrossRef] [PubMed]
5. Al-Samkari, H.; Karp Leaf, R.S.; Dzik, W.H.; Carlson, J.C.T.; Fogerty, A.E.; Waheed, A.; Goodarzi, K.; Bendapudi, P.K.; Bornikova, L.; Gupta, S.; et al. COVID-19 and coagulation: Bleeding and thrombotic manifestations of SARS-CoV-2 infection. *Blood* **2020**, *136*, 489–500. [CrossRef] [PubMed]
6. Liakopoulos, V.; Roumeliotis, S.; Papachristou, S.; Papanas, N. COVID-19 and the kidney: Time to take a closer look. *Int. Urol. Nephrol.* **2022**, *54*, 1053–1057. [CrossRef] [PubMed]

7. Abo-Haded, H.M.; Alshengeti, A.M.; Alawfi, A.D.; Khoshhal, S.Q.; Al-Harbi, K.M.; Allugmani, M.D.; El-Agamy, D.S. Cytokine Profiling among Children with Multisystem Inflammatory Syndrome versus Simple COVID-19 Infection: A Study from Northwest Saudi Arabia. *Biology* **2022**, *11*, 946. [CrossRef] [PubMed]
8. Koffman, J.; Gross, J.; Etkind, S.N.; Selman, L.E. Clinical uncertainty and Covid-19: Embrace the questions and find solutions. *Palliat. Med.* **2020**, *34*, 829–831. [CrossRef] [PubMed]
9. Sayed, A.A.; Allam, A.A.; Sayed, A.I.; Alraey, M.A.; Joseph, M.V. The use of neutrophil-to-lymphocyte ratio (NLR) as a marker for COVID-19 infection in Saudi Arabia. *Saudi Med. J.* **2021**, *42*, 370–376. [CrossRef]
10. Sayed, A.A.; Nozha, O.M. AI Developing a COVID-19 Mortality Prediction (CoMPred) Indicator for ICU Diabetic Patients Treated with Tocilizumab in Saudi Arabia: A Proof-of-Concept Study. *Biomedicines* **2023**, *11*, 2649. [CrossRef]
11. Ministry of Health. Saudi MoH Protocol for Patients Suspected of/Confirmed with COVID-19. Available online: https://www.moh.gov.sa/Ministry/MediaCenter/Publications/Documents/MOH-therapeutic-protocol-for-COVID-19.pdf (accessed on 5 August 2022).
12. Armstrong, R.A.; Kane, A.D.; Kursumovic, E.; Oglesby, F.C.; Cook, T.M. Mortality in patients admitted to intensive care with COVID-19: An updated systematic review and meta-analysis of observational studies. *Anaesthesia* **2021**, *76*, 537–548. [CrossRef] [PubMed]
13. Weiskopf, D.; Weinberger, B.; Grubeck-Loebenstein, B. The aging of the immune system. *Transpl. Int.* **2009**, *22*, 1041–1050. [CrossRef] [PubMed]
14. Chen, Y.; Klein, S.L.; Garibaldi, B.T.; Li, H.; Wu, C.; Osevala, N.M.; Li, T.; Margolick, J.B.; Pawelec, G.; Leng, S.X. Aging in COVID-19: Vulnerability, immunity and intervention. *Ageing Res. Rev.* **2021**, *65*, 101205. [CrossRef] [PubMed]
15. Alhoufie, S.T.; Mumena, W.A.; Alsharif, N.; Makhdoom, H.M.; Almutawif, Y.A.; Alfarouk, K.O.; Alharbi, M.Z.; Aljabri, K.; Aljifri, A. Epidemiological Characteristics and Outcomes Predictors for Intensive Care Unit COVID-19 Patients in Al-Madinah, Saudi Arabia. Retrospective Cohort Study. *Infect. Drug Resist.* **2023**, *16*, 5573–5586. [CrossRef] [PubMed]
16. Mobarki, A.A.; Dobie, G.; Saboor, M.; Madkhali, A.M.; Akhter, M.S.; Hakamy, A.; Humran, A.; Hamali, Y.; Jackson, D.E.; Hamali, H.A. MPR and NLR as Prognostic Markers in ICU-Admitted Patients with COVID-19 in Jazan, Saudi Arabia. *Infect. Drug Resist.* **2021**, *14*, 4859–4864. [CrossRef] [PubMed]
17. Wei, Y.-Y.; Wang, R.-R.; Zhang, D.-W., Chen, S.-H.; Tan, Y.-Y.; Zhang, W.-T.; Han, M.-F.; Fei, G.-H. Differential Characteristics of Patients for Hospitalized Severe COVID-19 Infected by the Omicron Variants and Wild Type of SARS-CoV-2 in China. *J. Inflamm. Res.* **2023**, *16*, 3063–3078. [CrossRef] [PubMed]
18. Wang, Y.; Zhao, J.; Yang, L.; Hu, J.; Yao, Y. Value of the Neutrophil-Lymphocyte Ratio in Predicting COVID-19 Severity: A Meta-analysis. *Dis. Markers* **2021**, *2021*, 2571912. [CrossRef] [PubMed]
19. Dymicka-Piekarska, V.; Dorf, J.; Milewska, A.; Łukaszyk, M.; Kosidło, J.W.; Kamińska, J.; Wolszczak-Biedrzycka, B.; Naumnik, W. Neutrophil/Lymphocyte Ratio (NLR) and Lymphocyte/Monocyte Ratio (LMR)—Risk of Death Inflammatory Biomarkers in Patients with COVID-19. *J. Inflamm. Res.* **2023**, *16*, 2209–2222. [CrossRef] [PubMed]
20. Regolo, M.; Vaccaro, M.; Sorce, A.; Stancanelli, B.; Colaci, M.; Natoli, G.; Russo, M.; Alessandria, I.; Motta, M.; Santangelo, N.; et al. Neutrophil-to-Lymphocyte Ratio (NLR) Is a Promising Predictor of Mortality and Admission to Intensive Care Unit of COVID-19 Patients. *J. Clin. Med.* **2022**, *11*, 2235. [CrossRef]
21. Regolo, M.; Sorce, A.; Vaccaro, M.; Colaci, M.; Stancanelli, B.; Natoli, G.; Motta, M.; Isaia, I.; Castelletti, F.; Giangreco, F.; et al. Assessing Humoral Immuno-Inflammatory Pathways Associated with Respiratory Failure in COVID-19 Patients. *J. Clin. Med.* **2023**, *12*, 4057. [CrossRef]
22. Buonacera, A.; Stancanelli, B.; Colaci, M.; Malatino, L. Neutrophil to Lymphocyte Ratio: An Emerging Marker of the Relationships between the Immune System and Diseases. *Int. J. Mol. Sci.* **2022**, *23*, 3636. [CrossRef]
23. Sette, A.; Crotty, S. Adaptive immunity to SARS-CoV-2 and COVID-19. *Cell* **2021**, *184*, 861–880. [CrossRef]
24. Sayed, A.A. The Cost-Effectiveness of Requesting a Complete Blood Count (CBC) in the Management of COVID-19 in Saudi Arabia. *Healthcare* **2022**, *10*, 1780. [CrossRef] [PubMed]
25. Semple, J.W.; Italiano, J.E.; Freedman, J. Platelets and the immune continuum. *Nat. Rev. Immunol.* **2011**, *11*, 264–274. [CrossRef]
26. Singh, S.; Sharma, R.; Singh, J.; Jain, K.; Paul, D. Thrombocytopenia in COVID-19: Focused Summary of Current Understanding of Mechanisms and Clinical Implications. *J. Pediatr. Hematol. Oncol.* **2021**, *43*, 243–248. [CrossRef]
27. Xu, P.; Zhou, Q.; Xu, J. Mechanism of thrombocytopenia in COVID-19 patients. *Ann. Hematol.* **2020**, *99*, 1205–1208. [CrossRef] [PubMed]
28. Lazarus, R.; Baos, S.; Cappel-Porter, H.; Carson-Stevens, A.; Clout, M.; Culliford, L.; Emmett, S.R.; Garstang, J.; Gbadamoshi, L.; Hallis, B.; et al. Safety and immunogenicity of concomitant administration of COVID-19 vaccines (ChAdOx1 or BNT162b2) with seasonal influenza vaccines in adults in the UK (ComFluCOV): A multicentre, randomised, controlled, phase 4 trial. *Lancet* **2021**, *398*, 2277–2287. [CrossRef]
29. Yasmin, F.; Najeeb, H.; Naeem, U.; Moeed, A.; Atif, A.R.; Asghar, M.S.; Nimri, N.; Saleem, M.; Bandyopadhyay, D.; Krittanawong, C.; et al. Adverse events following COVID-19 mRNA vaccines: A systematic review of cardiovascular complication, thrombosis, and thrombocytopenia. *Immun. Inflamm. Dis.* **2023**, *11*, e807. [CrossRef] [PubMed]
30. Elrashdy, F.; Tambuwala, M.M.; Hassan, S.S.; Adadi, P.; Seyran, M.; Abd El-Aziz, T.M.; Rezaei, N.; Lal, A.; Aljabali, A.A.A.; Kandimalla, R.; et al. Autoimmunity roots of the thrombotic events after COVID-19 vaccination. *Autoimmun. Rev.* **2021**, *20*, 102941. [CrossRef]

31. Cines, D.B.; Greinacher, A. Vaccine-induced immune thrombotic thrombocytopenia. *Blood* **2023**, *141*, 1659–1665. [CrossRef]
32. Fois, A.G.; Paliogiannis, P.; Scano, V.; Cau, S.; Babudieri, S.; Perra, R.; Ruzzittu, G.; Zinellu, E.; Pirina, P.; Carru, C.; et al. The Systemic Inflammation Index on Admission Predicts In-Hospital Mortality in COVID-19 Patients. *Molecules* **2020**, *25*, 5725. [CrossRef]
33. Yuan, X.; Huang, W.; Ye, B.; Chen, C.; Huang, R.; Wu, F.; Wei, Q.; Zhang, W.; Hu, J. Changes of hematological and immunological parameters in COVID-19 patients. *Int. J. Hematol.* **2020**, *112*, 553–559. [CrossRef] [PubMed]
34. Ghobadi, H.; Mohammadshahi, J.; Javaheri, N.; Fouladi, N.; Mirzazadeh, Y.; Aslani, M.R. Role of leukocytes and systemic inflammation indexes (NLR, PLR, MLP, dNLR, NLPR, AISI, SIR-I, and SII) on admission predicts in-hospital mortality in non-elderly and elderly COVID-19 patients. *Front. Med.* **2022**, *9*, 916453. [CrossRef] [PubMed]
35. Gutiérrez-Pérez, I.A.; Buendía-Roldán, I.; Pérez-Rubio, G.; Chávez-Galán, L.; Hernández-Zenteno, R.d.J.; Aguilar-Duran, H.; Fricke-Galindo, I.; Zaragoza-García, O.; Falfán-Valencia, R.; Guzmán-Guzmán, I.P. Outcome predictors in COVID-19: An analysis of emergent systemic inflammation indices in Mexican population. *Front. Med.* **2022**, *9*, 1000147. [CrossRef] [PubMed]
36. Yılmaz, A.; Taşkın, Ö.; Demir, U.; Soylu, V.G. Predictive Role of Biomarkers in COVID-19 Mortality. *Cureus* **2023**, *15*, e34173. [CrossRef] [PubMed]
37. Cakirca, G.; Cakirca, T.D.; Bindal, A.; Olcen, M. Inflammation-based Indices Predicting Mortality in COVID-19. *J. Coll. Physicians Surg. Pak.* **2023**, *33*, 112–114. [CrossRef] [PubMed]
38. Citu, C.; Gorun, F.; Motoc, A.; Sas, I.; Gorun, O.M.; Burlea, B.; Tuta-Sas, I.; Tomescu, L.; Neamtu, R.; Malita, D.; et al. The Predictive Role of NLR, d-NLR, MLR, and SIRI in COVID-19 Mortality. *Diagnostics* **2022**, *12*, 122. [CrossRef] [PubMed]
39. Al-kuraishy, H.M.; Al-Gareeb, A.I.; Kaushik, A.; Kujawska, M.; Batiha, G.E.-S. Hemolytic anemia in COVID-19. *Ann. Hematol.* **2022**, *101*, 1887–1895. [CrossRef] [PubMed]
40. Abu-Ismail, L.; Taha, M.J.J.; Abuawwad, M.T.; Al-Bustanji, Y.; Al-Shami, K.; Nashwan, A.; Yassin, M. COVID-19 and Anemia: What Do We Know So Far? *Hemoglobin* **2023**, *47*, 122–129. [CrossRef]
41. Bergamaschi, G.; Borrelli de Andreis, F.; Aronico, N.; Lenti, M.V.; Barteselli, C.; Merli, S.; Pellegrino, I.; Coppola, L.; Cremonte, E.M.; Croce, G.; et al. Anemia in patients with Covid-19: Pathogenesis and clinical significance. *Clin. Exp. Med.* **2021**, *21*, 239–246. [CrossRef]
42. Oh, S.M.; Skendelas, J.P.; Macdonald, E.; Bergamini, M.; Goel, S.; Choi, J.; Segal, K.R.; Vivek, K.; Nair, S.; Leff, J. On-admission anemia predicts mortality in COVID-19 patients: A single center, retrospective cohort study. *Am. J. Emerg. Med.* **2021**, *48*, 140–147. [CrossRef] [PubMed]
43. Setia, M. Methodology series module 3: Cross-sectional studies. *Indian J. Dermatol.* **2016**, *61*, 261. [CrossRef] [PubMed]
44. Wolszczak-Biedrzycka, B.; Dorf, J.; Wojewódzka-Żelezniakowicz, M.; Żendzian-Piotrowska, M.; Dymicka-Piekarska, V.; Matowicka-Karna, J.; Maciejczyk, M. Unveiling COVID-19 Secrets: Harnessing Cytokines as Powerful Biomarkers for Diagnosis and Predicting Severity. *J. Inflamm. Res.* **2023**, *16*, 6055–6070. [CrossRef] [PubMed]
45. Wolszczak-Biedrzycka, B.; Dorf, J.; Milewska, A.; Łukaszyk, M.; Naumnik, W.; Kosidło, J.W.; Dymicka-Piekarska, V. The Diagnostic Value of Inflammatory Markers (CRP, IL6, CRP/IL6, CRP/L, LCR) for Assessing the Severity of COVID-19 Symptoms Based on the MEWS and Predicting the Risk of Mortality. *J. Inflamm. Res.* **2023**, *16*, 2173–2188. [CrossRef]

medicina

MDPI

Article

Factors Associated with Length of Hospitalization in Patients with Diabetes and Mild COVID-19: Experiences from a Tertiary University Center in Serbia

Vojislav M. Ciric [1,2], Natasa Krsto Rancic [1,3,*], Milica M. Pesic [1,2], Danijela B. Radojkovic [1,2] and Nikola Milenkovic [2]

1 Faculty of Medicine Nis, University of Nis, 18000 Nis, Serbia; ciricv@yahoo.com (V.M.C.); pesic@medfak.ni.ac.rs (M.M.P.); danijela.radojkovic@medfak.ni.ac.rs (D.B.R.)

2 Universital Clinical Center Nis, Clinic for Endocrinology, Diabetes and Metabolic Diseases, 18000 Nis, Serbia; milenkovic@dr.com

3 Institute for Public Health Nis, Center for Diseases Control and Prevention, 18000 Nis, Serbia

* Correspondence: drrancicnatasa@gmail.com

Abstract: *Background and Objectives*: During the COVID-19 pandemic, there was an increased number of hospitalized COVID-19-positive patients suffering from type 2 diabetes mellitus (T2DM). The objective of this research study was to explore factors associated with the length of hospitalization of patients with T2DM and the mild form of COVID-19. *Material and Methods*: This retrospective cohort study involved all patients who tested positive for COVID-19 and those who were treated in the dedicated COVID-19 department of the University Clinical Center (UCC) in Nis between 10 September 2021 and 31 December 2021. Upon admission, patients underwent blood tests for biochemical analysis, including blood count, kidney and liver function parameters (C-reactive protein (CRP), creatinine kinase, and D-dimer), and glycemia and HbA1c assessments. Additionally, all patients underwent lung radiography. Univariate and multivariate regression analyses were employed to assess the impact of specific factors on the length of hospitalization among patients with T2DM. *Results*: Out of a total of 549 treated COVID-19-positive patients, 124 (21.0%) had T2DM, while 470 (79.0%) did not have diabetes. Among patients with T2DM, men were significantly younger than women (60.6 ± 16.8 vs. 64.2 ± 15.3, $p < 0.01$). The average hospitalization length of patients with diabetes was 20.2 ± 9.6 (5 to 54 days), and it was significantly longer than for patients without diabetes, at 15.0 ± 3.4, which ranged from 3 days to 39 (t-test ≈ 5.86, $p < 0.05$). According to the results of the univariate regression analysis, each year of age is associated with an increase in the length of hospital stay of 0.06 days (95% CI: 0.024 to 0.128, $p = 0.004$). Patients who received oxygen therapy were treated for 2.8 days longer than those who did not receive oxygen treatment (95% CI: 0.687 to 4988, $p = 0.010$), and each one-unit increase in CRP level was associated with a 0.02-day reduction in the length of hospitalization (95% CI: 0.004 to 0.029, $p = 0.008$). Based on the results of the multivariate regression analysis, each year of age is associated with an increase in the length of hospitalization by 0.07 days (95% CI: 0.022 to 0.110, $p = 0.003$). Patients who received oxygen therapy were treated for 3.2 days longer than those who did not receive oxygen therapy (95% CI: 0.653 to 5726, $p = 0.014$), and each unit increase in CRP level was associated with a 0.02-day reduction in the length of hospitalization (95% CI: 0.005 to 0.028, $p = 0.004$). *Conclusions*: Based on the presented results, COVID-19-positive patients with diabetes had, on average, longer hospitalizations than COVID-19 patients without diabetes. The hospital treatment of patients with T2DM and a milder form of COVID-19 was associated with older age, the use of oxygen therapy, and elevated CRP values. Patients who received oxygen therapy were treated approximately 3 days longer than those who did not receive this therapy.

Keywords: type 2 diabetes mellitus; COVID-19; length of hospitalization

1. Introduction

COVID-19 is a global health crisis that has placed a significant burden on healthcare systems worldwide [1]. Patients with diabetes mellitus (DM) are a particularly vulnerable population facing an increased risk of severe outcomes from COVID-19 infection, including prolonged hospitalization periods. DM, a chronic condition affecting the body's metabolic balance, can compromise the immune response and hinder the recovery process from infections [2].

In December 2019, cases of severe pneumonia with unknown etiology appeared in the human population in China [2]. The confirmation on 7 January 2020 was related to the identification of SARS-CoV-2 as the new causative agent of coronavirus disease 2019 (COVID-19). COVID-19 rapidly spread from China to the entire world; the World Health Organization (WHO) confirmed the human–human transmission of the SARS-CoV-2 virus on 23 January 2020 and declared a pandemic on 11 March 2020 [3,4]. Based on data from the WHO, there are cumulatively over 762 million confirmed cases of COVID-19 and more than 6.9 million deaths worldwide [5]. During the same period, according to the European Centre for Disease Prevention and Control in the EU/EEA territory, over 275 million confirmed cases of infection have been reported [6].

According to one meta-analysis, an overall pooled prevalence of 31% of DM in hospitalized COVID-19 patients [7] and those with type 2 diabetes mellitus (T2DM) is estimated. DM has been identified as the major comorbidity of hospitalized patients with COVID-19 [8–10]. The prevalence of DM in COVID-19 patients ranges from 5% to 36% [11,12]. People with diabetes are a particularly vulnerable group of patients regarding infections [13], and during COVID-19, it was demonstrated that DM is a pro-inflammatory syndrome characterized by an inadequate cytokine response, with significantly higher concentrations of interleukin-6 (IL-6), ferritin, and C-reactive proteins in the blood compared with COVID-19-positive patients without diabetes [14–16]. It has been shown that uncontrolled glycemia in patients with diabetes increases their vulnerability to inadequate immune responses relative to infection, further exacerbating the disease and leading to the development of acute respiratory distress syndrome (ARDS) and shock. The determined and increased secretion of proinflammatory cytokines in patients with diabetes may change the nature of the immune response related to SARS-CoV-2 infection into inflammation, increasing the probability of a severe course of COVID-19 and resulting in a cytokine storm and tissue and respiratory damage [15,16]. Good glycemic control may be important for maintaining the balance of the immune system [17].

Several studies have found associations between diabetes and greater odds of adverse clinical outcomes in COVID-19, including a longer length of hospitalization, higher mortality rates and intensive care unit (ICU) admissions, and the use of mechanical ventilation [18–20]. Moreover, based on the results of one retrospective analysis of 211,003 medical records, COVID-19-positive patients with T2DM had twice the risk of hospitalization [19]. Gottlieb et al. [20] and Martos-Benirez et al. [21] reported similar results. In a large cross-sectional study in Mexico, COVID-19-positive patients with DM were 38.4% more likely to be hospitalized; moreover, the estimated probability was higher if associated diseases were present. Halalau et al. [22] conducted a multicenter study to show a significant increase in the hospitalization of COVID-19-positive patients suffering not only from DM but also from pre-diabetes.

Based on the findings from a study from the United States of America (USA) with almost a million participants, 20.5% of COVID-19 hospitalizations were attributable to DM. It is estimated that a 10% reduction in DM prevalence could reduce hospital admissions for COVID-19 infection by 2.7% [23]. Based on the results of a large study from the USA, DM was the second most frequent comorbidity, corresponding to 15% of COVID-19-infected individuals, while the prevalence of DM in the same region was 9.7% [24]. T2DM was also reported as an independent risk factor for ICU admission after adjustments for age, sex, comorbidities, and insurance status [25]. Moreover, in a large cohort of hospitalized COVID-

19 participants, patients with T2DM had higher rates of intensive care unit (ICU) admission and intubation and longer hospital stays compared with patients without diabetes [26].

DM has not been proven to be an independent factor in the hospitalization of COVID-19-positive patients [20]. The heterogeneity in the design of the aforementioned studies and differences in local policies for COVID-19 spread prevention may be responsible for the lack of consensus. In addition to associated diseases, factors contributing to the hospitalization of patients with diabetes include older age, male sex, and delayed medical care and treatment [18–22].

The first confirmed case of COVID-19 in Serbia was registered on 6 March 2020, and the epidemic of greater epidemiological significance was declared on 19 March 2020. By the end of 2022, a total of 2,446,253 cases and 17,519 deaths were confirmed [27]. According to the Center for Disease Control (CDC) [28], the dominant strain of the virus in 2021 was the Delta variant. The Delta variant was initially identified in India and quickly spread to other countries. It was a significant factor in the increase in COVID-19 cases in many regions, as it was considered to be highly contagious. Omicron was first identified in Botswana and South Africa in late November 2021, and cases quickly began to surface and multiply in other countries. By December 2021, the original Omicron strain (BA.1) was no longer circulating, and Omicron subvariants are now driving most SARS-CoV-2 infections.

The main objective of this research study was to explore factors associated with the length of hospitalization in patients with T2DM and the mild form of COVID-19 in one tertiary university center in Serbia.

2. Material and Methods

2.1. Study Design

A retrospective cohort study in a single tertiary center was performed, and it included all COVID-19-positive patients treated in the COVID-19 department of the University Clinical Center (UCC) in Nis from 10 September 2021 to 31 December 2021. The total number of COVID-19 patients with a milder form of COVID-19 was 549 (according to the criteria in Table 1), and they were not hospitalized in the intensive care unit (ICU) of the hospital. After obligatory testing for SARS-CoV-2 polymerase chain reaction (PCR), the values of glycemia were checked using the oral glucose tolerance test (OGTT). Based on the results of this test and other medical documentation of the patients, all patients were divided into two groups: T2DM COVID-19-positive and only COVID-19-positive patients.

Table 1. Criteria of the mild form of COVID-19 based on the World Health Organization: COVID-19 disease severity [29].

Mild COVID-19 Illness
• Symptomatic patients satisfying the case definition for COVID-19 without evidence of hypoxia or pneumonia.
• Common symptoms include fever, cough, fatigue, anorexia, dyspnea, and myalgia. Other non-specific symptoms include sore throat, nasal congestion, headache, diarrhea, nausea/vomiting, and loss of smell/taste. Additional neurological manifestations reported include dizziness, agitation, weakness, seizures, or findings suggestive of stroke. Children may not report fever or cough as frequently as adults.
• Older people and immunosuppressed people may present atypical symptoms (e.g., fatigue, reduced alertness, reduced mobility, diarrhea, loss of appetite, delirium, and absence of fever).
• Symptoms due to physiological adaptations of pregnancy, adverse pregnancy events (e.g., dyspnea, fever, gastrointestinal symptoms, and fatigue), or other diseases (e.g., malaria) may overlap with COVID-19 symptoms.

The study was carried out following the Declaration of Helsinki and the decisions of the University Clinical Center's (UCC's) Ethics Committee (decision number 28827/2; dated 20 October 2020).

2.2. Data Sources and Patient Admission Procedure

Epidemiological, descriptive, clinical, and laboratory data were taken from the electronic records of hospitalized patients with COVID-19. Upon admission to the COVID-19 department, patients' medical histories were taken, and all patient characteristics, clinical symptoms of COVID-19, and the method of taking samples for COVID-19 testing were recorded. Moreover, upon admission, patients with COVID-19 had their blood taken for biochemical analysis, and the determination of blood counts and kidney and liver function parameters was carried out: C-reactive protein, creatinine kinase, D-dimer, glycemia, and HbA1c. The oral glucose tolerance test was carried out in some patients with specific symptoms: dry mouth, polydipsia, and high blood glucose. Medical documentation was obtained. All patients underwent lung radiography. The patients were administered specific COVID-19 therapy and oxygen therapy, and the vaccination status against COVID-19 was checked.

2.3. Statistical Analysis

All collected data were entered into the electronic database, and the software package SPPS version 22.0 was used for data processing. Univariate and multivariate regression analyses were used to determine the influence of certain factors on the length of hospitalization with respect to patients with T2DM.

3. Results

Of the total number of treated COVID-19-positive patients, there were 124 (21.0%) with T2DM and 470 (79.0%) without diabetes. Men with T2DM were significantly younger than women (60.6 ± 16.8 vs. 64.2 ± 15.3, $p < 0.01$). Patients with T2DM had no significant differences in gender and age with respect to patients without diabetes ($p > 0.01$). There were significantly more patients with T2DM who were vaccinated against COVID-19, at 70 patients (56.5%), than patients without diabetes, at 142 patients (30.1%). The average hospitalization length in patients with diabetes was 20.2 ± 9.6 (5 to 54 days), and it was significantly longer than in patients without diabetes, at 15.0 ± 3.4, which ranged from 3 days to 39. The serum levels of CRP were much higher in patients with diabetes, ranging from 2.2 to 325.0 (and creatinine ranged from 45.0 to 771.4) than in those without diabetes (CRP ranged from 1.0 to 224.0; creatinine ranged from 42.0 to 663.0). The diabetes group had significantly higher average serum levels of CRP than the group without diabetes ($p = 0.008$). Patients with diabetes had a significantly higher rate of pre-existing comorbidities (65.0% vs. 48%) than patients without diabetes.

Table 2 shows the univariate analysis results of the most significant factors impacting the length of hospitalization of patients with T2DM and a mild form of COVID-19.

Table 2. Correlations between the length of hospitalization and other investigated characteristics; the results of univariate and multivariate regression analyses.

Characteristics	R	95% CI Limits		*p*
		Lower	Upper	
	Univariate regression analysis			
Men	−1.004	−2.700	0.692	0.245
Age (years)	0.076	0.024	0.128	0.004
T2DM	1.189	−1.073	3.451	0.302
Vaccine	0.803	−0.916	2.522	0.359
Oxygen therapy	2.837	0.687	4.988	0.010
COVID-19-specific Th	0.180	−3.930	4.289	0.932
HbA1c	−1.864	−4.261	0.533	0.122
CRP	−0.017	−0.029	−0.004	0.008

Table 2. *Cont.*

Characteristics	R	95% CI Limits		*p*
		Lower	Upper	
		Univariate regression analysis		
Creatinine	−0.009	−0.019	0.002	0.100
DM duration	−0.244	−0.885	0.396	0.422
		Multivariate regression analysis		
Men	−0.175	−1.572	1.222	0.805
Age (years)	0.066	0.022	0.110	0.003
T2DM	−0.952	−3.592	1.687	0.479
Vaccine	0.605	−0.920	2.130	0.436
Oxygen therapy	3.189	0.653	5.726	0.014
COVID-19-specific Th	−1.347	−5.078	2.383	0.478
HbA1c	−1.496	−3.011	0.020	0.053
CRP	−0.016	−0.028	−0.005	0.004
Creatinine	−0.008	−0.017	0.001	0.083
T2DM duration	−0.192	−0.759	0.375	0.507

According to the results of the univariate regression analysis, each year of age is associated with an increase in the length of hospitalization by 0.07 days (95% CI: 0.024 to 0.128 days, $p = 0.004$). Patients who received oxygen therapy were treated 2.8 days longer than those who did not receive oxygen treatment (95% CI: 0.687 to 4.988, $p = 0.010$), and each one-unit increase in CRP level was associated with a 0.02-day reduction in the length of hospitalization (95% CI: 0.4 to 0.029, $p = 0.008$).

Based on the results of the multivariate regression analysis, each year of age is associated with an increase in the length of hospitalization by 0.07 days (95% CI: 0.022 to 0.110, $p = 0.003$). Patients who received oxygen therapy were treated 3/2 days longer than those who did not (95% CI: = 0.653 to 5.726, $p = 0.014$), and each unit increase in CRP level was associated with a 0.02-day reduction in the length of hospitalization (95% CI: 0.005 to 0.028, $p = 0.004$).

Only 5% of the variability in hospitalization duration was determined using the characteristics examined in this research study (coefficient of determination: $R^2 = 0.050$).

4. Discussion

Based on the results of our study, COVID-19-positive patients with diabetes had, on average, longer hospitalization durations than COVID-19 patients without diabetes. The length of hospitalization of T2DM patients with mild COVID-19 was associated with older age, the use of oxygen therapy, and elevated CRP values. Women with T2DM were significantly older than men.

Based on the findings of Al-Salameh et al., COVID-19 patients with diabetes had a higher risk of death, higher ICU admission rates, and prolonged hospital stays [30]. Our results correspond to these results and the findings from COVID-19 hospitals in Serbia. According to the findings of the COVID-19 hospital in Batajnica, Serbia, better metabolic control upon admission was associated with shorter hospital stay durations and lower mortality rates in COVID-19-positive patients with diabetes, which implies the importance of prior glycemic control among patients with T2DM and CKD [31]. In a COVID-19 hospital in Zvezdara, out of 3664 patients, 960 (26.2%) had DM, which accounted for more than a quarter of the patients; moreover, in over half of them, DM persisted for longer than 10 years [32].

There are also different findings available.

According to Kisic et al., among the total number of examined COVID-19-positive patients, 68.6% exhibited a comorbid condition, whereas 57.5% had pre-existing cardiovascular disease (CVD). Statistical analyses confirmed that comorbidities did not significantly influence the duration of hospitalization [33]. According to the findings of Alabai et al. (2024), $SatO_2$, glycemia at hospital admission, and HbA1c had the highest sensitivity and specificity in predicting the prognosis of T2DM patients with SARS-CoV-2 infection. Glycemic control is essential in the prognosis of patients with DM and COVID-19 infection [34]. Our results indicated that age was one of the factors influencing longer hospitalization durations among COVID-19-positive patients with diabetes.

In our study, women were significantly older than men and had longer hospitalization durations. Although the pathophysiological mechanisms are still not understood, they may be explained by the dysfunction of the immune system with aging. Age-specific rates per 100,000 inhabitants by gender during 2022 in the Republic of Serbia, as a result of COVID-19, were higher in all age categories among females, with the exception of those in the age categories of 0–14 and 60 and above, where a higher rate was observed among males. The highest age-specific rates of COVID-19 incidence in the general population in Serbia were observed in the age group of 60 and above (13,556.91/100,000 inhabitants), while the lowest age-specific rate was recorded in the age group of 0–14 years, at 6525.68 per 100,000 inhabitants [35].

In a single-center descriptive study conducted over a period of 2 years (April 2020 to April 2022) in Turkey among 3050 COVID-19 patients treated in the ICU, there were findings of a potential association between age and sex, and biomarkers such as D-dimer, CRP, liver enzymes, ferritin, lactate dehydrogenase were associated with the severity of COVID-19 and prolonged hospitalization of patients [36].

During COVID-19, there were significantly fewer hospitalized children and young people with type 1 diabetes mellitus (T1DM), which indirectly suggests that they were at lower risk of severe clinical presentation and that hospitalization was not necessary [7,11,12]. An increased risk of COVID-19 in children and adults with T1DM has not been identified [34], and there is also no documented evidence of increased mortality among these patients during the COVID-19 pandemic. According to previous studies, older patients with diabetes are at a higher risk for severe COVID-19 and could eventually require ICU admission; their condition may even result in death [12,21,22,35,36].

In a study conducted in China, it was determined that COVID-19-positive patients were mostly men (60%), but more often, women exhibited elevated body temperatures and prolonged hospitalization. There were more women in the elderly population; thus, they were hospitalized more often, and the observed factor was older age with a high body temperature [37].

According to our results, one reason for prolonged hospitalization was elevated CRP levels among patients with diabetes. Similar data can be found in the literature. According to the findings of Liu et al., increased CRP levels and lymphopenia are independent risk factors for COVID-19 severity, while lymphopenia is also a risk factor for prolonged hospital stay [18].

In a study on COVID-19-positive patients with an asymptomatic clinical picture and those with mild symptoms, which was conducted by Wu et al., it was determined that patients with diabetes had elevated body temperatures upon admission, and this was the main reason for prolonged hospitalization [37]. The results of a retrospective study conducted in Vietnam reported that age, the place of permanent residence, and sources of infection were significantly associated with the prolonged hospitalization of patients with T2DM and COVID-19 during the second wave of COVID-19 [38].

Based on our findings, patients with diabetes who received oxygen therapy were treated approximately 3 days longer than those who did not receive this form of therapy. According to the results of a study conducted in Korea, DM was not an independent predictor of the severity of the clinical picture of the disease, which was defined as the need for oxygen therapy and/or artificial ventilation [19]. DM was a predictor of ICU admission, the occurrence of COVID-19 complications, and prolonged hospitalization duration [39–42]. A study in western Sydney reported that patients with diabetes had a 6% increase in mortality, an 8% increase in ICU requirement, and a 6.6-day increase in the length of stay ($p < 0.01$) [43]. Based on the finding of a study by Luviano-Garcı'a et al. (2024), the variables associated with a greater risk of requiring intubation after high-flow therapy were age (HR = 1.018, 95% CI: 1.003–1.034, $p = 0.022$) and body mass index (BMI) (HR = 1.071, 95% CI: 1.024–1.120, $p = 0.003$) [44].

The control measures during COVID-19 and the illness itself have impacted the deterioration of the health of patients with T2DM in several ways: reduced mobility due to restrictions on outings in some countries due to lockdowns, the irregular supply of dietary food and medication for diabetes and associated conditions, and disruptions in regular medical check-ups and glycemic control. Many patients with COVID-19 symptoms delayed seeking medical attention and testing due to the fear of isolation, hospitalization, and separation from their families. There has been an increase in anxiety and depression among this group of patients and the entire population.

Limitations of the study: Limitations commonly observed in studies on the length of hospitalization due to COVID-19 include small sample sizes, insufficient data, and temporal constraints.

The limitations of our small sample include insufficient representativeness, an increased risk of chance effects, and difficulty in identifying rare events. The other limitations of the study are that laboratory biochemical tests were not performed for all patients, and it was not possible to evaluate all important parameters. There is a lack of data on COVID-19 vaccination statuses for all hospitalized individuals. The interpretation of the results can also be affected by the sample size. In order to avoid mistakes, we took a sample of patients with diabetes who were treated in the largest healthcare facility in the city of Nis and the entire territory of southeastern and southern Serbia.

Power of the study: This is the first study to determine factors that contribute to hospitalization and the length of hospitalization of patients with diabetes and a mild clinical form of COVID-19.

5. Conclusions

Based on the presented results, the length of hospital treatment of patients with diabetes and a milder form of COVID-19 was associated with older age, the use of oxygen therapy, and elevated CRP values. Patients who received oxygen therapy were treated approximately 3 days longer than those who did not receive therapy. Understanding these factors is crucial for adjusting medical care and improving outcomes for these patients during the pandemic.

Author Contributions: V.M.C.: investigation, data curation, writing—original draft; N.K.R.: conceptualization; formal analysis, methodology; M.M.P.: supervision; D.B.R.: investigation, data curation; N.M.: software, investigation; data curation. All authors have read and agreed to the published version of the manuscript.

Funding: This research received no external funding.

Institutional Review Board Statement: This study was reviewed and approved by the Ethics Committee Decision of the UCC number 28827/2 dated 20 October 2020. Written informed consent was not obtained.

Informed Consent Statement: This study complied with the guidelines for human studies and included evidence that the research was conducted ethically in accordance with the World Medical Association Declaration of Helsinki.

Data Availability Statement: The dataset underlying this study is available upon reasonable request from the first author or the corresponding author.

Conflicts of Interest: The authors have no conflicts of interest to declare.

References

1. World Health Organization (WHO). Weekly Epidemiological Update on COVID-19. 7 June 2023. Available online: https://www.who.int/publications/m/item/weekly-epidemiological-update-on-covid-19-23-august-202 (accessed on 7 June 2023).
2. Sharma, P.; Behl, T.; Sharma, N.; Singh, S.; Grewal, A.S.; Albarrati, A.; Albratty, M.; Meraya, A.M.; Bungau, S. COVID-19 and diabetes: Association intensify risk factors for morbidity and mortality. *Biomed. Pharmacother.* **2022**, *151*, 113089. [CrossRef]
3. Report of Clustering Pneumonia of Unknown Etiology in Wuhan City. Wuhan Municipal Health Commission. 2019. Available online: http://wjw.wuhan.gov.cn/front/web/showDetail/2019123108989 (accessed on 21 February 2024).
4. World Health Organization. Transmission of SARS-CoV-2: Implications for Infection Prevention Precautions, Scientific Brief. 9 July 2020. Available online: https://www.who.int/publications/i/item/modes-of-transmission-of-virus-causing-covid-19-implications-for-ipc-precaution-recommendations (accessed on 29 March 2020).
5. World Health Organization. Coronavirus (COVID-19) Dashboard. Available online: https://covid19.who.int/ (accessed on 21 February 2024).
6. ECDC. COVID-19 Situation Update Worldwide. 6 April 2023. Available online: https://www.ecdc.europa.eu/en/covid-19/situation-updates (accessed on 14 April 2024).
7. Bradley, S.A.; Banach, M.; Alvarado, N.; Ivica Smokovski, I.; Bhaska, S.M.M. Prevalence and impact of diabetes in hospitalized COVID-19 patients: A systematic review and meta-analysis. *J. Diabetes* **2022**, *14*, 144–157. [CrossRef]
8. Singh, A.K.; Gupta, R.; Ghosh, A.; Misra, A. Diabetes in COVID-19: Prevalence, pathophysiology, prognosis and practical considerations. *Diabetes Metab Syndr.* **2020**, *14*, 303–310. [CrossRef]
9. Alguwaihes, A.M.; Al-Sofiani, M.E.; Megdad, M.; Albader, S.S.; Alsari, M.H.; Alelayan, A.; Alzahrani, S.H.; Sabico, S.; Al-Daghri, N.M.; Jammah, A.A. Diabetes and COVID-19 among hospitalized patients in Saudi Arabia: A single-centre retrospective study. *Cardiovasc. Diabetol.* **2020**, *19*, 205. [CrossRef] [PubMed]
10. Guo, M.; Li, Y.; Dong, H.; Zhou, Z.; Zhang, C.; Tian, R.; Qin, H.; Wang, Y.; Shen, K.; Du, L.; et al. Diabetes is a risk factor for the progression and prognosis of COVID-19. *Diabetes Metab. Res Rev.* **2020**, *31*, e3319. [CrossRef]
11. Rees, E.M.; Nightingale, E.S.; Jafari, Y.; Waterlow, N.R.; Clifford, S.; Pearson, C.A.B.; CMMID Working Group; Jombart, T.; Procter, S.R.; Knight, G.M. COVID-19 length of hospital stay: A systematic review and data synthesis. *BMC Med.* **2020**, *18*, 270. [CrossRef] [PubMed]
12. Pijls, B.G.; Jolani, S.; Atherley, A.; Derckx, R.T.; Dijkstra, J.I.; Franssen, G.H.; Hendriks, S.; Richters, A.; Venemans-Jellema, A.; Zalpuri, S.; et al. Demographic risk factors for COVID-19 infection, severity, ICU admission and death: A meta-analysis of 59 studies. *BMJ Open* **2021**, *11*, e044640. [CrossRef] [PubMed]
13. Knapp, S. Diabetes and infection: Is there a link?—A mini-review. *Gerontology* **2013**, *59*, 99–104. [CrossRef] [PubMed]
14. Petrie, J.R.; Guzik, T.J.; Touyz, R.M. Diabetes, hypertension, and cardiovascular disease: Clinical insights and vascular mechanisms. *Can. J. Cardiol.* **2018**, *34*, 575–584. [CrossRef]
15. Geerlings, S.E.; Hoepelman, A.I. Immune dysfunction in patients with diabetes mellitus (DM). *FEMS Immunol. Med. Microbiol.* **1999**, *26*, 259–265. [CrossRef] [PubMed]
16. Moutschenm, M.P.; Scheenm, A.J.; Lefebvrem, P.J. Impaired immune responses in diabetes mellitus: Analysis of the factors and mechanisms involved. Relevance to the increased susceptibility of diabetic patients to specific infections. *Diabete Metab.* **1992**, *18*, 187–201.
17. Geza, T.; Wojtowicz, K.; Guzik, P.; Góra, T. Increased Risk of COVID-19 in Patients with Diabetes Mellitus—Current Challenges in Pathophysiology, Treatment and Prevention. *Int. J. Environ. Res. Public Health* **2022**, *19*, 6555. [CrossRef] [PubMed]
18. Liu, X.; Zhou, H.; Zhou, Y.; Wu, X.; Zhao, Y.; Lu, Y.; Tan, W.; Yuan, M.; Ding, X.; Zou, J.; et al. Risk factors associated with disease severity and length of hospital stay in COVID-19 patients. *J. Infect.* **2020**, *81*, e95–e97. [CrossRef] [PubMed]
19. You, J.H.; Lee, S.A.; Chun, S.Y.; Song, S.O.; Lee, B.W.; Kim, D.J.; Boyko, E.J. Clinical Outcomes of COVID-19 Patients With Type 2 Diabetes: A Population-Based Study in Korea. *Endocrinol. Metab.* **2020**, *35*, 901–908. [CrossRef] [PubMed]
20. Hernández-Galdamez, D.R.; González-Block, M.Á.; Romo-Dueñas, D.K.; Lima-Morales, R.; Hernández-Vicente, I.A.; Lumbreras-Guzmán, M.; Mendez-Hernandez, P. Increased Risk of Hospitalization and Death in Patients With COVID-19 and Pre-Existing Noncommunicable Diseases and Modifiable Risk Factors in Mexico. *Arch. Med. Res.* **2020**, *51*, 683–689. [CrossRef]
21. Gottlieb, M.; Sansom, S.; Frankenberger, C.; Ward, E.; Hota, B. Clinical Course and Factors Associated With Hospitalization and Critical Illness Among COVID-19 Patients in Chicago, Illinois. *Acad. Emerg. Med.* **2020**, *27*, 963–973. [CrossRef]
22. Martos-Benitez, F.D.; Soler-Morejon, C.D.; Garcia-Del Barco, D. Chronic Comorbidities and Clinical Outcomes in Patients With and Without COVID-19: A Large Population-Based Study Using National Administrative Healthcare Open Data of Mexico. *Intern. Emerg. Med.* **2021**, *16*, 1507–1517. [CrossRef] [PubMed]
23. Halalau, A.; Odish, F.; Imam, Z.; Sharrak, A.; Brickner, E.; Lee, P.B.; Foglesong, A.; Michel, A.; Gill, I.; Qu, L.; et al. Epidemiology, Clinical Characteristics, and Outcomes of a Large Cohort of COVID-19 Outpatients in Michigan. *Int. J. Gen. Med.* **2021**, *14*, 1555–1563. [CrossRef] [PubMed]
24. O'Harem, M.; Liu, J.; Cudhea, F.; Micha, R.; Mozaffarin, D. Coronavirus Disease 2019 Hospitalizations Attributable to Cardiometabolic Conditions in the United States: A Comparative Risk Assessment Analysis. *J. Am. Heart Assoc.* **2021**, *10*, eo19259. [CrossRef]
25. Xu, G.; Liu, B.; Sun, Y.; Du, Y.; Snetselaar, L.G.; Hu, F.B.; Bao, W. Prevalence of Diagnosed Type 1 and Type 2 Diabetes Among US Adults in 2016 and 2017: Population Based Study. *BMJ* **2018**, *362*, k1497. [CrossRef]

26. Huang, J.F.; Wang, X.B.; Zheng, K.I.; Liu, W.Y.; Chen, J.J.; George, J.; Zheng, M.H. Obesity hypoventilation syndrome and severe COVID-19. *Metabol. Clin. Exp.* **2020**, *108*, 154249. [CrossRef] [PubMed]
27. Huang, A.A.; Huang, Y.S. Hospitalized COVID-19 patients with diabetes have an increased risk for pneumonia, intensive care unit requirement, intubation, and death: A cross-sectional cohort study in Mexico in 2020. *Health Sci Rep.* **2023**, *6*, e1222. [CrossRef]
28. Centers for Disease Control and Prevention. *Epidemiological Triad. Atlanta, Georgia: Centers for Disease Control and Prevention*; Centers for Disease Control and Prevention: Atlanta, GA, USA, 2020.
29. World Health Organization. Living Guidance for Clinical Management of COVID-19. 2021. Available online: https://apps.who.int/iris/handle/10665/338882 (accessed on 25 January 2021).
30. Al-Salameh, A.; Lanoix, J.P.; Bennis, Y. Characteristics and outcomes of COVID-19 in hospitalized patients with and without diabetes. *Diabetes Metab. Res Rev.* **2021**, *37*, e3388. [CrossRef] [PubMed]
31. Stoiljkovic, M.; Lalic, N.; Macesic, M.; Stanarcic Gajovic, J.; Mina Milovacevic, M.; Spurnic, A.; Adzic-Vukicevic, T. Type 2 Diabetes and Chronic Kidney Disease: COVID-19 Outcomes. In Proceedings of the First World Conference "Fighting COVID-19 Pandemic—Health Challenges", Belgrade, Serbia, 26–28 March 2022; Volume 235.
32. Kisic, G.; Petrovic, T.; Peric, V. Impact of Comorbidities on the Length and Course Hospitalisation in Patients with COVID-19. In Proceedings of the First World Conference "Fighting COVID-19 Pandemic—Health Challenges", Belgrade, Serbia, 26–28 March 2022; Volume 237.
33. Vuksanovic, M.; Jojic, B.; Marjanovic Petkovic, M.; Stojanovic, J.; Andjelic Jelic, M.; Beljic Zivkovic, T. Glycemic Control and Vaccinal Status of Hospitalized Patients with Diabetes in Covid Hospital KBC Zvezdara. In Proceedings of the First World Conference "Fighting COVID-19 Pandemic—Health Challenges", Belgrade, Serbia, 26–28 March 2022; Volume 254.
34. Albai, O.; Braha, A.; Timar, B.; Sima, A.; Deaconu, L.; Timar, R. Assessment of the Negative Factors for the Clinical Outcome in Patients with SARS-CoV-2 Infection and Type 2 Diabetes Mellitus. *Diabetes Metab. Syndr. Obes.* **2024**, *17*, 271–282. [CrossRef] [PubMed]
35. Institute of Public Health of Serbia 'Dr. Milan Jovanović Batut'. *Report on Infectious Diseases in the Republic of Serbia for the Year 2022; COVID-19*; Institute of Public Health of Serbia 'Dr. Milan Jovanović Batut': Belgrade, Serbia, 2023; pp. 25–38.
36. Genc, S.; Taghizadehghalehjoughi, A.; Naldan, M.E.; Gülcü, O.; Caglayan, C.; Spanakis, M.; Nikolouzakis, T.K.; Alegakis, A.; Docea, A.O.; Drocas, A.I.; et al. Evaluation of various blood biomarkers associated with the outcomes of patients with COVID-19 treated in intensive care units. *Exp. Ther. Med.* **2024**, *27*, 82. [CrossRef] [PubMed]
37. Wu, S.; Xue, L.; Legido-Quigley, H.; Khan, M.; Wu, H.; Peng, X.; Li, X.; Li, P. Understanding factors influencing the length of hospital stay among non-severe COVID 19 patients: A retrospective cohort study in a Fangcang shelte hospital. *PLoS ONE* **2020**, *15*, e0240959. [CrossRef] [PubMed]
38. Do, T.V.; Manabe, T.; Vu, G.V.; Nong, V.M.; Fujikura, Y.; Phan, D.; Pham, T.T.; Do, C.D.; Doan, T.T.; Nguyen, N.T.; et al. Clinical characteristics and mortality risk among critically ill patients with COVID-19 owing to the B.1.617.2 (Delta) variant in Vietnam: A retrospective observational study. *PLoS ONE* **2023**, *18*, e0279713. [CrossRef] [PubMed]
39. O'Malley, G.; Ebekozien, O.; Desimone, M.; Pinnaro, C.T.; Roberts, A.; Polsky, S.; Noor, N.; Aleppo, G.; Basina, M.; Tansey, M.; et al. COVID-19 hospitalization in adults with type 1 diabetes: Results from the T1DM Exchange Multicenter Surveillance Study. *J. Clin. Endocrinol. Metab.* **2021**, *106*, e936–e942. [CrossRef]
40. Corrao, S.; Argano, C.; Natoli, G.; Nobili, A.; Corazza, G.R.; Mannucci, P.M.; Perticone, F.; RePoSi Investigators. Sex Differences in the Pattern of Comorbidities, Functional Independence, and Mortality in Elderly Inpatients: Evidence from the RePoSI Register. *J. Clin. Med.* **2019**, *8*, 81. [CrossRef]
41. Richardson, S.; Hirsch, J.S.; Narasimhan, M.; Crawford, J.M.; McGinn, T.; Davidson, K.W.; Barnaby, D.P.; Becker, L.B.; Chelico, J.D.; Cohen, S.L.; et al. Presenting Characteristics, Comorbidities, and Outcomes Among 5700 Patients Hospitalized with COVID-19 in the New York City Area. *JAMA* **2020**, *323*, 2052–2059. [CrossRef]
42. Moon, S.J.; Rhee, E.J.; Jung, J.H.; Han, K.D.; Kim, S.R.; Lee, W.Y.; Yoon, K.H. Independent Impact of Diabetes on the Severity of Coronavirus Disease 2019 in 5307 Patients in South Korea: A Nationwide Cohort Study. *Diabetes Metab. J.* **2020**, *44*, 737–746. [CrossRef] [PubMed]
43. Cheung, N.W.; Gilroy, N.; Hor, A.; Jose, S.; Kairaitis, K.; Nayyar, V.; O'Sullivan, M.V.; Wheatley, J.; Chipps, D.R. Diabetes and hyperglycaemia among hospitalizeed patients with COVID-19 in Western Sydney: A retrospective cohort study. *Intern. Med. J.* **2022**, *53*, 194–201. [CrossRef] [PubMed]
44. Luviano-García, J.A.; Loose-Esparza, A.; Hernández-Ruíz, Y.G.; Sanz-Sánchez, M.Á.; Maheda-García, H.J.; Sosa-Medellin, M.A.; Garza-Silva, A.; Romero-Ibarguengoitia, M.E. Risk factors for intubation and mortality in patients treated with high flow nasal cannula due to COVID-19 infection. Survival Analysis Study in a Northern Mexican Population. *PLoS ONE* **2024**, *19*, e0296931. [CrossRef] [PubMed]

medicina

MDPI

Article

Colliding Challenges: An Analysis of SARS-CoV-2 Infection in Patients with Pulmonary Tuberculosis versus SARS-CoV-2 Infection Alone

Camil Mihuta [1,2], Adriana Socaci [2,3,*], Patricia Hogea [2,4,5], Emanuela Tudorache [2,4,5], Monica Simina Mihuta [6] and Cristian Oancea [2,4,5]

1 Department of Doctoral Studies, "Victor Babes" University of Medicine and Pharmacy, 300041 Timisoara, Romania; camil.mihuta@umft.ro
2 Clinical Hospital for Infectious Diseases and Pneumology "Dr. Victor Babes", 300041 Timisoara, Romania; hogea.patricia@umft.ro (P.H.); emanuela.tudorache@umft.ro (E.T.); oancea@umft.ro (C.O.)
3 Department of Biology and Life Sciences, Faculty of Medicine, "Vasile Goldis" Western University of Arad, 310025 Arad, Romania
4 Center for Research and Innovation in Precision Medicine of Respiratory Diseases (CRIPMRD), "Victor Babes" University of Medicine and Pharmacy, 300041 Timisoara, Romania
5 Department of Pulmonology, "Victor Babes" University of Medicine and Pharmacy, 300041 Timisoara, Romania
6 Center of Molecular Research in Nephrology and Vascular Disease, Faculty of Medicine, "Victor Babes" University of Medicine and Pharmacy, 300041 Timisoara, Romania; simina.mihuta@umft.ro
* Correspondence: socaci.adriana@uvvg.ro

Abstract: *Background and Objectives*: The concurrent occurrence of tuberculosis and COVID-19 coinfection poses significant clinical complexities, warranting a nuanced approach to diagnosis, management, and patient care. *Materials and Methods*: A retrospective, cross-sectional study was conducted on two groups: one comprising 32 patients with pulmonary TB (PTB) and COVID-19 co-infection, and one including 100 patients with COVID-19 alone. Data was collected from medical records, including patient history, clinical parameters, laboratory, imaging results, and patient outcome. *Results*: A lower BMI emerges as a significant marker suggesting underlying PTB in patients with *SARS-CoV-2* co-infection. Type 2 diabetes mellitus increases the risk of death in PTB-*SARS-CoV-2* co-infection. Co-infected patients show lymphocytopenia and higher neutrophil levels, CRP, transaminases, and D-dimer levels. Elevated CRP and ALT levels are linked to increased co-infection likelihood. Certain parameters like SpO2, CRP, ALT, AST, and D-dimer effectively differentiate between co-infected and COVID-19 patients. Platelet-to-lymphocyte ratio is notably higher in co-infected individuals. Lesion severity on imaging is significantly associated with co-infection, highlighting imaging's diagnostic importance. Longer hospital stays are linked to co-infection but not significantly to death risk. *Conclusions*: Certain clinical and biological factors may serve as potential indicators of PTB co-infection in patients with *SARS-CoV-2*.

Keywords: COVID19 outcomes; immunocompromised in *SARS-CoV-2* infection; *SARS-CoV-2* and tuberculosis co-infection; pulmonary tuberculosis

1. Introduction

Tuberculosis (TB) is an infectious disease with profound implications for human health. *Mycobacterium tuberculosis* primarily invades the lungs, but it can also disseminate to other organs and tissues, including the intestines, liver, lymph nodes, skin, brain, and various systems such as musculoskeletal and reproductive [1].

The year 2020 is likely to be etched in memory as the "COVID-19 year", marked by the emergence of the severe acute respiratory syndrome coronavirus 2 (*SARS-CoV-2*) responsible for the pandemic. While COVID-19 continues to dominate both scientific literature and the media, it is crucial not to overlook other communicable diseases, including TB [2–6]. Since 2019, the genetic makeup of the *SARS-CoV-2* reference sequence has undergone alterations, leading to speculations about the emergence of variants capable of evading immune responses and resisting treatments and vaccines [7–9]. Phylogenetic analysis indicated that the Romanian epidemic commenced with numerous introduction events from various European countries, succeeded by localized transmission [10]. Roughly all variants ultimately have circulated on Romanian territory, but the most prominent at the time of our study (the initial months of the pandemic) were variants pertaining to lineage B, subtype B.1.5 and B.1.1 [10,11]. These variants produced a high variability in symptomatology and severity. Diabetes and arterial hypertension are comorbidities which were shown to be associated with a more severe disease form [11].

Amid the World Health Organization's (WHO) declaration of COVID-19 as a Public Health Emergency of International Concern, considerable attention has been devoted to exploring the potential interactions between *SARS-CoV-2* and TB infection. The prevailing view, shared by the WHO and specialized scientific sources, suggests that the COVID-19 pandemic could exacerbate the global TB epidemic. This anticipated worsening is attributed to various factors, including additional strains on health systems from COVID-19, leading to the weakening of National TB programs. The potential biological effects of the interaction between the two infections are also emphasized, reminiscent of the historical concept of a 'cursed duet', previously applied to TB and HIV [7–16].

Unlike COVID-19, TB is an ancient menace that has plagued humanity for millennia, with 25% of the global population harboring latent *Mycobacterium tuberculosis* infection, and within this group, 5–15% may progress to develop active TB during their lifetime. The risk of reactivation varies both geographically and individually [12,17]. Hence, the convergence of COVID-19 and TB poses grave challenges, impacting TB diagnosis, treatment, and control programs [18,19]. Individuals with active TB are often immunocompromised, making them more vulnerable to COVID-19's severe effects. Consequently, the synergistic relationship between TB, HIV, and COVID-19 has created a global syndemic, underscoring the urgent need for comprehensive research on TB/COVID-19 co-infection [20]. The two pathogens, *Mycobacterium tuberculosis* and *HIV*, can mutually potentiate each other, accelerating the deterioration of immune functions. Each of these diseases holds significance and can notably impact lung function through distinctive cytokine storms, immunosuppression, and respiratory failure. Reported co-infections of *SARS-CoV-2* with *HIV* and *Mycobacterium tuberculosis* can alter their pathogenesis and disease advancement. Individuals with pulmonary tuberculosis and *HIV*/AIDS might exhibit heightened susceptibility to *SARS-CoV-2* infection, potentially resulting in lethal synergistic effects and increased disease severity [21]. Moreover, worldwide, it is estimated that between 10 to 25% of TB infections occur extrapulmonarily, infecting virtually any organ, thus definitive diagnosis usually requires invasive procedures and complex imaging examinations, as symptoms can be very heterogeneous [22].

Both lung TB and COVID-19 share similarities in their airborne transmission, lung-centric effects, symptoms, and social determinants. However, their pathogenesis differs significantly, suggesting that understanding their interactions could inform new prevention and treatment strategies for TB/COVID-19 co-infection. Common clinical manifestations of COVID-19 include fever, respiratory symptoms such as dispnoea, tachypnea, cough, and even hemoptysis, along with less severe symptoms such as fatigue, headache, myalgia, and gastrointestinal symptoms like vomiting and diarrhea. Prolonged cough is a primary symptom for both lung TB and COVID-19 [20,23–25]. While limited information exists on the risk and severity of concurrent TB and COVID-19, previous studies suggest the potential exacerbation of TB in co-infection with certain viruses, such as measles. TB patients face a potential risk of co-infection with *SARS-CoV-2* and vice-versa [17,25,26].

With regard to biomarkers, COVID-19 and TB present elevated levels of C-reactive protein, D-Dimer, and interleukin 6, but also alterations such as leukopenia, neutrophilia or even platelet dysfunctions. These shared clinical parameters and underlying immunological reactions imply that co-infection may not only complicate diagnostic processes but also lead to a potentially fatal convergence in immunopathogenesis [27]. Macrostructural pulmonary changes caused by TB, such as fibrosis and bronchial obstructions, compromise lung function and defense mechanisms, potentially worsening COVID-19 outcomes. These insights underscore the importance of addressing TB/COVID-19 co-infection comprehensively [28].

Hence, the need for additional research specifically addressing the TB-COVID-19 co-infection is evident. This study aims to better understand and mitigate the impact of this novel pathogenic combination. We assessed differences in several clinical, biological and imagistic markers in order to better understand the impact of moderate and severe forms of *SARS-CoV-2* infection on patients with recently diagnosed lung TB.

2. Materials and Methods

The present retrospective, cross-sectional, randomized study involved 132 adult patients aged 39 to 81, hospitalized at the Victor Babeș Hospital of Infectious Diseases and Pneumoftiziology from Timișoara. We analyzed data from March to June 2020. The design of the study was based on the comparison of two groups of patients, one with lung tuberculosis and *SARS-CoV-2* co-infection ($n = 32$), and a control group including age-matched patients with a diagnosis of only moderate or severe *SARS-CoV-2* infection ($n = 100$). The main objective was to determine the impact of *SARS-CoV-2* on an already tarred organism due to TB.

Inclusion criteria:

- ☐ pulmonary TB (PTB) diagnosed 1 month prior to the confirmation of *SARS-CoV-2* infection at most, through solid or liquid cultures (Gene-Xpert) in the TB ambulatory service from Timișoara [29];
- ☐ moderate or severe *SARS-CoV-2* forms of infection at the moment of hospital admittance, confirmed by nasopharyngeal exudate RT-PCR analysis in an acreditted laboratory. A moderate form was considered that in which the individual was exhibiting signs of lower respiratory disease during clinical evaluation or imaging, with oxygen saturation measured by pulse oximetry SpO2 $\geq$ 94% on room air.

A severe form is characterized by an SpO2 < 94% on room air, a respiratory rate exceeding 30 breaths/min, or lung infiltrates exceeding 50% [30].

- ☐ normal renal function (normal GFR, creatinine and urea levels) [31];
- ☐ BCG vaccination completed in all participants [32].

Exclusion criteria:

- ☐ extrapulmonary TB, including pleural TB efussions, TB lymphadenopaties, miliar TB, osteoarticular TB, intestinal TB, urogenital TB, meningitis TB, and other forms.
- ☐ overweight (BMI = 25 to 30 kg/m^2) or obesity (BMI $\geq$ 30 kg/m^2) [33];
- ☐ pre-existing severe or uncontrolled arterial hypertension [34];
- ☐ lung cancer [35] or other neoplasies [36];
- ☐ idiopathic lung fibrosis [37,38];
- ☐ pre-existing advanced chronic heart failure [39];
- ☐ hepatic, renal, or digestive chronic conditions that may result in weight loss and *HIV* infection

The Ethics Council for Scientific Research at the Victor Babeș University of Medicine and Pharmacy Timisoara granted approval for the study, which adheres to the principles of the Helsinki Declaration (04/19 January 2021). Before enrollment in the study, informed consent was obtained from all patients after comprehensive explanations about the nature of the data analysis.

2.1. Data Collection

The data was collected from personal medical files and included anamnestic information, clinical parameters and biological and imagistic investigations.

The medical history revealed the BCG vaccination status. Comorbidities such as COPD and type 2 DM were noted. A part of the patients diagnosed with TB were observed to have had a history of TB prior to the present infection (all of them underwent appropriate therapy at the time and were deemed cured). The smoking status of each patient was determined: never smoked, smoker. Three social groups were analyzed as per employment: unemployed, employed, and retired.

The BMI was calculated using the standard formula Weight (kg)/Height^2 (m^2) [40]. The SpO2 (%) values obtained using calibrated pulse oximeters in the COVID-19 unit [41] were recorded from charts at two points: first, at the time of *SARS-CoV-2* infection diagnosis, and second, the lowest value recorded during hospitalization. Peripheral systolic and diastolic blood pressures (SBP, DBP, mmHg) were obtained from charts at diagnosis. The *SARS-CoV-2* symptoms noted in all patients were: fever, coughing, dispnoea, fatigue, abdominal pain, chest pain, myalgia, vomiting/nausea, diarrhea, headache, olfactory/taste disorders. The symptomatology was classified as more severe if any of these symptoms associated tachypnea (respiratory rate $\geq$ 30 breaths/min) [42].

We analyzed the following blood markers: C-reactive protein (CRP, mg/L), procalcitonin (PCT), aspartate aminotransferase (AST, U/L), alanine aminotransferase (ALT, U/L), lactate dehydrogenase (LDH, U/L), inteleukin-6 (IL-6, pg/mL), D-dimer levels (mg/L), neutrophil, lymphocyte and platelet count (/µL) [40]. We calculated the neutrophil to lymphocyte ratio (NLR) [43], the platelet to lymphocyte ratio (PLR) [44], and the systemic immuno-inflammatory index (SII), calculated as platelet count x NLR [45].

X-ray images were analyzed and the following lesions were noted at the moment of *SARS-CoV-2* infection:

- ☐ unilateral pulmonary infiltrate, no cavities;
- ☐ bilateral pulmonary infiltrates, no cavities;
- ☐ unilatsiral pulmonary cavitary lesions;
- ☐ bilateral pulmonary cavitary lesions.

We considered bilateral pulmonary cavitary lesions the most severe lesions.

An experienced radiology specialist (over 10-year experience) reviewed all CT scans completed at the confirmation of *SARS-CoV-2* infection

The chest CT interpretation focused on detecting lesions such as: ground-glass opacifications, consolidations, crazy paving pattern, linear opacities combined, air bronchogram sign, tree in bud [46], and cavitary lesions [47]. To quantify the extent of lung lesions, each of the five lung lobes was visually scored from 0 to 5, with the following classification:

0 points: no involvement;
1 point: less than 5% involvement;
2 points: 5–25% involvement;
3 points: 26–49% involvement;
4 points: 50–75% involvement;
5 points: more than 75% involvement.

The total chest CT involvement score was then determined by summing the individual scores from each lobe, yielding a range from 0 to 25. This approach provides a comprehensive view of the disease's impact on the lungs [48,49].

Cavitary lesions were included in calculating the lung involvement score, but were also noted separately, as an aggravating factor suggestive for lung TB.

The number of total hospitalization days and the outcome (resolved-PCR converted or death) were also determined in each case.

2.2. Data Analysis

Data collection was conducted using Microsoft Excel for Microsoft 365 MSO (Version 2404 build 16.0.17531.20140) and statistical analyses were performed with MedCalc Statistical Software version 20.111 (MedCalc Software Ltd., Ostend, Belgium). The primary focus of the analysis was to examine the impact of *SARS-CoV-2* infection on patients with and without PTB co-infection. Clinical, imagistic and biologic parameters were assessed in comparison. Significance was determined by *p*-values below 0.05. To assess the normality of the data distribution, the Shapiro–Wilk test was employed. Subsequently, appropriate statistical tests were chosen based on the normality of the data: medians and the Mann–Whitney test were used for non-normal variables. The AUC-ROC analysis was employed in order to evaluate the significance of various parameters in discerning between the presence and absence of co-infection. Cut-off values for such discrimination were determined with the ultimate scope of highlighting the significance of certain parameters in evaluating these medical conditions. Logistic regressions were employed to identify independent predictors of co-infection and fatal outcome. The Fisher's exact test was used to evaluate the associations between sets of binary data.

3. Results

This study included 132 patients, divided in 2 study groups comprising 32 patients with PTB and *SARS-CoV-2* co-infection, and 100 patients with *SARS-CoV-2* infection alone.

Out of the co-infected patients, 21 (65%) were male and 11 (34%) female. In the *SARS-CoV-2* group, 52 patients were male and 48 were female. The mean age in the co-infected group was 62.8 years, SD = 12.82, while the median age in the *SARS-CoV-2* group was 57 years; a significant difference in age between the two groups was not detected, $p = 0.07$ (Mann–Whitney test).

The BMI was significantly lower in the co-infection group, with a median value of 21.88 vs. 24.82, $p = 0.0002$ (Mann–Whitney test); see Figure 1.

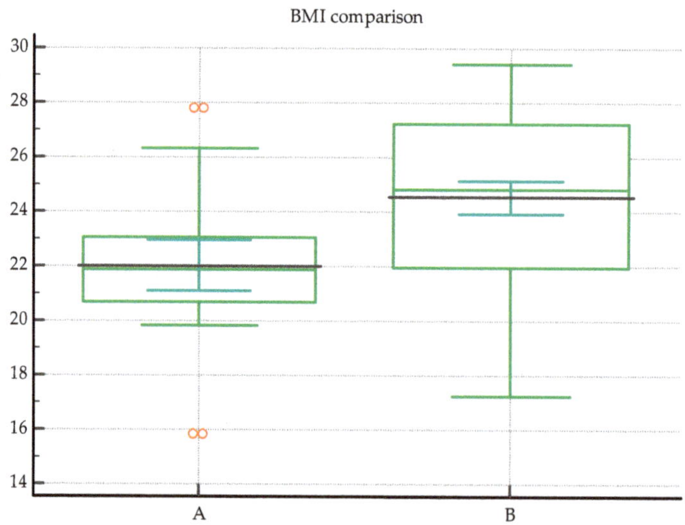

Figure 1. BMI comparison between the two groups: A = the co-infection group, B = the *SARS-CoV-2* group; $p = 0.0002$.

The comparison between co-infected and *SARS-CoV-2* infected patients showed that there are significant differences between the two groups in the majority of the analyzed parameters. The co-infected group revealed significantly lower SpO2 both at diagnosis, and with regard the lowest value registered, lower neutrophil and lymphocyte counts, and higher SBP levels, CRP, transaminase, and D-dimer levels. The chest CT involvement score was also significantly higher in the co-infection group. PLR was higher in the PTB-*SARS-CoV-2* group (Table 1).

Table 1. Comparison between co-infected and *SARS-CoV-2* infected patients with regard to multiple parameters (Mann–Whitney test).

Parameter	Co-Infection Group Median Value	*SARS-CoV-2* group Median Value	*p*
SpO2 at diagnosis	90	94	**0.0009**
Lowest SpO2	83.5	89.5	**0.004**
Peripheral SBP at diagnosis	138	133	**0.04**
Peripheral DBP at diagnosis	92	87	0.07
CRP	89.5	55.5	**0.0001**
LDH	288	243.5	0.51
IL-6	4.2	1.2	0.08
AST	36	29	**0.003**
ALT	38.5	30	**0.0002**
D-dimer	1.91	0.91	**0.01**
Neutrophils *	6758.75 (SD = 3733.15)	5878.3 (SD = 1162.67)	**<0.001**
Lymphocytes	2210	3010	**0.003**
Thrombocytes	242.5×10^3	252×10^3	0.42
NLR	2	1.83	0.67
PLR	128.85	77.95	**0.03**
SII	538,198.71	459,783.69	0.7
Chest CT involvement score	16	12	0.002

* The T-student test was employed for neutrophil count. The bolded data in this table represents statistically significant results.

A multiple parameter logistic regression was employed with the dependent variable being the presence/absence of PTB-*SARS-CoV-2* co-infection and the independent variables being clinical and anamnestic parameters: age, sex, BMI, employment status, associating COPD, type 2 DM, the severity of symptoms and the status of previously having TB. The BMI and the severity of symptoms emerged as significant predictors of PTB-*SARS-CoV-2* co-infection. The lower the BMI levels, the higher the odds of co-infection. Severe symptomatology is associated with a higher probability of co-infection. The rest of the variables were not included in the model. See Table 2.

Table 2. Logistic regression depicting significant predictors of TB-*SARS-CoV-2* co-infection (part 1).

Parameter	Odds Ratio	95% CI	Coefficient	Std. Err.	Constant	*p*
BMI	0.76	0.65–0.89	−0.26	0.08	4.9	**0.001**
Symptoms severity	1.16	1.19–8.56	1.16	0.5	4.9	**0.02**

The bolded data in this table represents statistically significant results.

The logistic regression employed for the paraclinical and biological parameters, with the dependent variable being the presence/absence of PTB-*SARS-CoV-2* co-infection and the independent variables being: SpO2 at diagnosis, lowest SpO2, SBP, DBP, CRP, LDH, PCT, IL-6, AST, ALT, D-dimer, neutrophil count, lymphocyte count, thrombocyte count, NLR, PLR, SII, and the chest CT involvement score. The model revealed as significant predictors ($p < 0.0001$) the SpO2 levels at diagnosis, LDH, ALT, neutrophil count, and the CT score (see Table 3). The higher the ALT levels and CT score, the higher the odds of co-infection, and the higher the SpO2 at diagnosis and LDH levels, the lower the probability of co-infection. The rest of the variables were not included in the model.

Table 3. Logistic regression depicting significant predictors of PTB-*SARS-CoV-2* co-infection (part 2).

Parameter	Odds Ratio	95% CI	Coefficient	Std. Err.	*p*
SpO2 at diagnosis	0.58	0.55–0.91	−0.33	0.12	**0.007**
LDH	0.98	0.98–0.99	−0.01	0.003	**0.0005**
ALT	1.05	1.01–1.11	0.05	0.02	**0.01**
Neutrophil count	0.99	0.99–1	−0.0002	0.0001	**0.03**
Chest CT involvement score	1.35	1.14–1.61	0.3	0.08	**0.0005**

The constant was 47.62. The bolded data in this table represents statistically significant results.

Further on, AUC-ROC analyses were employed in order to determine the significance of multiple parameters in discriminating between the presence and absence of PTB co-infection (Table 4).

Table 4. AUC-ROC analysis for the clinical and anamnestic parameters, as discriminators between the presence and the absence of PTB co-infection in *SARS-CoV-2* patients (n = 132).

Parameter	AUC	*p*	Se%	95% CI	Sp%	95% CI	PPV %	NPV %
Age	0.6	0.058	81.25	63.6–92.8	39	29.4–49.3	29.9	87.7
Sex	0.58	0.08	68.75	50.0–83.9	48	37.9–58.2	29.7	82.8
BMI	**0.72**	**<0.0001**	84.37	67.2–94.7	67	56.9–76.1	43	93.1
Employment status	0.5	0.97	75	56.6–88.5	10	4.9–17.6	21.1	55.6
Smoking	0.51	0.72	37.5	21.1–56.3	66	55.8–75.2	26.1	76.7
COPD	0.5	0.97	81.25	63.6–92.8	19	11.8–28.1	24.3	76
Type 2 DM	0.59	0.052	37.5	21.1–56.3	81	71.9–88.2	38.7	80.2

The bolded data in this table represents statistically significant results.

The AUC-ROC analysis showed that sex (Figure A1) and age are not reliable discriminators, $p = 0.08$, and $p = 0.058$, respectively. The analysis revealed that a cut-off value for the BMI ≤ 23.23 was significant for discriminating between the presence of PTB co-infection and its absence ($p < 0.0001$), see Figure 2 and Table 4. Hence, the smaller the value of BMI, the higher the probability of TB co-infection.

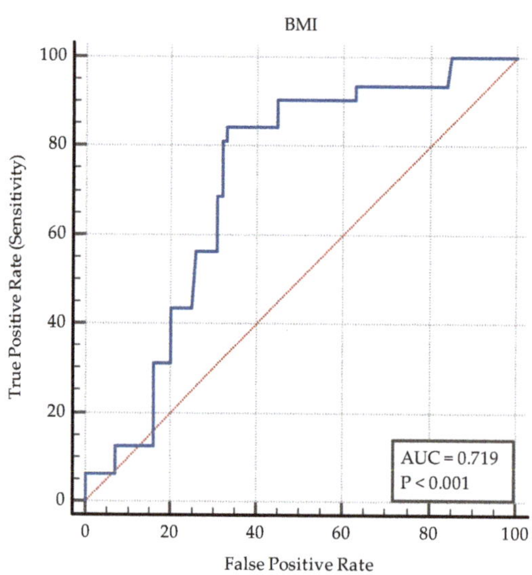

Figure 2. ROC curve for BMI.

With regard to employment status, in the co-infection group 25% were unemployed, 31.2% employed, and 43.8%, retired. In the *SARS-CoV-2* group, 10% were unemployed, 58% employed, and 32% retired. See Figure 3. The employment status does not seem to be significant for acquiring PTB-*SARS-CoV-2* co-infection, $p = 0.97$. Despite a relatively good sensibility, it revealed a very low specificity, according to the AUC-ROC analysis (Table 2, Figure A2).

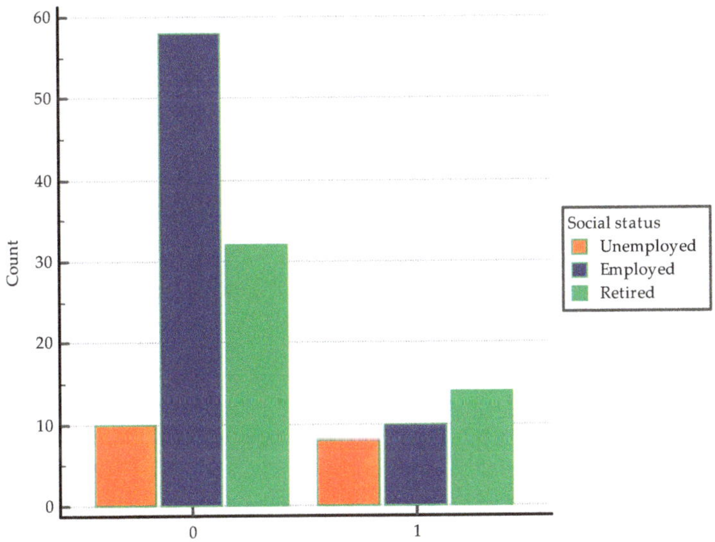

Figure 3. Distribution of cases according to the social status. 0 = *SARS-CoV-2* group, 1 = co-infection group.

With regard to smoking, 37.5% patients in the co-infection group were smokers, while in the *SARS-CoV-2* group, 34%. The AUC-ROC analysis did not reveal a significant power of discrimination between the two groups of study, with relatively low sensitivity and specificity (Table 4, Figure A3).

In the co-infection group, 18.7% patients associated COPD, and 59.4% associated type 2 DM. In the *SARS-CoV-2* group, 19% also presented COPD, and 19%, diabetes. As for associating both conditions, 3 patients were detected in the co-infection group and 6 patients in the *SARS-CoV-2* group. Neither the association of COPD nor type 2 DM were significant factors for aquiring PTB-*SARS-CoV-2* co-infection, although in the case of diabetes, the analysis almost reached significance, with a $p = 0.052$ and a good specificity (Table 4, Figures A4 and A5).

Further on, the AUC-ROC analysis focused on clinical and biological parameters presented in Table 5. The following cut-off values were determined as significant for distinguishing between the presence and absence of PTB: SpO2 at diagnosis $\leq$89%, worst SpO2 $\leq$ 85%, CRP > 81 mg/L, IL-6 > 0.8 pg/mL, ALT > 35 U/L, AST > 40 U/L, D-dimer > 1.44 mg/L, lymphocyte count $\leq$ 2880/µL, PLR > 139.3, and the chest CT involvement score >14 (Figures 4 and 5). The analysis revealed that SpO2 at diagnosis and the lowest SpO2 value have very good specificities, but relatively lower sensibilities. The gravity of the symptoms also has a good specificity, but quite a low sensibility. The CRP, ALT, AST and D-dimer levels revealed the same pattern. So do the imagistic parameters-chest X-ray and CT involvement score (Figure 5). In contrast, IL-6 and the lymphocytopenia revealed good sensibilities, with lower specificities (Table 5). See also Figures A6–A11.

Table 5. AUC-ROC analysis for the clinical, biologic and imagistic parameters, as discriminators between the presence and the absence of PTB co-infection in *SARS-CoV-2* patients (n = 132).

Parameter	AUC	p	Se%	95% CI	Sp%	95% CI	PPV %	NPV %
SpO2 at diagnosis	**0.69**	**0.002**	46.88	29.1–65.3	94	87.4–97.8	71.4	84.7
Lowest SpO2	**0.67**	**0.007**	62.5	43.7–78.9	72	62.1–80.5	41.7	85.7
Symptoms severity	**0.62**	**0.01**	43.75	26.4–62.3	80	70.8–87.3	41.2	81.6
CRP	**0.73**	**<0.001**	65.62	46.8–81.4	75	65.3–83.1	45.7	87.2
PCT	0.56	0.17	28.12	13.7–46.7	84	75.3–90.6	36	78.5
LDH	0.54	0.52	62.5	43.7–78.9	50	39.8–60.2	28.6	80.6
IL-6	**0.6**	**0.04**	81.25	63.6–92.8	45	35–55.3	32.1	88.2
AST	**0.67**	**0.006**	46.88	29.1–65.3	93	86.1–97.1	68.2	84.5
ALT	**0.72**	**0.0001**	65.62	46.8–81.4	78	68.6–85.7	48.8	87.6
D-dimer	**0.64**	**0.01**	56.25	37.7–73.6	69	59.0–77.9	36.7	83.1
Neutrophils	0.58	0.3	46.88	29.1–65.3	92	84.8–96.5	65.2	84.4
Lymphocytes	**0.67**	**0.002**	78.12	60–90.7	59	48.7–68.7	37.8	89.4
Thrombocytes	0.54	0.48	37.5	21.1–56.3	88	80–93.6	50	81.5
NLR	0.71	0.52	43.75	26.4–62.3	80	70.8–87.3	41.2	81.6
PLR	0.62	**0.04**	50	31.9–68.1	79	69.7–86.5	43.2	83.2
SII	0.52	0.74	43.75	26.4–62.3	76	66.4–84	36.8	86.9
Chest Rx	**0.7**	**<0.001**	62.5	43.7–78.9	75	65.3–83.1	44.4	86.2
Chest CT involvement score	**0.67**	**0.001**	62.5	43.7–78.9	73	63.2–81.4	42.6	85.9

The bolded data in this table represents statistically significant results.

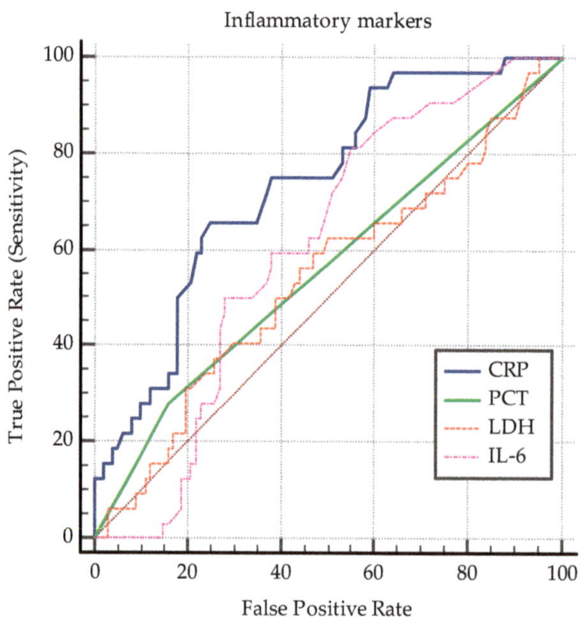

Figure 4. ROC curves for the inflammatory markers.

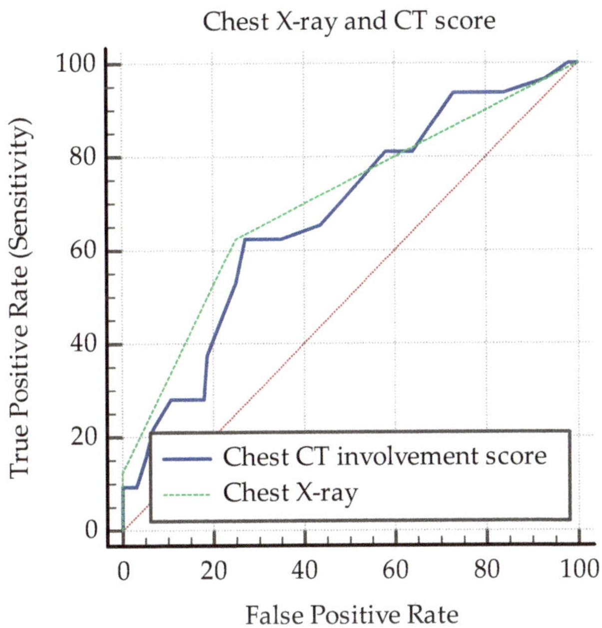

Figure 5. ROC curves for chest X-ray and CT involvement score.

Fisher's exact test was used to evaluate the connection between associating PTB infection and several instances presented in Table 6. Having TB prior to the present episode and having a more severe symptomatology were revealed as significantly associated with the likelihood of associating a TB infection.

Table 6. Associations between the probability of having TB co-infection and several parameters (Fisher's exact test).

	Parameter	Fisher's Exact Test *p*
Presence of PTB	Smoking	0.83
	COPD	0.99
	Type 2 DM	0.053
	TB prior to present episode	**<0.0001**
	Severe symptoms	**0.01**
	PCT	0.19
	Outcome	0.31

The bolded data in this table represents statistically significant results.

The Chi-squared test was used to analyze associations between the imagistic lesions shown on chest X-ray and chest CT. The severity of the lesions on X-ray were significantly associated with co-infection (Chi-squared = 22.55, DF = 2, $p < 0.0001$), see Figure 6.

With regard to the presence of ground glass opacities and cavitary lesions on chest CT, the following analysis involved only their presence. Ground glass and bilateral cavitary lesions were considered the most severe finds and were significantly associated with co-infection (Chi-squared = 29.1, DF = 3, $p < 0.0001$), see

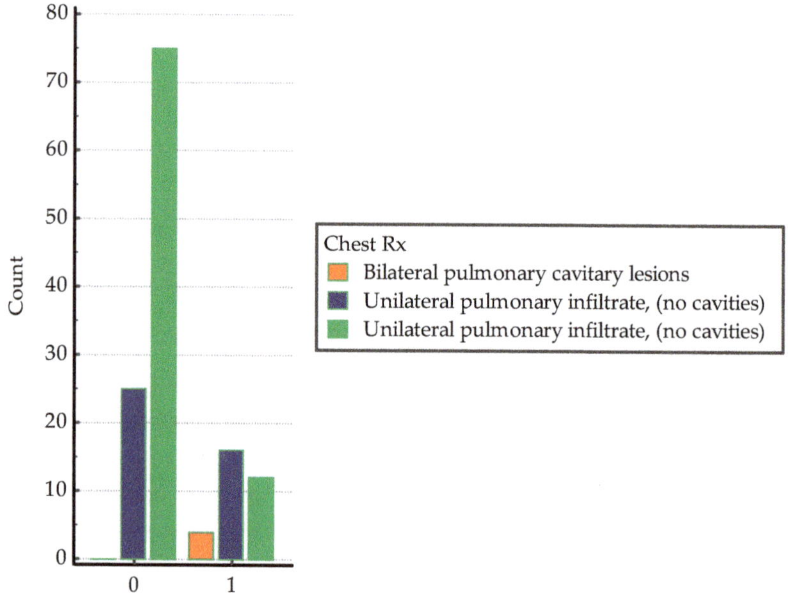

Figure 6. Distribution of X-ray pulmonary lesions in the two groups; 0 = *SARS-CoV-2* group, 1 = co-infection group.

Figure 7.

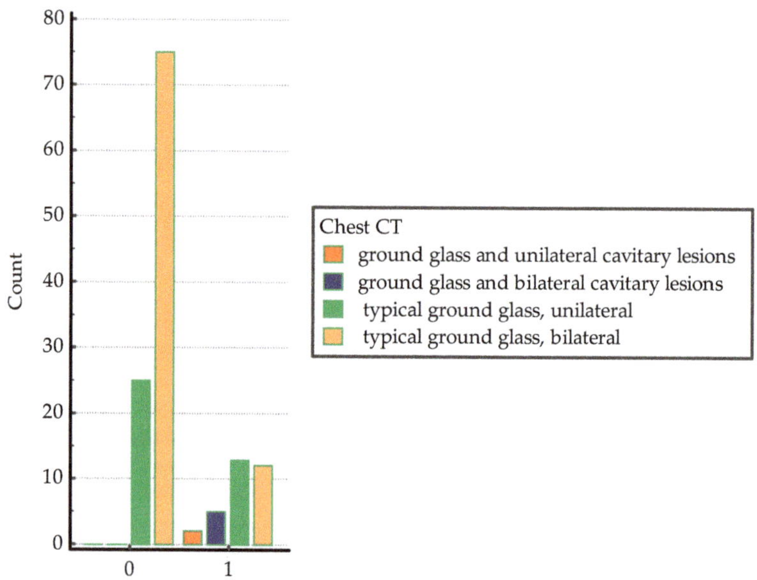

Figure 7. Distribution of CT pulmonary lesions in the two groups; 0 = *SARS-CoV-2* group, 1 = co-infection group.

However, according to the chest CT involvement score, we divided the subjects into two groups according to the previous AUC-ROC analysis result showing that a cut-off >14 is significant for the likelihood of co-infection, in our cohort (Table 7).

Table 7. Distribution of subjects according to the chest CT involvement score cut-off.

Chest CT Involvement Score	PTB-*SARS-CoV-2* Co-Infection *n*	Associated Cavitary Lesions *n*	*SARS-CoV-2* Co-Infection *n*
>14	20	2	27
≤14	12	2	73

Within the two categories of chest CT involvement score, there were no differences between coinfected and subjects with COVID-19 alone in neither >14 category (p = 0.8, Mann–Whitney test), nor ≤ 14 (p = 0.85, T-test).

The length of hospitalization is also a reliable parameter that discerns between the two groups, with a cut-off (criterion) of >10 days, AUC = 0.69, p = 0.001, Se% = 65.62, 95% CI = 46.8–81.4, Sp% = 78, 95% CI = 68.6–85.7, PPV% = 48, NPV% = 87.6 (see Figure 8).

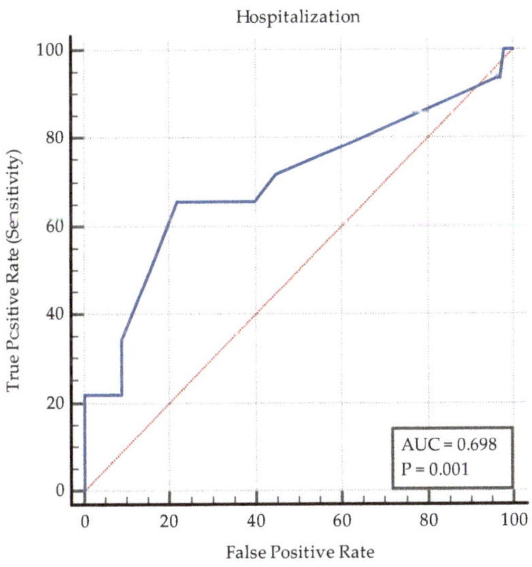

Figure 8. ROC curve for the days of hospitalization.

With regard fatal outcomes, 25% (n = 8) of the patients in the co-infection group and 17% in the *SARS-CoV-2* group died. The AUC-ROC analysis did not show that a fatal outcome is a reliable discriminator between the two instances (AUC = 0.54, p = 0.35, Se% = 25, 95% CI = 11.5–43.4, Sp% = 83, 95% CI = 74.2–89.8, PPV% = 32, NPV% = 76.6), see Figure 9.

The logistic regression analysis did not retain the presence of PTB-*SARS-CoV-2* co-infection as a significant predictor of fatality. A multiple parameter logistic regression was employed to evaluate the effects of several markers (independent variables: severe symptoms, smoking, COPD, type 2 DM, prior TB infection) on outcome (dependent variable). The result showed that the presence of type 2 DM, severe symptomatology and longer hospitalization are significant independent predictors of fatal outcome (Table 8).

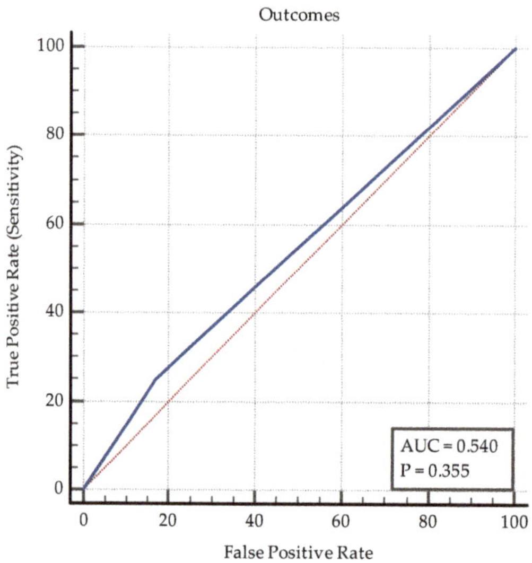

Figure 9. ROC curve for outcomes.

Table 8. Logistic regression depicting significant predictors of fatal outcome.

Parameter	Odds Ratio	95% CI	Coefficient	Std. Err.	Constant	*p*
Type 2 DM	7.03	1.8–27.3	1.9	0.69	−4.78	**0.004**
Severe symptoms	12.17	3.1–47.75	2.49	0.69	−4.78	**0.0003**
Hospitalization	1.16	1.02–1.32	0.15	0.006	−4.78	**0.02**

The bolded data in this table represents statistically significant results.

4. Discussion

This study aimed to analyze the impact of *SARS-CoV-2* infection on patients with PTB. To achieve that we compared two groups: one with PTB and *SARS-CoV-2* co-infection and a group with only *SARS-CoV-2* infection. The discussion will focus on the key findings and their implications in understanding the interaction between these two infectious diseases.

The demographic characteristics of the study population revealed a predominance of males in the co-infected group, with a 1.9:1 male to female ratio, whereas the *SARS-CoV-2* group had a more balanced sex distribution (52% males). Globally, tuberculosis affects a significantly higher number of men than women. The exact reason for this sex disparity remains uncertain, with epidemiological factors traditionally regarded as the primary drivers. One common explanation suggests that the male bias observed in TB cases stems from systematic underreporting and underdiagnosis of the disease in women [50]. A comprehensive meta-analysis of 29 surveys across 14 countries revealed a consistent male bias in both notification and prevalence rates [51], hence, considering the consistent reports about sex bias around the world, it is strongly suggested that biological sex differences do exist [52].

Furthermore, although age is a significant risk factor for both TB [53] and a more severe form of COVID-19 [54], this study did not detect significant differences in age between the two studied groups, due to the design of the study, which ensured that the selection of patients in the *SARS-CoV2* group is as similar as possible to the co-infection group.

This study confirms lower BMI as a significant marker of a probable PTB-*SARS-CoV-2* co-infection. Low BMI represents a risk factor for developing lung TB due to an immunomodulatory effect on cytokine and chemokine response [55]. It has been known for decades that a BMI 10% lower than the ideal body weight increases the risk of developing lung TB three times in young men [56], and that the lowest BMI category is associated with a fivefold risk of lung TB compared to the highest BMI category [57], as shown in two very large cohort studies. The inverse link between BMI and the risk of developing lung TB has been reconfirmed multiple times [58–60]. In contrast, COVID-19 is associated with a higher risk of severe outcomes in overweight and obese individuals [61,62]. On the other hand, however, frailty, a common characteristic of TB patients, represents a major risk factor for mortality or longer hospitalization in COVID-19 patients [63]. Frailty is associated with both extremes of the BMI spectrum, and is often observed in both underweight [64] and severely obese individuals [65]. A healthy BMI may reduce the prevalence of frailty [64], leading to better outcomes in both acute and chronic ailments. Nevertheless, BMI is not a clinical marker with reliable specificity to TB infection, as numerous other pulmonary and extrapulmonary pathologies might associate weight loss. In situations where these pathologies are excluded, such as our study, a lower BMI could bring additional information for the diagnostic effort.

Social determinants such as poverty, living conditions, population density, and economic status play a role in influencing the incidence of COVID-19 and TB [66,67]. Employment status did not emerge as significantly impactful for the likelihood of co-infection in our study. However, the proportion of unemployed individuals reached 25% in the TB group, compared to 10% in the *SARS-CoV-2* group. Unemployment in TB patients poses a significant challenge, as they seem to exhibit more severe radiographic abnormalities and increased occurrences of treatment discontinuations and elevated mortality rates during hospitalization [68].

More than a third of both studied groups were smokers, but smoking did not emerge as a significant marker or predictor of co-infection. Smoking is connected to TB through its potential of damaging the immune response through defects in macrophages, monocytes and CD4 lymphocytes function, and hence, making the organism more susceptible to TB infection [69]. Most studies agree that smoking also increases the susceptibility to *SARS-CoV-2* infection, about 1.5 times according to a comprehensive literature review [61], although differences in populations and tobacco products (e-cigarettes) have been invoked as less harmful or even protective in a few studies [70]. A further impactful risk factor can be heavy alcohol consumption. Its toxic impact on the immune system heightens the risk of developing active illness. Alcohol intake stands as one of the foremost modifiable risk factors for tuberculosis, with alcohol use disorders prevalent in 30% of TB cases and contributing to 11.4% (9.3–13%) of TB-related mortality [71]. Regarding the subjects of our study, 90% declared no alcohol consumption at all, with the remaining occasionally consuming small amounts.

Comorbidities such as COPD and type 2 DM are aggravating factors for both TB and *SARS-CoV-2* infection. COPD is characterized by a combination of emphysema and chronic bronchitis, leading to chronic systemic inflammation that weakens the immune system. People with COPD are prone to various additional health problems, including heart failure, diabetes, atherosclerosis, osteoporosis, muscle loss, and co-infections. Among these complications, active TB poses a significant risk for individuals with COPD. Recent research indicates that individuals with COPD are three times more likely to develop active TB compared to those without. Moreover, once infected, individuals with COPD and TB face twice the risk of mortality compared to those without these conditions [72]. On the other hand, COPD is associated with worse outcomes in *SARS-CoV-2* infection, although data is unclear on whether COPD increases the susceptibility to coronavirus infection [73]. This study has not shown that COPD increases the probability of co-infection or the risk of fatal outcome. In contrast, associating type 2 DM has been significantly more prevalent in our study (59.4% of the subjects in the co-infection group presented type 2 DM, versus 18.7%, COPD). Diabetes heightens the susceptibility to TB and correlates with the manifestation of severe cavitating disease as well as unfavorable treatment outcomes, including mortality [74–77]. An underlying cause is the exacerbation of insulin resistance and stress-induced hyperglycemia by TB, which may ameliorate during the course of treatment [78,79]. It is even advisable to screen TB patients for DM after 2–3 months of initiating TB treatment [80]. Furthermore, diabetic patients with *SARS-CoV-2* infection are expected to present worse symptomatology and even worse outcomes. SpO2 at hospital admission, along with glycemia and glycosylated hemoglobin, seem to have the highest sensitivity and specificity in predicting the prognosis of type 2 DM patients with *SARS-CoV-2* infection [81]. Associating TB and type 2 DM in the context of *SARS-CoV-2* has not been studied sufficiently. Our study shows that type 2 DM increases the likelihood of a fatal outcome, but the analysis did not confirm it as significant for predicting co-infection. Further studies of this grave trio should be encouraged in larger samples. Another very significant comorbidity which was excluded from this particular study is represented by an impaired kidney function. Chronic kidney disease (CKD) can predispose individuals to TB due to impaired immune function and reduced ability to fight infections. In contrast, TB can exacerbate kidney function impairment in patients with CKD, leading to worsening renal outcomes. Additionally, CKD and COVID-19 are considered significant risk factors for severe COVID-19 outcomes. Patients with CKD often have underlying conditions such as diabetes and hypertension, which further increase their vulnerability to severe COVID-19. COVID-19 can directly affect kidney function through various mechanisms, including direct viral invasion of renal cells, systemic inflammation, and cytokine release syndrome. Acute kidney injury is a common complication of severe COVID-19 and can exacerbate pre-existing CKD or lead to new-onset kidney dysfunction [82].

A greater severity of acute symptomatology in COVID-19 at hospital admission is associated with a higher probability of co-infection with PTB [16,83–85]. In this regard, our study aligns with other findings. These results should be taken into consideration specifically in TB-endemic regions, especially in these post-pandemic times when *SARS-CoV-2* infection has become less concerning. Moreover, severe symptoms are also connected with higher odds of fatal outcome.

In comparing patients with co-infection to those with *SARS-CoV-2* infection alone, significant differences emerge across various parameters. Co-infected individuals exhibited notably lower levels of SpO2 at both diagnosis and at their lowest recorded value, and higher levels of systolic blood pressure. The logistic regression connected lower SpO2 levels to a greater probability of co-infection. A systematic review of case reports of TB-COVID-19 co-infections has placed SpO2 levels at 90–97% room air in most cases [86]; the lower the SpO2, the worse the outcome [87]. Contrary to our results, the aforementioned review reported that about a third of the cases presented hypotension [86]. Among individuals with COVID-19 alone, arterial hypertension is considered a prevalent comorbidity. Due to the involvement of angiotensin converting enzyme 2 in *SARS-CoV-2* infection, there is speculation regarding the potential role of hypertension in the pathogenesis of COVID-19 [88]. Hypertension correlates with a 2.5-fold heightened risk of elevated disease severity and mortality among COVID-19 patients. Moreover, this association was predominantly observed among individuals aged over 60 years [89].

The present study reported diminished lymphocyte count and higher levels of C-reactive protein, transaminases, and D-dimer in the co-infection group. Lymphopenia is consistently identified as a characteristic observed in cases of COVID-19 [86,90–92]. It has been suggested that in addition to the specific clinical signs and symptoms, lymphopenia could be helpful in suspecting and isolating cases [90]. Neutrophilia is more typical in COVID-19, with severe neutrophilia being correlated to severe disease [93,94]. Our study reported normal median neutrophil count in the *SARS-CoV2* group, and significantly higher neutrophil levels in the co-infection group. Neutrophilia is a protective immune response in active TB infection, with neutrophil counts normalizing usually within 6 months of treatment [95]. Neutropenia is a rare complication of anti-tuberculous treatment, such as isoniazid [96]. Referring again to the previously mentioned review of case reports, the rise in serum inflammatory markers such as CRP, D-dimer, and IL-6 was reported to have a significant association with unfavorable outcome [86]. Moreover, when substantially elevated, these markers predict mortality and are used as a main indicator of intensive care need [97]. Liver enzymes are typically elevated due to activation of immune responses and represent markers of systemic inflammation [86,98]. Our study showed that higher ALT and neutrophil count levels are associated with increased odds of co-infection. With regard to the AUC-ROC analysis, parameters such as SpO2, CRP, ALT, AST, and D-dimer levels exhibited good discriminatory power between co-infected and COVID-19 patients alone, while others like IL-6 and lymphocyte count showed higher sensitivity but lower specificity.

Systemic inflammation was also analyzed via three surrogate markers: the neutrophil to lymphocyte ratio (NLR), the platelet to lymphocyte ratio (PLR), and the systemic immune-inflammation index (SII). These are markers usually utilized to determine the prognosis of viral or bacterial infections. They are considered more feasible, cost-effective, and accessible markers, that can be readily conducted within any healthcare facility setting [99,100].

High NLR accurately predicts disease severity and mortality in COVID-19 [101,102]. The pre-treatment NLR upon admission could serve as a valuable biomarker for predicting mortality and the onset of acute respiratory distress syndrome in individuals with miliary tuberculosis [103]. A recent meta-analysis has shown that NLR has a reliable power to discriminate between PTB infection and bacterial community acquired pneumonia—the lower the NLR, the higher the chances of PTB infection [104]. Our study has not showed significant differences in NLR between the two groups.

Blood hypercoagulability is a prevalent condition observed among hospitalized COVID-19 patients, often accompanied by elevated D-dimers [105]. Thrombocytopenia has been associated with disease severity in several studies [106], while others have noted that patients with significantly elevated platelet counts tend to experience longer hospitalization stays. This latter observation is thought to be linked to the correlation between platelet count and the cytokine storm associated with *SARS-CoV-2* infection. Specifically, IL-6 promotes megakaryocyte generation by stimulating thrombopoietin levels, leading to elevated platelet counts [107]. The PLR, particularly during the peak of the platelet count, has emerged as an independent prognostic factor for prolonged hospitalization [108]. Moreover, an increased PLR is associated with increased risk of fatal outcome [108,109]. Elevated PLR levels have also been examined in several studies regarding TB. It has been shown to discriminate between TB infection and non-infection in COPD patients [110]. Our study showed that PLR is significantly higher in the case of PTB-*SARS-CoV-2* co-infected patients. Moreover, it showed that a PLR > 139.3 can distinguish between the two groups with a specificity of 79% ($p = 0.04$).

Like the NLR and PLR, the SII serves as a proinflammatory marker of systemic inflammation and holds potential for independently predicting mortality in COVID-19 cases [111]. SII is also a reliable marker of inflammation in TB patients [112]. Our study revealed more elevated SII in the co-infection group, but the difference was not statistically significant. Further studies should be employed on larger samples in order to clarify the role of these three surrogate markers in PTB-*SARS-CoV-2* co-infection.

Additionally, our study showed that the severity of lesions on chest X-ray and CT scans was significantly associated with co-infection, highlighting the importance of imaging modalities in diagnosis and prognosis. Chest X-rays are typically the initial imaging modality of choice due to their widespread availability and cost-effectiveness. However, chest CT scans offer greater sensitivity compared to conventional X-rays. They allow for the detection of complications beyond pulmonary involvement and can also indicate alternative diagnoses. In COVID-19 cases, the predominant radiological findings often include bilateral airspace opacities, such as consolidations and/or ground-glass opacities [113]. Imaging plays a crucial role in diagnosing and managing tuberculosis also. While chest X-rays serve as the primary imaging tool for pulmonary tuberculosis, CT is invaluable for evaluating both pulmonary and extrapulmonary manifestations of the disease [114]. Our study focused on the chest CT involvement score, which was significantly higher in co-infected subjects. Moreover, this score was shown to serve both as a significant independent predictor of co-infection, and as a significant discriminator between co-infection and

COVID-19 alone, with a cut-off >14. One of the first studies to evaluate a PTB-*SARS-CoV-2* co-infected cohort showed that on chest CT evaluations, about 43% of patients presented multifocal ground-glass opacities distributed peripherally, specific to COVID-19, and about 47% presented lesions associated to TB such as cavitary lesions, branching micronodules, and consolidations [16]. Other studies have supported more or less the same findings, suggestive of both diseases [115,116].

The length of hospitalization emerged as a reliable parameter for distinguishing between the two groups, with a longer duration associated with co-infection. The analysis did not reveal a significant difference in fatal outcomes between the co-infected and *SARS-CoV-2* groups.

An observation on extrapulmonary TB and *SARS-CoV-2* co-infection is important, although our study did not explore this issue. Studies conducted during the same time-frame of the pandemic indicate a slight increase in extrapulmonary tuberculosis cases. The similarity in symptoms between pulmonary TB and COVID-19 may have skewed suspicions towards TB lung disease, potentially contributing to the uptick in extrapulmonary tuberculosis diagnoses [22]. Further multicenter studies involving larger populations from diverse regions would provide greater clarity on diagnosing extrapulmonary TB amidst the COVID-19 pandemic.

The key strengths of this study are the valuable results concerning a multitude of parameters which show that the initial premise that *SARS-CoV-2* has an additive impact on TB patients than on those TB-free, is true. Although a few studies with somewhat similar designs have been completed before and thus have been cited here, we believe our input is valuable to the global information on *PTB-SARS-CoV-2* co-infection, as TB infection is still an important issue in many parts of our world. We bring forward accessible and cost-efficient markers which can be used to determine the probability of co-infection in questionable situations. We consider the single-center nature of our study and thus, the sample size of the co-infection group as a limitation for this study, but, according to our pre-statistical estimations, the ratios were sufficient to provide statistical significance. Further research directions could explore extrapulmonary TB-COVID-19 co-infections or the impact of HIV or CKD on the outcome of TB-*SARS-CoV-2* co-infection. From an epidemiological point of view, the impact of anti-*SARS-CoV-2* vaccines on co-infection should be explored. Our study collected data from a period when vaccines were not available. However, vaccines have played a crucial role in slowing down and stopping the pandemic, and demonstrated significant efficacy in preventing severe forms of the disease and deaths associated with COVID-19. With regard to TB-*SARS-CoV-2* co-infection, further research is needed to better understand the duration of protection provided by vaccines, and the adaptation of vaccines to new virus strains [117].

5. Conclusions

The study highlights the intricate relationship between *SARS-CoV-2* infection and pulmonary tuberculosis, indicating that certain demographic, clinical, and biological factors may serve as potential indicators of TB co-infection in patients with *SARS-CoV-2*.

A lower BMI emerges as a significant marker suggesting underlying pulmonary TB in patients with *SARS-CoV-2*.

The presence of type 2 diabetes mellitus increases the likelihood of a fatal outcome in patients with PTB-*SARS-CoV-2* co-infection.

Co-infected patients exhibit more pronounced lymphocytopenia and higher levels of neutrophils, C-reactive protein, transaminases, D-dimer levels, and a higher chest CT involvement score.

High ALT and chest CT score are associated with an increased likelihood of co-infection. Parameters including SpO2, CRP, ALT, AST, D-dimer levels, and the chest CT score demonstrate good discriminatory power between co-infected individuals and those with COVID-19 alone. The platelet-to-lymphocyte ratio is notably elevated in co-infected patients.

While longer hospitalization durations are linked to co-infection, they do not significantly increase the likelihood of a fatal outcome.

Author Contributions: Conceptualization, C.O. and C.M.; methodology, C.O., C.M. and A.S.; software, M.S.M.; validation, C.O. and A.S.; formal analysis, C.M. and A.S.; investigation, C.M. and A.S.; resources, A.S. and C.O.; data curation, M.S.M., P.H. and E.T.; writing—original draft preparation, C.M.; writing—review and editing, A.S. and C.O.; visualization, M.S.M., P.H. and E.T.; supervision, C.O.; project administration, A.S. and C.O. All authors have read and agreed to the published version of the manuscript.

Funding: We would like to acknowledge VICTOR BABES UNIVERSITY OF MEDICINE AND PHARMACY TIMISOARA for their support in covering the costs of publication for this research paper, according to the UMFVBT Senate Decision No. 24/7135/24.06.2020.

Institutional Review Board Statement: The study was conducted in accordance with the Declaration of Helsinki and approved by the Ethics Council for Scientific Research at the Victor Babeș University of Medicine and Pharmacy Timisoara, No. 04/19 January 2021.

Informed Consent Statement: Informed consent was obtained from all subjects involved in the study. Written informed consent has been obtained from the patients to publish this paper.

Data Availability Statement: The findings of this study are supported by data which can be obtained upon request from the corresponding author. However, ethical restrictions prevent the public availability of the data.

Acknowledgments: We express our gratitude to all the patients who participated in this study, wishing them continued good health. We also recognize the valuable contributions of each author and the support provided by our affiliated institutions in facilitating our research and publishing our results.

Conflicts of Interest: The authors declare no conflicts of interest.

Abbreviations

ALT	Alanine aminotransferase
AST	Aspartate aminotransferase
AUC	Area under the receiver operating characteristic curve
BMI	Body mass index
COPD	Chronic Obstructive Pulmonary Disease
CRP	C-reactive protein
CT	Computer tomography
DM	Diabetes Mellitus
HIV	Human Deficiency Virus
IL-6	Interleukin 6
LDH	Lactate Dehydrogenase
n	number of subjects
p	*p*-value
PCT	Procalcitonin
PTB	pulmonary tuberculosis
ROC	Receiver operating characteristic
RT-PCR	Reverse Transcription Polymerase Chain Reaction
SpO2	Saturation of peripheral oxygen
TB	Tuberculosis
X-ray	high-energy electromagnetic radiation
WHO	World Health Organization

Appendix A

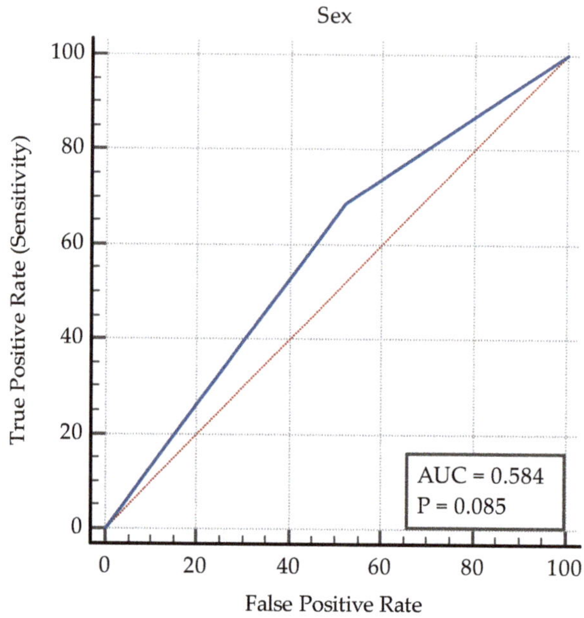

Figure A1. ROC curve for sex.

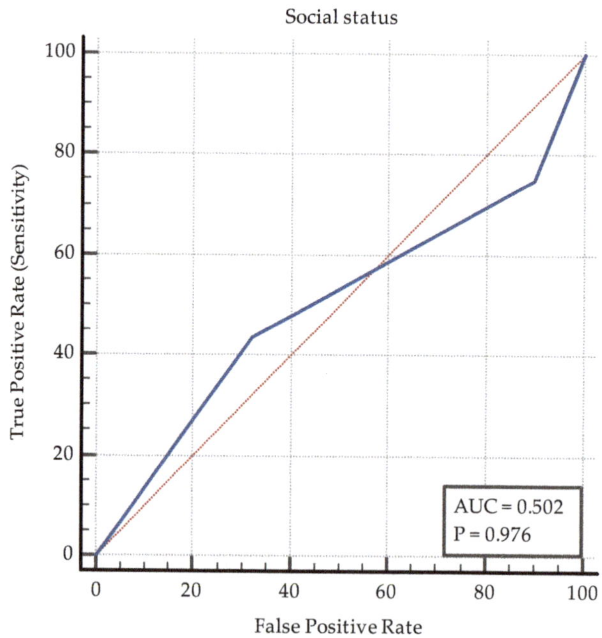

Figure A2. ROC curve for employment status.

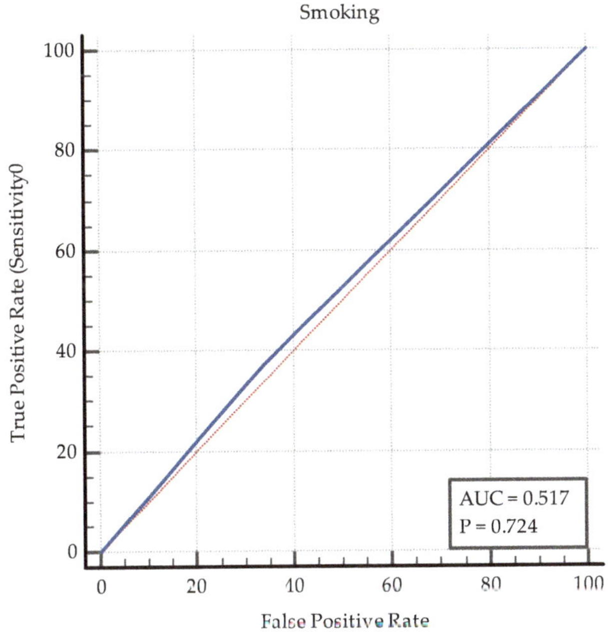

Figure A3. ROC curve for the status of smoking.

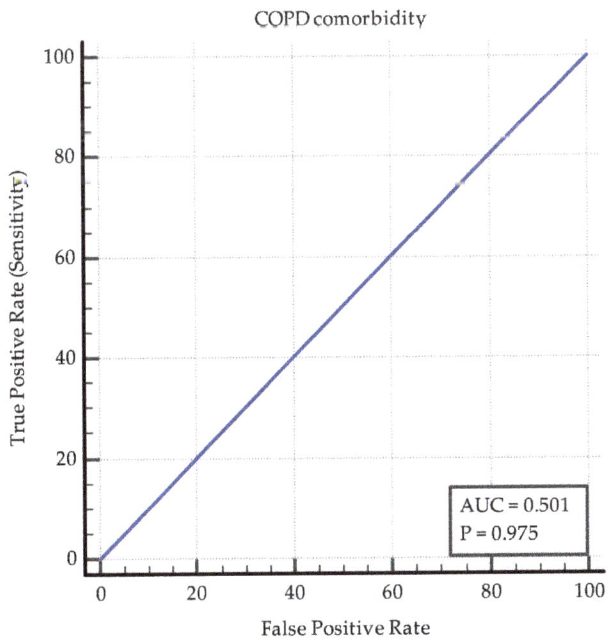

Figure A4. ROC curve for the association of COPD.

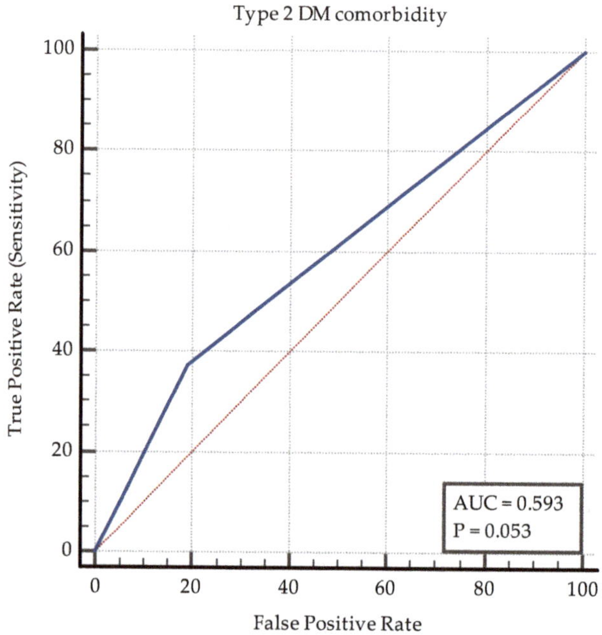

Figure A5. ROC curve for the association of type 2 DM.

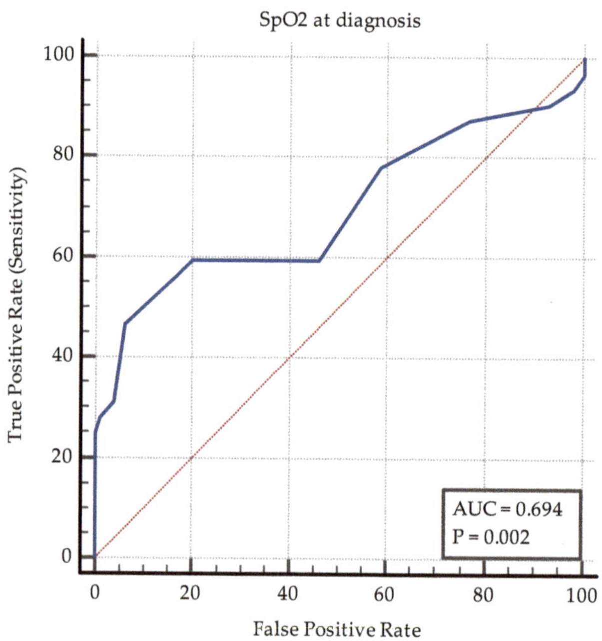

Figure A6. ROC curve for the values of SpO2 at diagnosis.

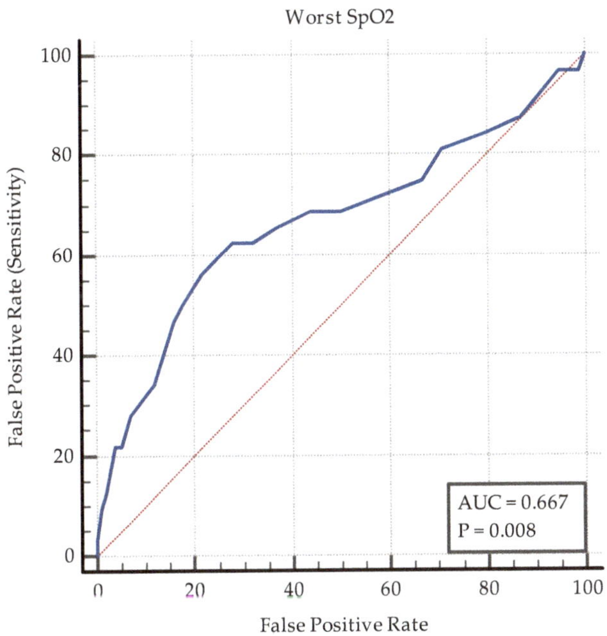

Figure A7. ROC curve for the lowest values of SpO2.

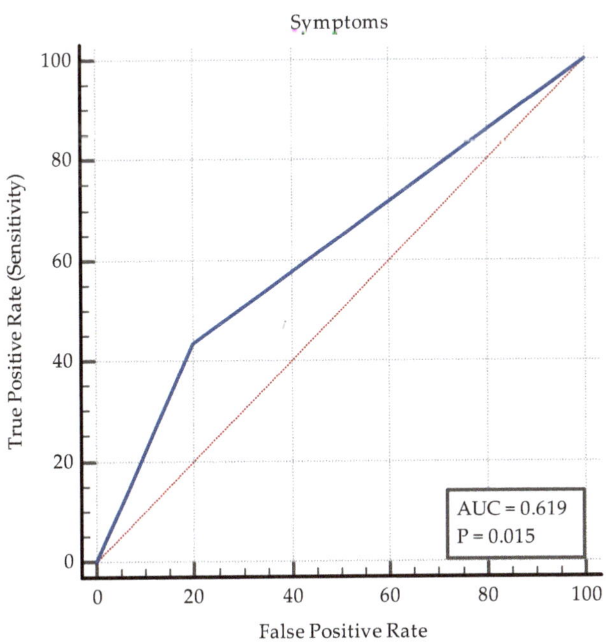

Figure A8. ROC curve for the severity of symptoms.

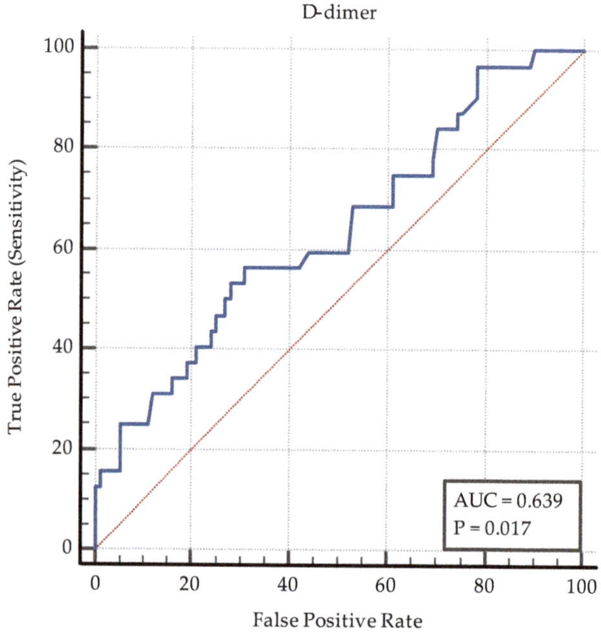

Figure A9. ROC curve for the value of D-dimer.

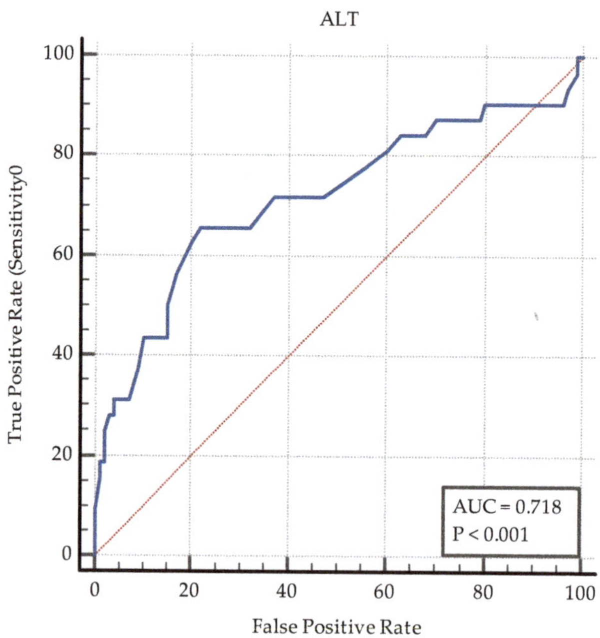

Figure A10. ROC curve for the value of ALT.

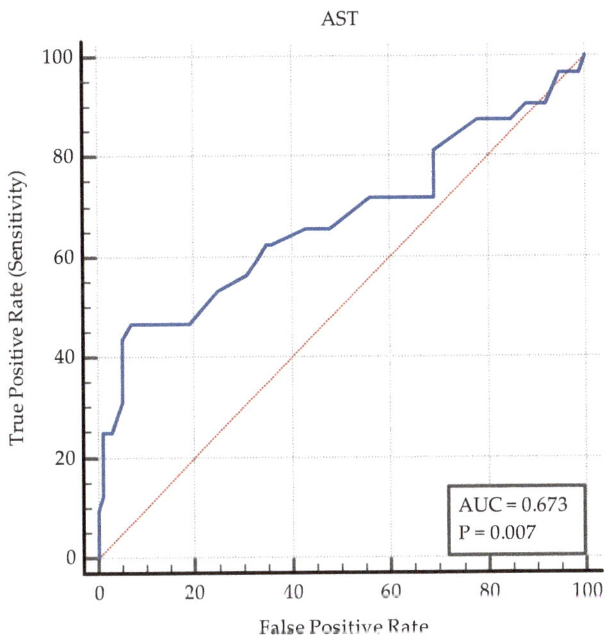

Figure A11. ROC curve for the value of AST.

References

1. Mathiasen, V.D.; Andersen, P.H.; Johansen, I.S.; Lillebaek, T.; Wejse, C. Clinical features of tuberculous lymphadenitis in a low-incidence country. *Int. J. Infect. Dis.* **2020**, *98*, 366–371. [CrossRef] [PubMed]
2. Visca, D.; Ong, C.W.M.; Tiberi, S. Tuberculosis and COVID-19 interaction: A review of biological, clinical, and public health effects. *Pulmonology* **2021**, *27*, 151–165. [CrossRef] [PubMed]
3. Wu, Z.; McGoogan, J.M. Characteristics of and important lessons from the coronavirus disease 2019 (COVID-19) outbreak in China: Summary of a report of 72,314 cases from the Chinese Center for Disease Control and Prevention. *JAMA* **2020**, *323*, 1239–1242. [CrossRef] [PubMed]
4. Chen, N.; Zhou, M.; Dong, X.; Qu, J.; Gong, F.; Han, Y. Epidemiological and clinical characteristics of 99 cases of 2019 novel coronavirus pneumonia in Wuhan, China: A descriptive study. *Lancet* **2020**, *395*, 507–513. [CrossRef]
5. Guan, W.J.; Ni, Z.Y.; Hu, Y.; Liang, W.H.; Ou, C.Q.; He, J.X.; China Medical Treatment Expert Group for COVID-19. Clinical Characteristics of Coronavirus Disease 2019 in China. *N. Engl. J. Med.* **2020**, *382*, 1708–1720. [CrossRef] [PubMed]
6. Ong, C.W.M.; Goletti, D. Impact of the global COVID-19 outbreak on the management of other communicable diseases. *Int. J. Tuberc. Lung Dis.* **2020**, *24*, 547–548. [CrossRef] [PubMed]
7. Kames, J.; Holcomb, D.D.; Kimchi, O.; DiCuccio, M.; Hamasaki-Katagiri, N.; Wang, T.; Komar, A.A.; Alexaki, A.; Kimchi-Sarfaty, C. Sequence analysis of SARS-CoV-2 genome reveals features important for vaccine design. *Nat. Sci. Rep.* **2020**, *10*, 15643. [CrossRef] [PubMed]
8. Harvey, W.T.; Carabelli, A.M.; Jackson, B.; Gupta, R.K.; Thomson, E.C.; Harrison, E.M.; Ludden, C.; Reeve, R.; Rambaut, A.; COVID-19 Genomics UK (COG-UK) Consortium; et al. SARS-CoV-2 variants, spike mutations and immune escape. *Nat. Rev. Microbiol.* **2021**, *19*, 409–424. [CrossRef] [PubMed]
9. Farinholt, T.; Doddapaneni, H.; Qin, X.; Menon, V.; Meng, Q.; Metcalf, G.; Chao, H.; Gingras, M.C.; Farinholt, P.; Agrawal, C.; et al. Transmission event of SARS-CoV-2 Delta variant reveals multiple vaccine breakthrough infections. *medRxiv* **2021**, *19*, 255. [CrossRef]
10. Surleac, M.; Banica, L.; Casangiu, C.; Cotic, M.; Florea, D.; Sandulescu, O.; Milu, P.; Streinu-Cercel, A.; Vlaicu, O.; Paraskevis, D.; et al. Molecular Epidemiology Analysis of SARS-CoV-2 Strains Circulating in Romania during the First Months of the Pandemic. *Life* **2020**, *10*, 152. [CrossRef]
11. Lobiuc, A.; Dimian, M.; Gheorghita, R.; Sturdza, O.A.C.; Covasa, M. Introduction and Characteristics of SARS-CoV-2 in North-East of Romania During the First COVID-19 Outbreak. *Front. Microbiol.* **2021**, *12*, 654417. [CrossRef]
12. World Health Organization. *Global Tuberculosis Report 2020*; World Health Organization: Geneva, Swizerland, 2020; Available online: https://apps.who.int/iris/bitstream/handle/10665/336069/9789240013131-eng.pdf (accessed on 14 February 2024).

13. Cilloni, L.; Fu, H.; Vesga, J.F.; Dowdy, D.; Pretorius, C.; Ahmedov, S. The potential impact of the COVID-19 pandemic on the tuberculosis epidemic: A modelling analysis. *EClinicalMedicine.* **2020**, *28*, 100603. [CrossRef]
14. Migliori, G.B.; Thong, P.M.; Akkerman, O.; Alffenaar, J.W.; Álvarez-Navascués, F.; Assao-Neino, M.M. Worldwide Effects of Coronavirus Disease Pandemic on Tuberculosis Services, January–April 2020. *Emerg. Infect. Dis.* **2020**, *26*, 2709–2712. [CrossRef] [PubMed]
15. Buonsenso, D.; Iodice, F.; Sorba Biala, J.; Goletti, D. COVID-19 effects on tuberculosis care in Sierra Leone. *Pulmonology* **2021**, *27*, 67–69. [CrossRef]
16. Tadolini, M.; Codecasa, L.R.; García-García, J.M.; Blanc, F.X.; Borisov, S.; Alffenaar, J.W. Active tuberculosis, sequelae and COVID-19 co-infection: First cohort of 49 cases. *Eur. Respir. J.* **2020**, *56*, 2001398. [CrossRef] [PubMed]
17. Mousquer, G.T.; Peres, A.; Fiegenbaum, M. Pathology of TB/COVID-19 co-infection: The phantom menace. *Tuberculosis* **2020**, *126*, 102020. [CrossRef]
18. Singh, A.; Prasad, R.; Gupta, A.; Das, K.; Gupta, N. Severe acute respiratory syndrome coronavirus-2 and pulmonary tuberculosis: Convergence can be fatal. *Monaldi Arch. Chest Dis.* **2020**, *90*, 441–450. [CrossRef] [PubMed]
19. Liao, M.; Liu, Y.; Yuan, J.; Wen, Y.; Xu, G.; Zhao, J.; Chen, L.; Li, J.; Wang, X.; Wang, F.; et al. The landscape of lung bron-choalveolar immune cells in COVID-19 revealed by single-cell RNA sequencing. *MedRxiv* **2020**, *26*, 842–844. [CrossRef]
20. Carlos, W.G.; Dela Cruz, C.S.; Cao, B.; Pasnick, S.; Jamil, S. Novel Wuhan (2019-nCoV) Coronavirus. *Am. J. Respir. Crit. Care Med.* **2020**, *201*, 7–8. [CrossRef]
21. Rolo, M.; González-Blanco, B.; Reyes, C.A.; Rosillo, N.; López-Roa, P. Epidemiology and factors associated with Extra-pulmonary tuberculosis in a Low-prevalence area. *J. Clin. Tuberc. Other Mycobact. Dis.* **2023**, *32*, 100377. [CrossRef]
22. Udoakang, A.J.; Djomkam Zune, A.L.; Tapela, K.; Nganyewo, N.N.; Olisaka, F.N.; Anyigba, C.A.; Tawiah-Eshun, S.; Owusu, I.A.; Paemka, L.; Awandare, G.A.; et al. The COVID-19, tuberculosis and HIV/AIDS: Ménage à Trois. *Front. Immunol.* **2023**, *14*, 1104828. [CrossRef] [PubMed]
23. Wang, W.; Xin, C.; Xiong, Z.; Yan, X.; Cai, Y.; Zhou, K. Clinical characteristics and outcomes of 421 patients with coronavirus disease 2019 treated in a mobile cabin hospital. *Chest* **2020**, *158*, 939–946. [CrossRef] [PubMed]
24. Wei, M.; Zhao, Y.; Qian, Z.; Yang, B.; Xi, J.; Wei, J. Pneumonia caused by Mycobacterium tuberculosis. *Microb. Infect.* **2020**, *22*, 278–284. [CrossRef] [PubMed]
25. Narjess, B.; Faramarz, M.J.; Shabnam, R. Mycobacterium tuberculosis and SARS-CoV-2 Coinfections: A Review. *Front. Microbiol.* **2021**, *12*, 747826. [PubMed]
26. Getnet, F.; Demissie, M.; Worku, A.; Gobena, T.; Tschopp, R.; Girmachew, M. Delay in diagnosis of pulmonary tuberculosis increases the risk of pulmonary cavitation in pastoralist setting of Ethiopia. *BMC Pulm. Med.* **2019**, *19*, 201. [CrossRef] [PubMed]
27. Kaftan, A.N.; Hussain, M.K.; Algenabi, A.A.; Naser, F.H.; Enaya, M.A. Predictive Value of C–reactive Protein, Lactate Dehydrogenase, Ferritin and D-dimer Levels in Diagnosing COVID-19 Patients: A Retrospective Study. *Acta Inform. Med.* **2021**, *29*, 45–50. [CrossRef] [PubMed]
28. Dheda, K.; Booth, H.; Huggett, J.F.; Johnson, M.A.; Zumla, A.; Rook, G.A.W. Lung remodeling in pulmonary tuberculosis. *J. Infect. Dis.* **2005**, *192*, 1201–1209. [CrossRef] [PubMed]
29. Prakash, A.K.; Datta, B.; Goyal, P.; Chatterjee, P.; Gupta, G. GENE-XPERT gives early diagnosis in early tuberculosis. *Eur. Respir. J.* **2016**, *48* (Suppl. S60), PA2775. [CrossRef]
30. COVID-19 Treatment Guidelines Panel. Coronavirus Disease 2019 (COVID-19) Treatment Guidelines. National Institutes of Health. Available online: https://www.covid19treatmentguidelines.nih.gov/ (accessed on 1 March 2024).
31. Gounden, V.; Bhatt, H.; Jialal, I. Renal Function Tests. [Updated 2023 Jul 17]. In *StatPearls*; StatPearls Publishing: Treasure Island, FL, USA, 2024. Available online: https://www.ncbi.nlm.nih.gov/books/NBK507821/ (accessed on 13 February 2024).
32. World Health Organization. BCG vaccines: WHO position paper—February 2018. *Wkly. Epidemiol. Rec.* **2018**, *93*, 73–96.
33. Purnell, J.Q. Definitions, Classification, and Epidemiology of Obesity. [Updated 4 May 2023]. In *Endotext*; Feingold, K.R., Anawalt, B., Blackman, M.R., Boyce, A., Chrousos, G., Corpas, E., de Herder, W.W., Dhatariya, K., Dungan, K., Hofland, J., et al., Eds.; MDText.com, Inc.: South Dartmouth, MA, USA, 2000. Available online: https://www.ncbi.nlm.nih.gov/books/NBK279167/ (accessed on 13 February 2024).
34. Akpek, M. Does COVID-19 Cause Hypertension? *Angiology* **2022**, *73*, 682–687. [CrossRef]
35. Parker, C.S.; Siracuse, C.G.; Litle, V.R. Identifying lung cancer in patients with active pulmonary tuberculosis. *JTD* **2018**, *10* (Suppl. S28), S3392–S3397. [CrossRef] [PubMed]
36. Ramamoorthy, S.; Srinivas, B.H.; Badhe, B.A.; Jinkala, S.; Ganesh, R.N. Coexistence of malignancy and tuberculosis: Is it double disease or double hit related to COVID-19?—Experience from a tertiary care center. *Int. J. Clin. Exp. Pathol.* **2023**, *16*, 1–7.
37. Chung, M.J.; Goo, J.M.; Im, J.-G. Pulmonary tuberculosis in patients with idiopathic pulmonary fibrosis. *Eur. J. Radiol.* **2004**, *52*, 175–179. [CrossRef] [PubMed]
38. Novikova, L.; Ilkovich, Y.; Speranskaya, A. Tuberculosis in patients with idiopathic pulmonary fibrosis. *Eur. Respir J.* **2015**, *46*, PA2046. [CrossRef]
39. Metra, M.; Dinatolo, E.; Dasseni, N. The New Heart Failure Association Definition of Advanced Heart Failure. *Card. Fail. Rev.* **2019**, *5*, 5–8. [CrossRef] [PubMed]
40. NHLBI Obesity Education Initiative Expert Panel on the Identification E and T of O in A (US). Clinical Guidelines on the Identification, Evaluation, and Treatment of Overweight and Obesity in Adults: The Evidence Report. In *Obesity Prevention*

and Management; National Heart, Lung, and Blood Institute, Ed.; NHLBI Obesity Education Initiative Expert Panel on the Identification, Evaluation, and Treatment of Obesity in Adults (US): Bethesda, MD, USA, 1998.
41. Seifi, S.; Khatony, A.; Moradi, G.; Abdi, A.; Najafi, F. Accuracy of pulse oximetry in detection of oxygen saturation in patients admitted to the intensive care unit of heart surgery: Comparison of finger, toe, forehead, and earlobe probes. *BMC Nurs.* **2018**, *17*, 15. [CrossRef] [PubMed]
42. Fukui, S.; Ikeda, K.; Kobayashi, M.; Nishida, K.; Yamada, K.; Horie, S.; Shimada, Y.; Miki, H.; Goto, H.; Hayashi, K.; et al. Predictive prognostic biomarkers in patients with COVID 19 infection. *Mol. Med. Rep.* **2023**, *27*, 15. [CrossRef]
43. Ali, E.T.; Jabbar, A.S.; Al Ali, H.S.; Hamadi, S.S.; Jabir, M.S.; Albukhaty, S. Extensive Study on Hematological, Immunological, Inflammatory Markers, and Biochemical Profile to Identify the Risk Factors in COVID-19 Patients. *Int. J. Inflam* **2022**, *2022*, 5735546. [CrossRef]
44. Ravindra, R.; Ramamurthy, P.; Aslam, S.S.M.; Kulkarni, A.; Suhail, K.; Ramamurthy, P.S. Platelet Indices and Platelet to Lymphocyte Ratio (PLR) as Markers for Predicting COVID-19 Infection Severity. *Cureus* **2022**, *14*, e28206. [CrossRef]
45. Mangoni, A.A.; Zinellu, A. Systemic inflammation index, disease severity, and mortality in patients with COVID-19: A systematic review and meta-analysis. *Front. Immunol.* **2023**, *14*, 1212998. [CrossRef]
46. Hansell, D.M.; Bankier, A.A.; MacMahon, H.; McLoud, T.C.; Müller, N.L.; Remy, J. Fleischner society: Glossary of terms for thoracic imaging. *Radiology* **2008**, *246*, 697–722. [CrossRef] [PubMed]
47. Hernandez-Romieu, A.C.; Little, B.P.; Bernheim, A.; Schechter, M.C.; Ray, S.M.; Bizune, D.; Kempker, R. Increasing Number and Volume of Cavitary Lesions on Chest Computed Tomography Are Associated With Prolonged Time to Culture Conversion in Pulmonary Tuberculosis. *Open Forum Infect Dis.* **2019**, *6*, ofz232. [CrossRef] [PubMed]
48. Chang, Y.-C.; Yu, C.-J.; Chang, S.-C.; Galvin, J.R.; Liu, H.-M.; Hsiao, C.-H.; Kuo, P.-H.; Chen, K.-Y.; Franks, T.J.; Huang, K.-M.; et al. Pulmonary sequelae in convalescent patients after severe acute respiratory syndrome: Evaluation with thin-section CT. *Radiology* **2005**, *236*, 1067–1075. [CrossRef] [PubMed]
49. Yazdi, N.A.; Ghadery, A.H.; SeyedAlinaghi, S.; Jafari, F.; Jafari, S.; Hasannezad, M.; Koochak, H.E.; Salehi, M.; Manshadi, S.A.D.; Meidani, M.; et al. Predictors of the chest CT score in COVID-19 patients: A cross-sectional study. *Virol. J.* **2021**, *18*, 225, Erratum in *Virol. J.* **2021**, *18*, 241. [CrossRef] [PubMed]
50. Nhamoyebonde, S.; Leslie, A. Biological Differences Between the Sexes and Susceptibility to Tuberculosis. *J. Infect. Dis.* **2014**, *209* (Suppl. S3), S100–S106. [CrossRef] [PubMed]
51. Borgdorff, M.W.; Nagelkerke, N.J.; Dye, C.; Nunn, P. Gender and tuberculosis: A comparison of prevalence surveys with notification data to explore sex differences in case detection. *Int. J. Tuberc. Lung Dis.* **2000**, *4*, 123–132.
52. Min, J.; Park, J.S.; Kim, H.W.; Ko, Y.; Oh, J.Y.; Jeong, Y.-J.; Na, J.O.; Kwon, S.-J.; Choe, K.H.; Lee, W.-Y.; et al. Differential effects of sex on tuberculosis location and severity across the lifespan. *Sci. Rep.* **2023**, *13*, 6023. [CrossRef]
53. Caraux-Paz, P.; Diamantis, S.; de Wazières, B.; Gallien, S. Tuberculosis in the Elderly. *J. Clin. Med.* **2021**, *10*, 5888. [CrossRef] [PubMed]
54. Bartleson, J.M.; Radenkovic, D.; Covarrubias, A.J.; Furman, D.; Winer, D.A.; Verdin, E. SARS-CoV-2, COVID-19 and the Ageing Immune System. *Nat. Aging* **2021**, *1*, 769–782. [CrossRef]
55. Nathella Pavan, K.; Arul, P.N.; Kadar, M.; Pradeep, A.M.; Vaithilingam, V.B.; Nair, D.; Sujatha, N.; Babu, S. Low Body Mass Index Is Associated with Diminished Plasma Cytokines and Chemokines in Both Active and Latent Tuberculosis. *Front. Nutr.* **2023**, *10*, 1194682. [CrossRef]
56. Edwards, L.B.; Livesay, V.T.; Acquaviva, F.A.; Palmer, C.E. Height, Weight, Tuberculous Infection, and Tuberculous Disease. *Arch. Environ. Health* **1971**, *22*, 106–112. [CrossRef] [PubMed]
57. Tverdal, A. Body Mass Index and Incidence of Tuberculosis. *Eur. J. Respir. Dis.* **1986**, *69*, 355–362. [PubMed]
58. Cho, S.H.; Lee, H.; Kwon, H.; Shin, D.W.; Joh, H.-K.; Han, K.; Park, J.H.; Cho, B. Association of Underweight Status with the Risk of Tuberculosis: A Nationwide Population-Based Cohort Study. *Sci. Rep.* **2022**, *12*, 16207. [CrossRef] [PubMed]
59. Choi, H.; Yoo, J.E.; Han, K.; Choi, W.; Rhee, S.Y.; Lee, H.; Shin, D.W. Body Mass Index, Diabetes, and Risk of Tuberculosis: A Retrospective Cohort Study. *Front. Nutr.* **2021**, *8*, 739766. [CrossRef] [PubMed]
60. Casha, A.R.; Scarci, M. The Link between Tuberculosis and Body Mass Index. *J. Pers. Med.* **2017**, *9*, 3. [CrossRef] [PubMed]
61. Gao, M.; Piernas, C.; Astbury, N.M.; Hippisley-Cox, J.; O'Rahilly, S.; Aveyard, P.; Jebb, S.A. Associations between Body-Mass Index and COVID-19 Severity in 6·9 Million People in England: A Prospective, Community-Based, Cohort Study. *Lancet Diabetes Endocrinol.* **2021**, *9*, 350–359. [CrossRef]
62. Lockhart, S.M.; O'Rahilly, S. When Two Pandemics Meet: Why Is Obesity Associated with Increased COVID-19 Mortality? *Med* **2020**, *1*, 33–42. [CrossRef]
63. Hewitt, J.; Carter, B.; Vilches-Moraga, A.; Quinn, T.J.; Braude, P.; Verduri, A.; Pearce, L.; Stechman, M.; Short, R.; Price, A.; et al. The Effect of Frailty on Survival in Patients with COVID-19 (COPE): A Multicentre, European, Observational Cohort Study. *Lancet Public Health* **2020**, *5*, e444–e451. [CrossRef] [PubMed]
64. Jayanama, K.; Theou, O.; Godin, J.; Mayo, A.; Cahill, L.; Rockwood, K. Relationship of Body Mass Index with Frailty and All-Cause Mortality Among Middle-Aged and Older Adults. *BMC Med.* **2022**, *20*, 404. [CrossRef]
65. Watanabe, D.; Yoshida, T.; Watanabe, Y.; Yamada, Y.; Kimura, M. A U-Shaped Relationship between the Prevalence of Frailty and Body Mass Index in Community-Dwelling Japanese Older Adults: The Kyoto–Kameoka Study. *J. Clin. Med.* **2020**, *9*, 1367. [CrossRef]

66. Koupaei, M.; Naimi, A.; Moafi, N.; Mohammadi, P.; Tabatabaei, F.S.; Ghazizadeh, S.; Heidary, M.; Khoshnood, S. Clinical Characteristics, Diagnosis, Treatment, and Mortality Rate of TB/COVID-19 Coinfected Patients: A Systematic Review. *Front. Med.* **2021**, *8*, 740593. [CrossRef] [PubMed]
67. Duarte, R.; Aguiar, A.; Pinto, M.; Furtado, I.; Tiberi, S.; Lönnroth, K.; Migliori, G.B. Different Disease, Same Challenges: Social Determinants of Tuberculosis and COVID-19. *Pulmonology* **2021**, *27*, 338–344. [CrossRef] [PubMed]
68. Przybylski, G.; Dabrowska, A.; Pilaczyńska-Cemel, M.; Krawiecka, D. Unemployment in TB Patients—Ten-Year Observation at Regional Center of Pulmonology in Bydgoszcz, Poland. *Med. Sci. Monit.* **2014**, *20*, 2125–2131. [CrossRef] [PubMed]
69. Altet, M.; Alcaide, J.; Plans, P.; Taberner, J.; Saltó, E.; Folguera, L.; Salleras, L. Passive Smoking and Risk of Pulmonary Tuberculosis in Children Immediately Following Infection. A Case-Control Study. *Tuberc. Lung Dis.* **1996**, *77*, 537–544. [CrossRef] [PubMed]
70. Chattopadhyay, S.; Malayil, L.; Kaukab, S.; Merenstein, Z.; Sapkota, A.R. The Predisposition of Smokers to COVID-19 Infection: A Mini-Review of Global Perspectives. *Heliyon* **2023**, *9*, e17783. [CrossRef] [PubMed]
71. Morojele, N.K.; Shenoi, S.V.; Shuper, P.A.; Braithwaite, R.S.; Rehm, J. Alcohol Use and the Risk of Communicable Diseases. *Nutrients* **2021**, *13*, 3317. [CrossRef]
72. Inghammar, M.; Ekbom, A.; Engström, G.; Ljungberg, B.; Romanus, V.; Lofdahl, C.G.; Egesten, A. COPD and the Risk of Tuberculosis—A Population-Based Cohort Study. *PLoS ONE* **2010**, *5*, e10138. [CrossRef] [PubMed]
73. Awatade, N.T.; Wark, P.A.B.; Chan, A.S.L.; Mamun, S.M.A.A.; Mohd Esa, N.Y.; Matsunaga, K.; Rhee, C.K.; Hansbro, P.M.; Sohal, S.S. The Complex Association between COPD and COVID-19. *J. Clin. Med.* **2023**, *12*, 3791. [CrossRef] [PubMed]
74. Shewade, H.D.; Jeyashree, K.; Mahajan, P.; Shah, A.N.; Kirubakaran, R.; Rao, R.; Kumar, A.M.V. Effect of Glycemic Control and Type of Diabetes Treatment on Unsuccessful TB Treatment Outcomes among People with TB-Diabetes: A Systematic Review. *PLoS ONE* **2017**, *12*, e0186697. [CrossRef]
75. Baker, M.A.; Harries, A.D.; Jeon, C.Y.; Hart, J.E.; Kapur, A.; Lönnroth, K.; Ottmani, S.-E.; Goonesekera, S.D.; Murray, M.B. The Impact of Diabetes on Tuberculosis Treatment Outcomes: A Systematic Review. *BMC Med.* **2011**, *9*, 81. [CrossRef]
76. Faurholt-Jepsen, D.; Range, N.; PrayGod, G.; Jeremiah, K.; Faurholt-Jepsen, M.; Aabye, M.G.; Changalucha, J.; Christensen, D.L.; Grewal, H.M.S.; Martinussen, T.; et al. Diabetes is a Strong Predictor of Mortality during Tuberculosis Treatment: A Prospective Cohort Study among Tuberculosis Patients from Mwanza, Tanzania. *Trop. Med. Int. Health* **2013**, *18*, 822–829. [CrossRef] [PubMed]
77. Moreira, J.; Castro, R.; Lamas, C.; Ribeiro, S.; Grinsztejn, B.; Veloso, V.G. Hyperglycemia during Tuberculosis Treatment Increases Morbidity and Mortality in a Contemporary Cohort of HIV-Infected Patients in Rio de Janeiro, Brazil. *Int. J. Infect. Dis.* **2018**, *69*, 11–19. [CrossRef] [PubMed]
78. Dungan, K.M.; Braithwaite, S.S.; Preiser, J.C. Stress Hyperglycaemia. *Lancet* **2009**, *373*, 1798–1807. [CrossRef]
79. Kubjane, M.; Berkowitz, N.; Goliath, R.; Levitt, N.S.; Wilkinson, R.J.; Oni, T. Tuberculosis, HIV and the Association with Transient Hyperglycaemia in Peri-Urban South Africa. *Clin. Infect. Dis.* **2020**, *71*, 1080–1088. [CrossRef] [PubMed]
80. Ottmani, S.E.; Murray, M.B.; Jeon, C.Y.; Baker, M.A.; Kapur, A.; Lönnroth, K.; Harries, A.D. Consultation Meeting on Tuberculosis and Diabetes Mellitus: Meeting Summary and Recommendations. *Int. J. Tuberc. Lung Dis.* **2010**, *14*, 1513–1517. [PubMed]
81. Albai, O.; Braha, A.; Timar, B.; Sima, A.; Deaconu, L.; Timar, R. Assessment for Clinical Outcome in Patient with SARS-CoV-2 Infection and Diabetes Mellitus. *Diabetes Metab. Syndr. Obes.* **2024**, *17*, 271–282. [CrossRef]
82. Mathur, S.B.; Saxena, R.; Pallavi, P.; Jain, R.; Mishra, D.; Jhamb, U. Effect of Concomitant Tuberculosis Infection on COVID-19 Disease in Children: A Matched, Retrospective Cohort Study. *J. Trop. Pediatr.* **2022**, *68*, fmac056. [CrossRef] [PubMed]
83. Habib, G.; Mahmood, K.; Ahmad, L.; Gul, H.; Hayat, A.; Ur Rehman, M. Clinical Manifestations of Active Tuberculosis Patients Coinfected with Severe Acute Respiratory Syndrome Coronavirus-2. *J. Clin. Tuberc. Other Mycobact. Dis.* **2023**, *31*, 100359. [CrossRef]
84. Daneshvar, P.; Hajikhani, B.; Sameni, F.; Noorisepehr, N.; Zare, F.; Bostanshirin, N.; Yazdani, S.; Goudarzi, M.; Sayyari, S.; Dadashi, M. COVID-19 and Tuberculosis Coinfection: An Overview of Case Reports/Case Series and Meta-Analysis of Prevalence Studies. *Heliyon* **2023**, *9*, e13637. [CrossRef]
85. Gou, J.; Zhang, G. Characteristics of COVID-19 and Tuberculosis Co-Infection: A Cross-Sectional Study in Henan Province. *J. Clin. Med. Img.* **2022**, *6*, 1–8.
86. Mollalign, H.; Chala, D.; Beyene, D. Clinical Features and Treatment Outcome of Coronavirus and Tuberculosis Co-Infected Patients: A Systematic Review of Case Reports. *Infect. Drug Resist.* **2022**, *15*, 4037–4046. [CrossRef] [PubMed]
87. Illg, Z.; Muller, G.; Mueller, M.; Nippert, J.; Allen, B. Analysis of the Absolute Lymphocyte Count in COVID-19 Patients. *Am. J. Emerg. Med.* **2021**, *46*, 16–19. [CrossRef] [PubMed]
88. Tadic, M.; Cuspidi, C.; Grassi, G.; Mancia, G. COVID-19 and Arterial Hypertension: Hypothesis or Evidence? *J. Clin. Hypertens.* **2020**, *22*, 1120–1126. [CrossRef] [PubMed]
89. Lippi, G.; Wong, J.; Henry, B.M. Hypertension in Patients with Coronavirus Disease 2019 (COVID-19): A Pooled Analysis. *Pol. Arch. Intern. Med.* **2020**, *130*, 304–309. [PubMed]
90. Härter, G.; Spinner, C.D.; Roider, J.; Bickel, M.; Krznaric, I.; Grunwald, S.; Schabaz, F.; Gillor, D.; Postel, N.; Mueller, M.C.; et al. A Case Series of 33 Patients with COVID-19 in People Living with Human Immunodeficiency Virus. *Infection* **2020**, *48*, 681–686. [CrossRef] [PubMed]
91. Huang, I.; Pranata, R. Lymphopenia in Severe Coronavirus Disease-2019 (COVID-19): A Systematic Review and Meta-Analysis. *J. Intensive Care* **2020**, *8*, 36. [CrossRef]

92. Anai, M.; Akaike, K.; Iwagoe, H.; Akasaka, T.; Higuchi, T.; Miyazaki, A.; Naito, D.; Tajima, Y.; Takahashi, H.; Komatsu, T.; et al. A Decrease in Hemoglobin Levels Predicts an Increased Risk for Severe Respiratory Failure in COVID-19 Patients with Pneumonia. *Respir. Res.* **2021**, *59*, 187–193. [CrossRef] [PubMed]
93. Li, J.; Zhang, K.; Zhang, Y.; Gu, Z.; Huang, C. Neutrophils in COVID-19: Recent Insights and Advances. *Virol. J.* **2023**, *20*, 169. [CrossRef] [PubMed]
94. Janiuk, K.; Jabłońska, E.; Garley, M. Significance of NETs Formation in COVID-19. *Cells* **2021**, *10*, 151. [CrossRef]
95. Moideen, K.; Kumar, N.P.; Nair, D.; Banurekha, V.V.; Bethunaickan, R.; Babu, S. Heightened Systemic Levels of Neutrophil and Eosinophil Granular Proteins in Pulmonary Tuberculosis and Reversal following Treatment. *Infect. Immun.* **2018**, *86*, e00008-18. [CrossRef]
96. Cormican, L.J.; Schey, S.; Milburn, H.J. G-CSF Enables Completion of Tuberculosis Therapy Associated with Iatrogenic Neutropenia. *Eur. Respir. J.* **2004**, *23*, 649–650. [CrossRef] [PubMed]
97. Noor, F.M.; Islam, M.M. Prevalence and Associated Risk Factors of Mortality Among COVID-19 Patients: A Meta-Analysis. *J. Commun. Health* **2020**, *45*, 1270–1282. [CrossRef] [PubMed]
98. Baj, J.; Karakuła-Juchnowicz, H.; Teresiński, G.; Buszewicz, G.; Ciesielka, M.; Sitarz, R.; Forma, A.; Karakuła, K.; Flieger, W.; Portincasa, P.; et al. Specific and Non-Specific Clinical Manifestations and Symptoms: The Current State of Knowledge. *J. Clin. Med.* **2020**, *9*, 1753. [CrossRef] [PubMed]
99. Zulfic, Z.; Weickert, C.S.; Weickert, T.W.; Liu, D.; Myles, N.; Galletly, C. Neutrophil-Lymphocyte Ratio—A Simple, Accessible Measure of Inflammation, Morbidity and Prognosis in Psychiatric Disorders? *Australas. Psychiatry* **2020**, *28*, 454–458. [CrossRef] [PubMed]
100. Li, Q.; Xie, J.; Huang, Y.; Liu, S.; Guo, F.; Liu, L.; Yang, Y. Leukocyte Kinetics During the Early Stage Acts as a Prognostic Marker in Patients with Septic Shock in Intensive Care Unit. *Medicine* **2021**, *100*, e26288. [CrossRef] [PubMed]
101. Sumardi, U.; Valentino, B.; Prasetya, D.; Debora, J.; Sugianli, A.K. The Diagnostic Value of Kinetics of NLR to Identify Secondary Pulmonary Bacterial Infection Among COVID-19 Patients at Single Tertiary Hospital in Indonesia. *Int. J. Gen. Med.* **2023**, *16*, 3281–3289. [CrossRef]
102. Toori, K.U.; Qureshi, M.A.; Chaudhry, A.; Safdar, M.F. Neutrophil to Lymphocyte Ratio (NLR) in COVID-19: A Cheap Prognostic Marker in a Resource Constraint Setting. *Pak. J. Med. Sci.* **2021**, *37*, 1435–1439. [CrossRef] [PubMed]
103. Han, Y.; Kim, S.J.; Lee, S.H.; Sim, Y.S.; Ryu, Y.J.; Chang, J.H.; Shim, S.S.; Kim, Y.; Lee, J.H. High Blood Neutrophil-Lymphocyte Ratio Associated with Poor Outcomes in Miliary Tuberculosis. *J. Thorac. Dis.* **2018**, *10*, 339. [CrossRef] [PubMed]
104. Shojaan, H.; Kalami, N.; Ghasempour Alamdari, M.; Alorizy, S.M.E.; Ghaedi, A.; Bazrgar, A.; Khanzadeh, M.; Lucke-Wold, B.; Khanzadeh, S. Diagnostic Value of the Neutrophil Lymphocyte Ratio in Discrimination between Tuberculosis and Bacterial Community Acquired Pneumonia: A Meta-Analysis. *J. Clin. Tuberc. Other Mycobact. Dis.* **2023**, *33*, 100395. [CrossRef]
105. Connors, J.M.; Levy, J.H. Thromboinflammation and the Hypercoagulability of COVID-19. *J. Thromb. Haemost.* **2020**, *18*, 1559–1561. [CrossRef]
106. Lippi, G.; Plebani, M.; Henry, B.M. Thrombocytopenia is Associated with Severe Coronavirus Disease 2019 (COVID-19) Infections: A Meta-Analysis. *Clin. Chim. Acta* **2020**, *506*, 145–148. [CrossRef] [PubMed]
107. Qu, R.; Ling, Y.; Zhang, Y.H.; Wei, L.Y.; Chen, X.; Li, X.M.; Liu, X.Y.; Liu, H.M.; Guo, Z.; Ren, H.; et al. Platelet-to-Lymphocyte Ratio is Associated with Prognosis in Patients with Coronavirus Disease-19. *J. Med. Virol.* **2020**, *92*, 1533–1541. [CrossRef]
108. Urbano, M.; Costa, E.; Geraldes, C. Hematological Changes in SARS-CoV-2 Positive Patients. *Hematol. Transfus. Cell Ther.* **2022**, *44*, 218–224. [CrossRef]
109. Simon, P.; Le Borgne, P.; Lefevbre, F.; Cipolat, L.; Remillon, A.; Dib, C.; Hoffmann, M.; Gardeur, I.; Sabah, J.; Kepka, S.; et al. Platelet-to-Lymphocyte Ratio (PLR) Is Not a Predicting Marker of Severity but of Mortality in COVID-19 Patients Admitted to the Emergency Department: A Retrospective Multicenter Study. *J. Clin. Med.* **2022**, *11*, 4903. [CrossRef] [PubMed]
110. Chen, G.; Wu, C.; Luo, Z.; Teng, Y.; Mao, S. Platelet-Lymphocyte Ratios: A Potential Marker for Pulmonary Tuberculosis Diagnosis in COPD Patients. *Int. J. Chron. Obstruct. Pulmon. Dis.* **2016**, *11*, 2737–2740. [CrossRef]
111. Karaaslan, T.; Karaaslan, E. Predictive Value of Systemic Immune-Inflammation Index in Determining Mortality in COVID-19 Patients. *J. Crit. Care Med.* **2022**, *8*, 156–164. [CrossRef] [PubMed]
112. Ştefanescu, S.; Cocoş, R.; Turcu-Stiolica, A.; Mahler, B.; Meca, A.-D.; Giura, A.M.C.; Bogdan, M.; Shelby, E.-S.; Zamfirescu, G.; Pisoschi, C.-G. Evaluation of Prognostic Significance of Hematological Profiles After the Intensive Phase Treatment in Pulmonary Tuberculosis Patients from Romania. *PLoS ONE* **2021**, *16*, e0249301. [CrossRef] [PubMed]
113. Martínez Chamorro, E.; Díez Tascón, A.; Ibáñez Sanza, L.; Ossaba Vélez, S.; Borruel Nacente, S. Radiologic Diagnosis of Patients with COVID-19. *Radiología Engl. Ed.* **2020**, *63*, 56–73. [CrossRef]
114. Bomanji, J.B.; Gupta, N.; Gulati, P.; Das, C.J. Imaging in Tuberculosis. *Cold Spring Harb. Perspect. Med.* **2015**, *5*, a017814. [CrossRef]
115. Tham, S.M.; Lim, W.Y.; Lee, C.K.; Loh, J.; Premkumar, A.; Yan, B.; Kee, A.; Chai, L.; Tambyah, P.A.; Yan, G. Four Patients with COVID-19 and Tuberculosis, Singapore, April-May 2020. *Emerg. Infect. Dis.* **2020**, *26*, 2764–2766. [CrossRef]

116. Mançano, A.D.; Zanetti, G.; Marchiori, E. Concomitant COVID-19 and Pulmonary Tuberculosis: Computed Tomography Aspects. *Radiol. Bras.* **2022**, *55*, 1–5. [CrossRef] [PubMed]
117. Chirico, F.; Teixeira da Silva, J.A.; Tsigaris, P.; Sharun, K. Safety & Effectiveness of COVID-19 Vaccines: A Narrative Review. *Indian J. Med. Res.* **2022**, *155*, 91–104. [CrossRef] [PubMed]

medicina

MDPI

Article

Colliding Challenges Part 2: An Analysis of SARS-CoV-2 Infection in Patients with Extrapulmonary Tuberculosis Versus SARS-CoV-2 Infection Alone

Camil Mihuta [1,2], Adriana Socaci [2,3,*], Patricia Hogea [2,4,5], Emanuela Tudorache [2,4,5], Monica Simina Mihuta [6,7] and Cristian Oancea [2,4,5]

1 Department of Doctoral Studies, "Victor Babes" University of Medicine and Pharmacy, 300041 Timisoara, Romania; camil.mihuta@umft.ro
2 Clinical Hospital for Infectious Diseases and Pneumology "Dr. Victor Babes", 300041 Timisoara, Romania; hogea.patricia@umft.ro (P.H.); emanuela.tudorache@umft.ro (E.T.); oancea@umft.ro (C.O.)
3 Department of Biology and Life Sciences, Faculty of Medicine, "Vasile Goldis" Western University of Arad, 310025 Arad, Romania
4 Center for Research and Innovation in Precision Medicine of Respiratory Diseases (CRIPMRD), "Victor Babes" University of Medicine and Pharmacy, 300041 Timisoara, Romania
5 Department of Pulmonology, "Victor Babes" University of Medicine and Pharmacy, 300041 Timisoara, Romania
6 Department of Pediatrics, Faculty of Medicine, "Victor Babes" University of Medicine and Pharmacy, 300041 Timisoara, Romania; simina.mihuta@umft.ro
7 Center of Molecular Research in Nephrology and Vascular Disease, Faculty of Medicine, "Victor Babes" University of Medicine and Pharmacy, 300041 Timisoara, Romania
* Correspondence: socaci.adriana@uvvg.ro

Abstract: *Background and Objectives*: Coinfection with SARS-CoV-2 and extrapulmonary tuberculosis (extraPTB) presents unique clinical challenges due to dual inflammatory responses and potential differences in patient profiles compared to those with SARS-CoV-2 infection alone. This study uniquely contributes to the underexplored interaction between extraPTB and SARS-CoV-2, focusing on systemic inflammation as a critical determinant of outcomes. *Materials and Methods:* This retrospective, cross-sectional study included 123 patients aged 19–91 years, hospitalized at Victor Babeș Hospital in Timișoara from March 2020 to March 2022. We compared 23 extraPTB and SARS-CoV-2 coinfected patients with 100 age-matched SARS-CoV-2-only patients. Clinical records were examined for demographic, clinical, and laboratory data. *Results*: The coinfected group was younger, with 65% under 40 years, and presented significantly higher IL-6, PCT, and transaminase levels. Coexisting COPD and type 2 diabetes were independent predictors of coinfection. A higher SpO2 at diagnosis was positively associated with coinfection likelihood (OR = 5.37), while CT scores indicated less pulmonary involvement in coinfected patients. Non-fatal outcomes were more frequent in the coinfection group (95.7% sensitivity), and only one coinfected patient had a fatal outcome versus 17 in the SARS-CoV-2-only group. Low SpO2 and elevated IL-6 were significant predictors of mortality, with severe symptoms tripling fatality odds. *Conclusions*: Coinfection with extraPTB and SARS-CoV-2 is associated with younger age, heightened systemic inflammation, and longer hospital stays but does not significantly increase mortality risk compared to SARS-CoV-2 alone. These findings underscore the importance of monitoring systemic inflammatory markers and developing tailored management strategies to improve long-term care outcomes for coinfected patients, especially in resource-limited settings.

Keywords: COVID-19 outcomes; extra-pulmonary tuberculosis; SARS-CoV-2; extra-pulmonary tuberculosis coinfection

1. Introduction

The COVID-19 pandemic has significantly affected tuberculosis control efforts, leading to a sharp decline in case notifications due to disruptions in services. For the first time in over a decade, the mortality rate associated with tuberculosis has risen, as outlined in the World Health Organization Global Tuberculosis Report [1].

SARS-CoV-2, first identified in China in December 2019, was declared a pandemic by the World Health Organization on 11 March 2020 [2]. As of early 2024, over 774 million confirmed cases and more than 7 million deaths have been reported globally [3]. Preventive measures like masking and social distancing not only reduced COVID-19 transmission but also led to a notable decline in other respiratory infections, such as influenza and pneumococcal diseases [4]. The COVID-19 pandemic significantly disrupted tuberculosis (TB) control programs, causing a global decline in case reporting and limited access to care. This hindered the achievement of TB targets set by the United Nations [1]. While most TB cases result from reactivation of latent infections years after the initial infection, the pandemic's immediate impact on TB rates was minimal [5].

It remains uncertain whether COVID-19 triggers the reactivation of latent TB or whether TB infection increases susceptibility to SARS-CoV-2. Some researchers hypothesize that SARS-CoV-2 may provoke an exaggerated inflammatory response, potentially activating latent or hidden infections. Additionally, immunosuppressive treatments for COVID-19 could unmask TB, as these medications are known to reactivate mycobacterial infections [6].

Roughly one-quarter of the global population is estimated to harbor a latent Mycobacterium tuberculosis infection, with 5–15% eventually progressing to active TB during their lifetime. The risk of reactivation varies depending on geographic and individual factors [7].

The ongoing SARS-CoV-2 pandemic continues to cause widespread illness and death, with COVID-19 primarily affecting the respiratory system but also potentially damaging other organs. Meanwhile, TB remains a prevalent disease, primarily affecting the lungs but occasionally manifesting in extrapulmonary forms, involving organs such as the meninges, lymph nodes, gastrointestinal tract, pleura, genitourinary system, and bones [8].

After the Mycobacterium tuberculosis (MTB) enters the body, the immune system launches a combination of innate and adaptive responses, which may clear the bacteria or allow the infection to persist, with or without T cell involvement. For MTB to establish an infection, it must first bypass the airway's protective barriers and reach the lungs, where it infects alveolar macrophages, neutrophils, and dendritic cells. These infected cells then activate and recruit innate and adaptive lymphocytes to assist in containing the bacteria [9]. Natural killer (NK) cells play a crucial role by recognizing and destroying MTB-infected macrophages, enhancing IFN-γ production, and secreting cytokines that attract CD8+ T cells and NK T cells. This process facilitates the formation of granulomas, which consist of macrophages, neutrophils, and Langhans giant cells (formed from fused macrophages) and are surrounded by lymphocytes and a fibrotic layer [10].

Approximately 25% of pulmonary TB cases progress to extrapulmonary TB, which can affect any organ. Diagnosis often requires invasive procedures and imaging studies due to the wide range of symptoms, leading to delays from symptom onset to microbiological confirmation [11]. There is limited research on the co-occurrence of extrapulmonary TB and COVID-19, highlighting a significant gap in our understanding [12]. Extrapulmonary TB (extraPTB) does not typically present with the common symptoms observed in pulmonary TB (PTB) patients, such as cough, weight loss, hemoptysis, and night sweats. Instead, symptoms vary based on the affected organ system and may include joint pain, abdominal discomfort, headaches, diarrhea, or lymphadenopathy. ExtraPTB frequently affects the lymphatic system, particularly in individuals with compromised immune systems. Moreover, patients with extraPTB may have normal chest radiographs, which can further complicate diagnosis [13]. Recent research has explored the relationship between SARS-CoV-2 and host protein interactions, revealing that MTB shares many of the same host protein interaction partners as SARS-CoV-2. This finding is particularly relevant given that both diseases primarily affect the lungs, increasing the risk of compounded respiratory complications [14].

After having previously analyzed the impact of SARS-CoV-2 infection on patients with pulmonary TB infection [15], this study comes as a continuation of our team's work to assess the consequences of SARS-CoV-2 infection in patients with extraTB. This work uniquely contributes to the literature by focusing on the clinical dynamics of SARS-CoV-2 coinfection in patients with extraPTB, which remains under-researched compared to the more commonly studied pulmonary TB.

2. Materials and Methods

The present retrospective, cross-sectional, randomized study involved 123 adult patients aged 19 to 91 years, hospitalized at the Victor Babeș Hospital of Infectious Diseases and Pneumoftiziology from Timișoara between March 2020 and March 2022, during the COVID-19 pandemic.

2.1. Study Design and Objectives

This study aimed to compare two groups of patients: one group with extrapulmonary tuberculosis (extraPTB) and SARS-CoV-2 coinfection (n = 23) and a control group of age-matched patients diagnosed only with moderate or severe SARS-CoV-2 infection (n = 100). The primary objective was to evaluate the impact of SARS-CoV-2 on patients already burdened by tuberculosis.

2.2. Inclusion Criteria

Patients in the following situations were included in this study:

- Diagnosed with extrapulmonary TB within one month of SARS-CoV-2 infection confirmation using solid or liquid cultures (Gene-Xpert) at the TB ambulatory service in Timișoara [16].
- Diagnosed with moderate or severe forms of SARS-CoV-2 at hospital admission, confirmed by RT-PCR from nasopharyngeal swabs in an accredited laboratory. Moderate infection was characterized by signs of lower respiratory disease or imaging findings with $SpO2 \geq 94\%$ on room air. Severe infection was defined by $SpO2 < 94\%$ on room air, a respiratory rate > 30 breaths/min, or >50% lung infiltrates [17].
- Normal renal function (normal GFR, creatinine, and urea levels) [18].
- Prior BCG vaccination [19].

2.3. Exclusion Criteria

Patients presenting the following were excluded:

- Overweight (BMI = 25–30 kg/m^2) or obesity (BMI $\geq$ 30 kg/m^2) [20].
- Pre-existing severe or uncontrolled arterial hypertension [21].
- Pre-existing advanced chronic heart failure [22].
- Any type of neoplasia [23,24].
- Chronic pulmonary, hepatic, renal, or digestive conditions and HIV infection.

Exclusions for obesity and chronic conditions were applied to reduce confounding effects on inflammatory markers, which are independently elevated in these conditions, as well as on COVID-19 outcomes. While these exclusions might limit the generalizability to populations with metabolic or chronic comorbidities, they allow for a clearer analysis of coinfection dynamics between SARS-CoV-2 and extraPTB [25].

Ethical Considerations: This study received approval from the Ethics Council for Scientific Research at the Victor Babeș University of Medicine and Pharmacy Timisoara, adhering to the principles of the Helsinki Declaration (04/19 January 2021). Informed consent was obtained from all participants after explaining the nature of the data analysis.

Data Collection: Data were collected from personal medical files, including anamnesis, clinical parameters, and biological and imaging investigations.

Medical History: BCG vaccination status, comorbidities such as COPD and type 2 diabetes, and smoking status (never smoked, smoker) were documented. Employment status was categorized into unemployed, employed, and retired. No subject included in this study had ever been diagnosed and treated for tuberculosis.

Measurements: BMI was calculated using the formula weight (kg)/height^2 (m^2) [26]. SpO2 (%) values at the time of SARS-CoV-2 diagnosis and the lowest SpO2 (%) values during hospitalization were recorded using calibrated pulse oximeters [27]. Peripheral systolic and diastolic blood pressures (SBP, DBP, mmHg) were noted at diagnosis.

Symptoms: The SARS-CoV-2 symptoms recorded included fever, coughing, dyspnea, fatigue, abdominal pain, chest pain, myalgia, vomiting/nausea, diarrhea, headache, and olfactory/taste disorders. The symptoms were classified as more severe if accompanied by tachypnea (respiratory rate $\geq$ 30 breaths/min) [28].

Blood Markers: C-reactive protein (CRP, mg/L); procalcitonin (PCT); aspartate aminotransferase (AST, U/L); alanine aminotransferase (ALT, U/L); lactate dehydrogenase (LDH, U/L); interleukin-6 (IL-6, pg/mL); D-dimer levels (mg/L); and neutrophil, lymphocyte, and platelet counts (/µL) were recorded. The ratios calculated included the neutrophil-to-lymphocyte ratio (NLR), platelet-to-lymphocyte ratio (PLR), and systemic immuno-inflammatory index (SII) [29–31].

Imaging: An experienced radiologist reviewed all CT scans at SARS-CoV-2 infection confirmation. CT scans were assessed for lesions such as ground-glass opacifications, consolidations, crazy paving pattern, linear opacities, air bronchogram sign, tree in bud, and cavitary lesions [32,33]. The extent of lung involvement was scored from 0 to 5 for each lobe, with a total possible score ranging from 0 to 25, providing a comprehensive view of lung disease impact [3,34,35].

Outcome: The number of hospitalization days and patient outcomes (resolved-PCR converted or deceased) were recorded for each case.

2.4. Data Analysis

Data collection was carried out using Microsoft Excel, while statistical analyses were performed with MedCalc Statistical Software version 20.111 (MedCalc Software Ltd., Ostend, Belgium). The primary aim of the analysis was to examine the impact of SARS-CoV-2 infection on patients with and without PTB coinfection. Clinical, imaging, and biological parameters were compared between the groups. Statistical significance was defined as p-values below 0.05. To assess the normality of the data distribution, the Shapiro–Wilk test was utilized. Based on the results of this test, appropriate statistical methods were chosen: medians and the Mann–Whitney test were used for non-normally distributed variables. AUC–ROC analysis was employed to evaluate the significance of various parameters in distinguishing between the presence and absence of coinfection, with cut-off values determined to highlight the importance of specific parameters in these medical conditions. Logistic regression models were used to identify independent predictors of coinfection and fatal outcomes. The associations between binary datasets were evaluated using Fisher's exact test. Variance inflation factors (VIFs) were calculated for all predictors in the logistic regression model. All VIFs were below 5, indicating no significant multicollinearity. Missing data were minimal (<5%) and were handled using complete case analysis, given the limited sample size. This approach ensures the integrity of the dataset while avoiding bias introduced by imputation methods.

3. Results

This study included 123 patients, divided into two study groups comprising 23 patients with extraPTB and SARS-CoV-2 coinfection and 100 patients with SARS-CoV-2 infection alone.

The patients were distributed relatively homogenous regarding sex in both groups. Regarding age, the younger subjects were in the majority in the coinfection group, 65% under 40 years old, while in the SARS-CoV-2 group, the subjects aged 40 years and older comprised 89% of cases (Table 1). The mean age in the coinfected group was 40.1 years (SD = 18.6), while the median age in the SARS-CoV-2 group was 56.5 years.

Table 1. The number of subjects by sex and age.

		Coinfection Group n = 23	SARS-CoV-2 Group n = 100
Sex	F	10 (43.5%)	48
	M	13 (56.5%)	52
Age	19–40 y	15 (65.2%)	8
	41–65 y	6 (26.1%)	53
	>66 y	2 (8.7%)	36

The subjects in the extraPTB group were diagnosed with different types of TB infections: a total of thirteen subjects (56%) presented TB pleural effusion, five subjects (22%) presented TB lymphadenitis, two subjects (9%) presented TB meningitis, two subjects (9%) presented bone TB, and one subject (4%) presented gastrointestinal TB (see Figure 1). Only four of all cases of extraTB had previously undergone immunosuppressive therapies: one with pleural effusion and two with lymphadenitis.

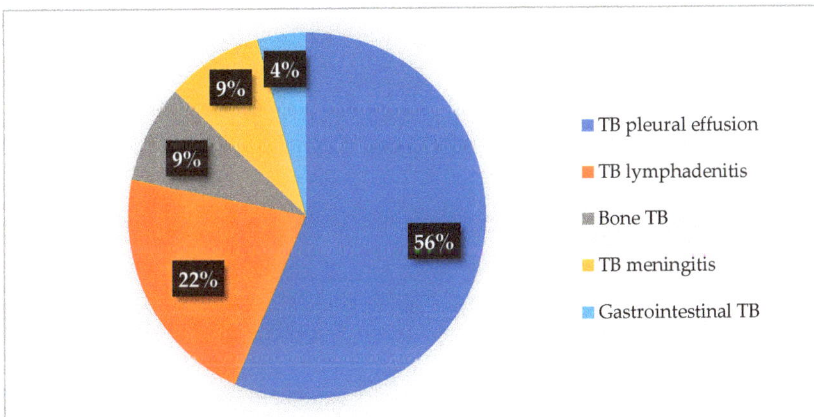

Figure 1. Types of extraPTB included in this study.

When analyzing sex-based differences regarding the proportion of extraPTB cases, in women, TB pleural effusion and TB lymphadenitis were the most predominant types of TB infections, with equal proportions of 40% (Figure 2), while in men, 69% of cases were of TB pleural effusion, followed by 15% TB meningitis (Figure 3).

A comparison between the extraPTB subtypes was performed in order to analyze the differences and understand subgroup dynamics: pleural effusion TB (thirteen subjects) vs. TB lymphadenitis (five subjects).

Patients with pleural TB were significantly older than those with lymphadenitis TB ($p = 0.03$, Mann–Whitney U test). There was no statistically significant difference in the proportion of smokers between patients with pleural TB and those with lymphadenitis TB ($p = 0.72$, Fisher's exact test).

Pleural TB patients had significantly lower SpO2 values at admission compared to lymphadenitis TB patients ($p = 0.03$). This suggests greater respiratory compromise in pleural TB cases. The median CRP levels ($p = 0.006$) and median IL-6 levels ($p = 0.04$) were significantly higher in patients with pleural TB compared to lymphadenitis TB. There was a statistically significant difference in the length of hospitalization between the two groups, with pleural TB patients having longer stays ($p = 0.002$). This may reflect the higher severity or more complex management of pleural TB cases. The Mann–Whitney U test was used for these continuous variables.

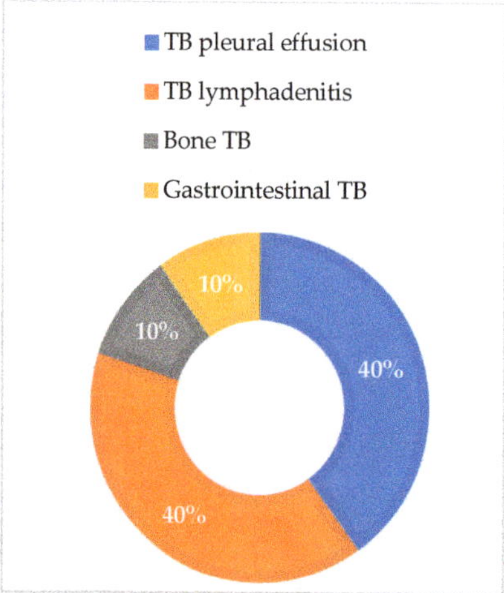

Figure 2. ExtraPTB cases in females.

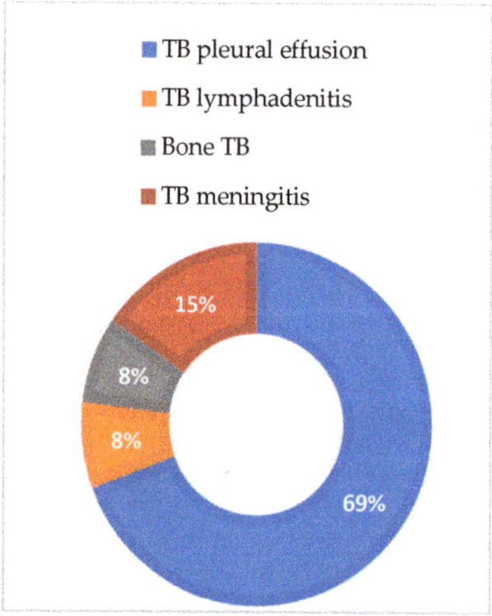

Figure 3. ExtraPTB cases in males.

No significant difference was observed in outcomes (resolved or deceased) between pleural TB and lymphadenitis TB patients ($p = 0.65$, Fisher's exact test). This indicates that the clinical outcome was not associated with the type of extrapulmonary TB in this dataset.

Regarding social status, 60.9% of the subjects in the coinfection group vs. 58% of the SARS-CoV-2 group were employed, and, respectively, 17.4% vs. 10% were unemployed, and 21.7% vs. 32% were retired (Figure 4).

Regarding smoking, the coinfection group consisted of similar proportions: a total of 47.8% of subjects having declared they were regular smokers and 52.2% having declared that they never had been smokers. In the SARS-CoV-2 group, approximately one-third of the subjects (34%) declared that they were smokers (Figure 5).

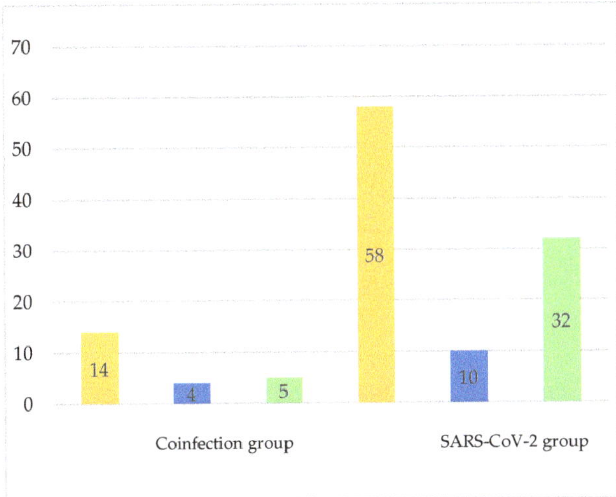

Figure 4. Distribution of cases according to the social status (yellow—no. of employed subjects; blue—no. of unemployed subjects; green—no. of retired subjects).

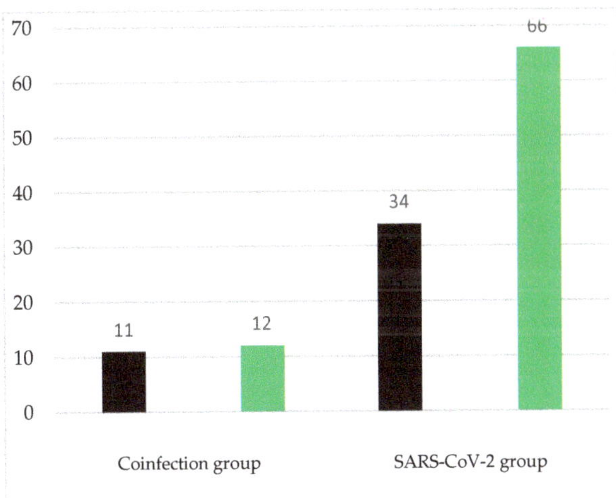

Figure 5. Distribution of cases according to smoking (black—no. of smokers; green—no. of non-smokers).

The comparison revealed significant differences between the two groups in most of the analyzed parameters. The SARS-CoV-2 group revealed significantly lower SpO2 both at diagnosis and with regard to the lowest value registered. Moreover, the chest CT involvement score revealed a significantly higher median score for the subjects pertaining to the SARS-CoV-2 infection group. In contrast, the coinfection group displayed higher IL-6, transaminase, and D-dimer median values and also higher NLR, PLR, and SII median values. No differences were detected with regard to blood pressure levels (Table 2).

A multiple parameter logistic regression was employed with the dependent variable being the presence/absence of extraPTB–SARS-CoV-2 coinfection and the independent variables being age, sex, BMI, employment status, smoking status, associating COPD, and type 2 DM. Age, employment status, associating COPD, and type 2 DM emerged as significant predictors of extraPTB–SARS-CoV-2 coinfection. As age increased, the likelihood of having extraPTB and COVID-19 coinfection slightly decreased (13%). The median age difference in the two study groups should be taken into consideration as per this result. Being employed was associated with 75% higher odds of having the coinfection. Individuals with COPD had 6.5 times higher odds of having the coinfection compared to those without COPD. Subjects with type 2 DM had over four times higher odds of having the coinfection compared to those without diabetes. We must mention, however, the large distribution of the data in the cases of coinfected subjects who associated COPD (95% CI 1.12–37.71) or type 2 DM (95% CI 1.1–39.66). We attribute these results to the small sample sizes and suggest this should be considered as a limit in interpreting the ORs. Sex, BMI, and the status of smoking were not retained by the model (see Table 3). In the coinfection group, four subjects (17.4%) associated COPD, and three (13%) associated type 2 DM. Only one subject associated both conditions. In the SARS-CoV-2 group, an equal proportion of 19% presented COPD and diabetes.

Table 2. Mann–Whitney comparative tests of multiple biological parameters between coinfected and SARS-CoV-2 infected subjects.

Parameter	Coinfection Group Median Value	SARS-CoV-2 Group Median Value	p
Age	36	56.5	**<0.001**
BMI	24.45	24.74	0.83
SpO2 at diagnosis	96	94	**0.001**
Lowest SpO2	92	89.5	**0.01**
Peripheral SBP at diagnosis	129	133	0.46
Peripheral DBP at diagnosis	85	87	0.52
CRP	66.1	55.5	0.36
LDH	203	243.5	0.3
IL-6	8.8	1.2	**0.0008**
AST	38	29	**0.005**
ALT	42	30	**0.003**
D-dimer	1.65	0.91	**0.01**
Neutrophils *	6194.8 (SD = 1837.6)	5878.3 (SD = 1162.7)	0.29
Lymphocytes	1460	3010	**<0.001**
Thrombocytes	351,000	252,000	**<0.001**
NLR	3.73	1.83	**<0.0001**
PLR	235.54	77.95	**<0.0001**
SII	1,255,888.88	459,784	**<0.0001**
Chest CT involvement score	6	12	**0.0001**

* The T-student test was employed for neutrophil count. The bolded data in this table represent statistically significant results.

The AUC–ROC analysis showed that younger age and being employed are significant discriminators. An SpO2 > 95% detects coinfection with a specificity of 77%. A positive PCT and an IL-6 > 3.6 pg/mL are both significant (Figure 6). While PCT has a high specificity of 84% and a relatively low sensibility (47.83%) in discriminating between coinfection and SARS-CoV-2 infection alone, IL-6 has an Se of 78.26% and an Sp of 69%. The transaminase levels also have significant value as discriminators: ALT having an Sp of 97% while AST having an Sp of 87% (Figure 7). High D-dimer levels also displayed significance: a level > 1.1 mg/L displaying an Se of 73.91% but a lower Sp (Figure 8). As per the blood cell count and the ratios calculated as inflammation markers, all are significant detectors of coinfection. High neutrophil and platelet counts and a lower lymphocyte count are associated with coinfection (Figure 9). High NLR, PLR, and SII are also associated with coinfection (Figure 10). As per the CT involvement score, as the extraTB group has displayed a lower pulmonary involvement, a CT score < 6 was associated with an Sp of 98% in detecting coinfection (Figure 11).

Table 3. Anamnestic data as predictors of extraPTB–SARS-CoV-2 coinfection (logistic regression).

Parameter	Odds Ratio	95% CI	Coefficient	Std. Err.	*p*
Age	0.87	0.82–0.93	−0.13	0.03	**0.0001**
Unemployment	0.25	0.08–0.75	−1.36	0.55	**0.01**
COPD	6.5	1.12–37.71	1.87	0.89	**0.03**
Type 2 DM	4.3	1.1–39.66	1.67	0.76	**0.001**

The bolded data in this table represent statistically significant results.

A logistic regression was also employed to include paraclinical parameters as independent variables. The presence/absence of extraPTB–SARS-CoV-2 coinfection was still considered the dependent variable, while the independent variables were represented by the SpO2 at diagnosis, lowest SpO2, SBP, DBP, CRP, LDH, PCT, IL-6, AST, ALT, D-dimer levels, neutrophil count, lymphocyte count, thrombocyte count, NLR, PLR, and SII. The SpO2 at diagnosis, the PCT, and the CT involvement score were deemed significant independent predictors for the presence of coinfection. Due to the fact that the coinfection group presented significantly higher SpO2 levels at diagnosis, the model revealed that a higher SpO2 at diagnosis is positively associated with the likelihood of having the coinfection (OR = 5.37). Moreover, also attesting to less pulmonary involvement in patients with coinfection, with each unit increase in the CT involvement score, the odds of having the coinfection decreased by 51%. This suggests that higher CT involvement scores are associated with higher odds of having the COVID-19 infection alone. A positive PCT is associated with an increased likelihood of having the coinfection, with patients presenting a positive PCT having a 6.5 times higher likelihood of being coinfected. The rest of the independent variables were not retained by the model (Table 4).

Table 4. Paraclinical parameters as predictors of extraPTB–SARS-CoV-2 coinfection (logistic regression).

Parameter	Odds Ratio	95% CI	Coefficient	Std. Err.	*p*
SpO2 at diagnosis	5.37	1.69–17.02	1.68	0.58	**0.004**
PCT	6.5	2.69–10.14	1.1	0.1	**0.01**
CT involvement score	0.49	0.3–0.8	−0.69	0.24	**0.004**

The bolded data in this table represent statistically significant results.

Further on, AUC–ROC analyses were employed in order to determine the significance of multiple parameters in discriminating between the presence and absence of extraPTB coinfection (Table 5).

Figure 6 demonstrates the diagnostic utility of inflammatory markers (PCT and IL-6) in distinguishing coinfection, with both markers showing moderate to high sensitivity.

Increased ALT and AST levels highlight the role of liver dysfunction in patients with coinfection, with both transaminases displaying high specificities (Figure 7).

Elevated D-dimer levels reflect enhanced coagulation activity in coinfected patients, with these levels displaying a moderately-high sensitivity (Figure 8).

Neutrophil and platelet counts are higher in coinfection, indicating enhanced systemic inflammation, while lymphocyte counts are reduced (Figure 9).

Table 5. AUC–ROC analysis for the clinical and anamnestic parameters as discriminators between the presence and the absence of PTB coinfection in SARS-CoV-2 patients (n = 132).

Parameter	AUC	*p*	Associated Criterion	Se%	95% CI	Sp%	95% CI	PPV %	NPV %
Age	**0.81**	**<0.0001**	**<38**	65.22	42.7–83.6	97	91.5–99.4	83.3	92.4
Sex	0.52	0.69	≤1 [a]	56.52	34.5–76.8	48	37.9–58.2	20	82.8
BMI	0.51	0.85	>18	86.96	66.4–97.2	1	0.03–5.4	16.8	25
Employment status	**0.74**	**0.0003**	≤1 [b]	60.87	38.5–80.3	90	82.4–95.1	58.3	90.9
Smoking status	0.57	0.23	≥1 [c]	47.83	26.8–69.4	66	55.8–75.2	24.4	84.6
Associated COPD	0.5	0.85	0 [d]	82.61	61.2–95.0	19	11.8–28.1	19	82.6
Associated type 2 DM	0.53	0.46	0 [e]	86.96	66.4–97.2	19	11.8–28.1	19.8	86.4
SpO2 at diagnosis	**0.71**	**0.0006**	**>95**	60.87	38.5–80.3	77	67.5–84.8	37.8	89.5
Lowest SpO2	0.66	0.02	>92	47.83	26.8–69.4	80	70.8–87.3	35.5	87
Symptoms severity	0.53	0.39	≤0 [f]	86.96	66.4–97.2	20	12.7–29.2	20	87
CRP	0.56	0.36	>80	43.48	23.2–65.5	74	64.3–82.3	27.8	85.1
PCT	**0.66**	**0.004**	**>0** [g]	47.83	26.8–69.4	84	75.3–90.6	40.7	87.5
LDH	0.56	0.23	≤321	95.65	78.1–99.9	36	26.6–46.2	25.6	97.3
IL-6	**0.72**	**<0.0001**	**>3.6**	78.26	56.3–92.5	69	59.0–77.9	36.7	93.2
AST	**0.69**	**0.007**	**>41**	52.17	30.6–73.2	87	78.8–92.9	48	88.8
ALT	**0.68**	**0.01**	**>44**	47.83	26.8–69.4	97	91.5–99.4	78.6	89
D-dimer	**0.66**	**0.01**	**>1.1**	73.91	51.6–89.8	58	47.7–67.8	28.8	90.6
Neutrophil count	**0.53**	**0.71**	**>7710**	30.43	13.2–52.9	96	90.1–98.9	63.6	85.7
Lymphocyte count	**0.82**	**<0.0001**	**≤2240**	91.3	72.0–98.9	75	65.3–83.1	45.7	97.4
Platelet count	**0.77**	**<0.0001**	**>285,000**	82.61	61.2–95.0	66	55.8–75.2	35.8	94.3
NLR	**0.78**	**<0.0001**	**>2.6**	86.96	66.4–97.2	73	63.2–81.4	42.6	96.1
PLR	**0.86**	**<0.0001**	**>142.63**	91.3	72.0–98.9	80	70.8–87.3	50	94.3
SII	**0.83**	**<0.0001**	**>946,666.66**	86.96	66.4–97.2	79	69.7–86.5	48.8	96.3
Chest CT involvement score	**0.76**	**0.0007**	**≤6**	60.87	38.5–80.3	98	93.0–99.8	87.5	91.6

The bolded data in this table represent statistically significant results. [a] (1 = M, 2 = F); [b] (1 = employed, 2 = retired, 3 = unemployed); [c] (0 = non-smoker, 1 = smoker); [d] (0 = no COPD, 1 = associated COPD); [e] (0 = no type 2 DM, 1 = associated type 2 DM); [f] (0 = non-severe symptoms, 1 = severe symptoms); [g] (0 = normal PCT, 1 = elevated PCT).

Higher NLR, PLR, and SII values demonstrate significant inflammatory and immune responses in coinfected patients (Figure 10).

Lower CT involvement scores in coinfection suggest reduced pulmonary involvement compared to SARS-CoV-2 infection alone (Figure 11).

Fisher's exact test determined that, out of the binary data analyzed, regarding the connection between coinfection and the following parameters, the presence of COPD, type 2 DM, and a positive PCT have been significantly associated with the increased likelihood of coinfection (Table 6).

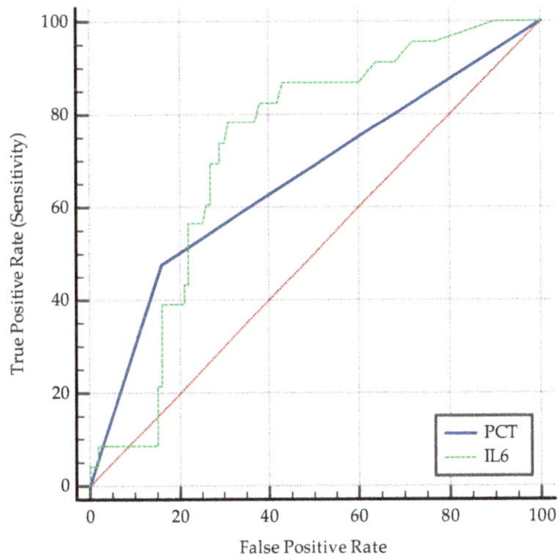

Figure 6. ROC curve for the significant inflammatory markers (PCT and IL6).

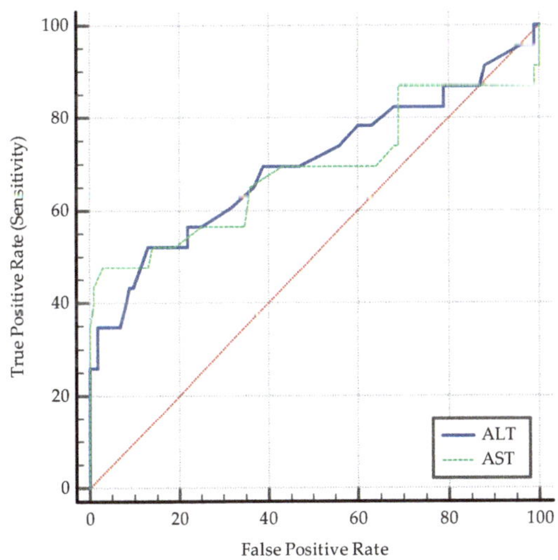

Figure 7. ROC curve for transaminase levels.

Table 6. Fisher's exact test: association between several parameters and the likelihood of coinfection.

	Parameter	Fisher's Exact Test p
Presence of extraPTB	Smoking	0.23
	COPD	**0.02**
	Type 2 DM	**0.01**
	Severe symptoms	0.56
	PCT	**0.001**
	Outcome	0.19

The bolded data in this table represent statistically significant results.

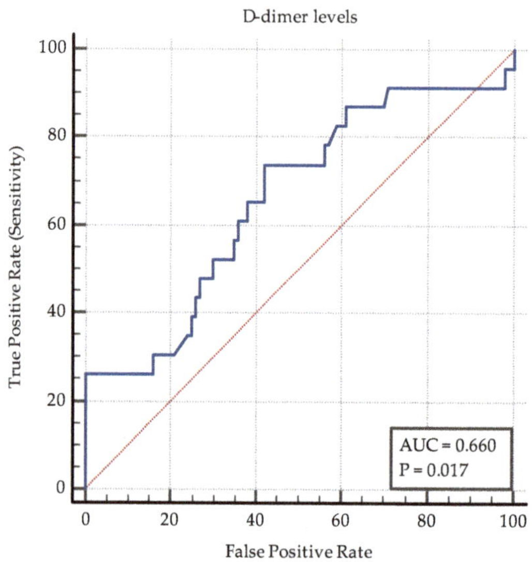

Figure 8. ROC curve for D-dimer levels.

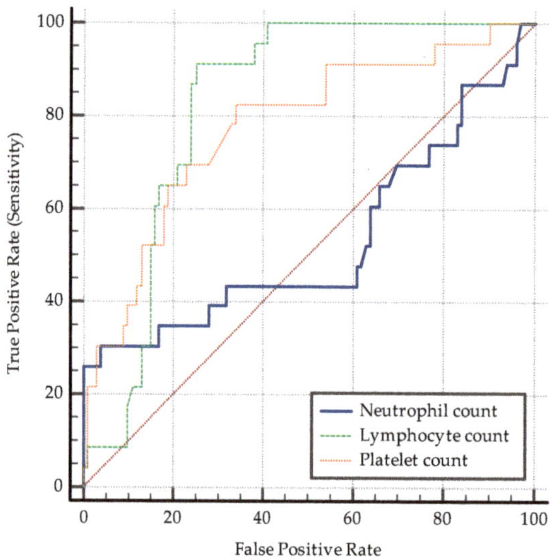

Figure 9. ROC curve for blood cell count.

The median hospitalization period was 30 days (limits: 15–60 days) for the subjects with coinfection and only 8 days (limits: 4–17 days) for the subjects with SARS-CoV-2 infection alone. A hospitalization period larger than 17 days can predict the coinfection status with a sensibility of 95.65% (95% CI = 78.1–99.9) and a specificity of 100% (95% CI = 96.4–100), AUC = 0.99, $p < 0.0001$, in our cohort (Figure 12).

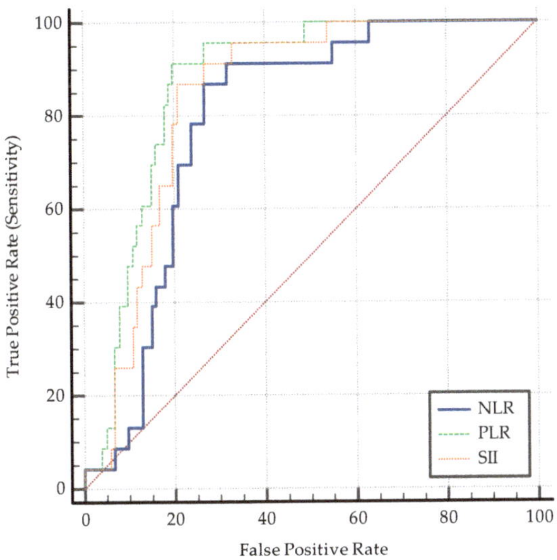

Figure 10. ROC curve for NLR, PLR, and SII.

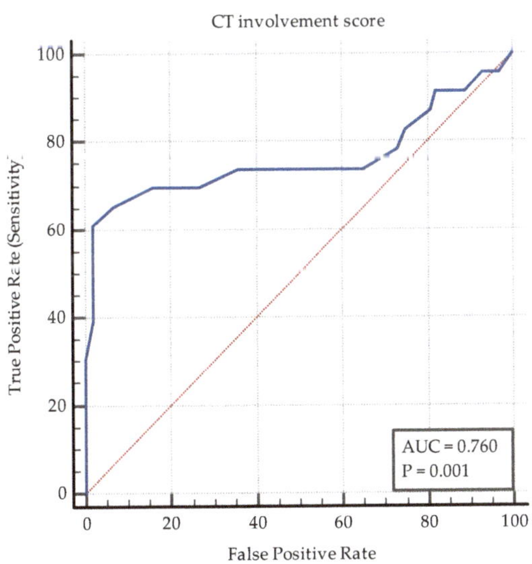

Figure 11. ROC curve for the CT involvement score.

While 17 subjects in the SARS-CoV-2 group had fatal outcomes, only one subject in the coinfection group had the same outcome. The AUC–ROC analysis showed that a non-fatal outcome is a reliable predictor of coinfection, with a very high sensitivity (Se = 95.65%, 95% CI = 78.1–99.9) but a low specificity (Sp = 17%, 95% CI = 78.1–99.9), AUC = 0.56, $p = 0.02$ (Figure 13).

A logistic regression was employed with the status of either coinfection or SARS-CoV-2 infection alone, sex, smoking status, COPD and type 2 DM association, and the gravity of symptoms as independent variables. The outcome represented the dependent variable. The results showed the severity of symptoms increases the probability of a fatal outcome by three-fold (OR = 3.21, $p < 0.0001$). The status of coinfection is not a predictor of fatality. The rest of the parameters were not retained by the model.

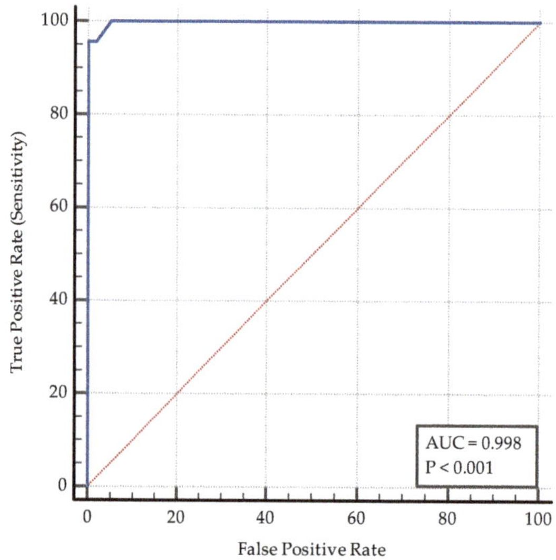

Figure 12. ROC curve for the hospitalization period.

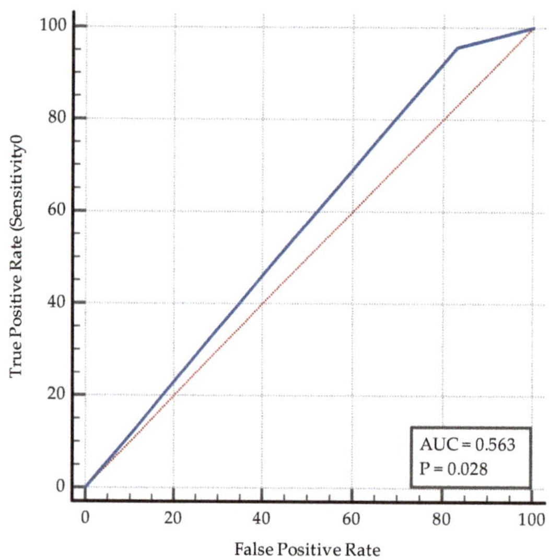

Figure 13. ROC curve for outcomes.

Another logistic regression was employed to evaluate the effects of several non-binary markers (independent variables: age, BMI, SpO2 at diagnosis and the lowest SpO2, CT involvement score, CRP, PCT, IL-6, LDH, ALT, AST, Ne count, Ly count, Tr count, D-dimer levels, NLR, PLR, SII, and hospitalization period) on outcome (dependent variable). The result showed that the lowest value of SpO2 registered and IL-6 are significant independent predictors of a fatal outcome. The rest of the variables were not retained by the model (Table 7).

Table 7. Logistic regression—predictors of fatal outcomes.

Parameter	Odds Ratio	95% CI	Coefficient	Std. Err.	Constant	*p*
Lowest SpO2	0.61	0.46–0.82	−0.48	0.14	38.3	**0.001**
IL-6	1.07	1.01–1.14	0.03	6.35	38.3	**0.01**

The bolded data in this table represent statistically significant results.

4. Discussions

This study builds on our prior research regarding the effects of SARS-CoV-2 on patients with pulmonary TB [15] by shifting the focus to those with extrapulmonary tuberculosis (extraPTB). It aims to examine how COVID-19 affects extraPTB patients compared to those infected only with SARS-CoV-2, contributing to the broader understanding of the interaction between TB and COVID-19, with an emphasis on these less-explored forms of TB. To our knowledge, a study focusing on precisely that has not been published before. Two groups were compared: one with extraPTB and SARS-CoV-2 coinfection and a group with only SARS-CoV-2 infection. The discussion will focus on the key findings and their implications in understanding the interaction between these two infectious diseases.

4.1. Key Findings

The results demonstrated significant differences between the coinfected group and the group with SARS CoV-2 infection alone, both in terms of clinical and laboratory parameters. Coinfected patients exhibited higher levels of inflammatory markers, such as IL-6, CRP, and systemic inflammatory indices (NLR, PLR, SII), as well as D-dimer and transaminase levels. The coinfected patients also displayed a significantly lower lymphocyte count. A positive PCT was associated with a 6.5 times increase in the likelihood of having coinfection. Although these results suggest an amplified inflammatory response in coinfected patients, the symptomatology and outcomes were contrary. Interestingly, the SARS-CoV-2 group presented with more severe hypoxemia (lower SpO2 levels at diagnosis and during hospitalization) and more extensive lung involvement, as evidenced by higher chest CT scores. An explanation could be that patients with extraPTB typically have less pulmonary involvement than those with pulmonary TB. This finding is consistent with studies that have identified less severe lung disease in patients with extrapulmonary forms of TB, particularly when coinfected with other respiratory pathogens [36].

These findings indicate that, while patients with extraPTB may present with less severe respiratory symptoms, they may still be at risk of severe systemic inflammation, which requires careful monitoring. Elevated PCT and IL-6 levels, in particular, have been previously identified as markers of severe COVID-19 outcomes, and their role in the coinfected population needs further exploration [37]. It has been shown that some of the markers of COVID-19 deterioration and the development of acute respiratory distress syndrome include elevated LDH, CRP, IL-6, D-dimer levels, lymphocytes, platelets, renal function, and also high-sensitive troponin. Moreover, critically ill patients often exhibit significant lymphopenia and neutrophilia, leading to an increased NLR [37].

One explanation for the less severe respiratory lesions in patients with coinfection could be the activity of anti-inflammatory regulatory T cells (Treg) in extraPTB. Treg cells tend to increase, especially in cases of active TB. These cells likely expand in response to heightened inflammation rather than causing the disease. Treg cells, a subset of CD4+ T lymphocytes (1–5% of circulating CD4+ cells), prevent autoimmunity and maintain immune balance [38–40]. Treg cells may help limit excessive immune responses, which could prevent tissue damage, but this suppression also allows for the pathogen to persist. Studies show that patients with latent TB infection may have higher Treg levels, which could protect against progression to active TB, while those with active TB show an increase in Treg cells over time [41]. Depleting Treg cells enhances immune responses to pathogens like Helicobacter pylori, HIV, hepatitis C virus, MTB [42], and also SARS-CoV-2 [43].

For instance, Treg depletion experiments in mouse models of TB have demonstrated increased production of pro-inflammatory cytokines, such as TNF-α and IFN-γ, resulting in heightened bacterial clearance but at the cost of increased tissue pathology [41]. Similarly, in SARS-CoV-2, lower Treg activity has been linked to excessive cytokine storms, contributing to respiratory failure in severe COVID-19 cases. This reduction may affect patients by weakening inflammatory control, disrupting the Treg/Th17 balance, and increasing the risk of respiratory failure [43,44]. Interestingly, the Treg/Th17 balance is a key factor in immune regulation during coinfections. Th17 cells promote inflammation, which is crucial for pathogen clearance but can also lead to tissue damage if unchecked. An imbalance skewed toward Th17 dominance, as observed in some severe COVID-19 cases, has been associated with worse outcomes [44,45]. In contrast, Treg predominance, as is often observed in extraPTB, might suppress this excessive inflammatory response, potentially explaining the less severe respiratory lesions in coinfected patients. However, it remains unclear whether reduced Tregs lead to poor outcomes or if higher Treg levels are beneficial. Many researchers agree that maintaining a balanced Treg count is crucial in mitigating the adverse effects of severe SARS-CoV-2 infection [44–46].

Further, the role of Tregs in mediating systemic versus localized immune responses is increasingly recognized. In the case of extraPTB, Tregs may preferentially act on systemic inflammation, sparing the lungs from excessive immune-mediated damage while controlling the extrapulmonary spread of Mycobacterium tuberculosis. This systemic modulation may offer partial protection against the widespread pulmonary inflammation characteristic of severe SARS-CoV-2 infection [41,44,45].

4.2. Demographic Factors, Age, and Comorbidities

The key factors traditionally linked to the development of extraPTB are being at either end of the age spectrum, female sex, migration from countries with high TB prevalence, and having a compromised immune system [47]. Global epidemiology studies place extraPTB at 20–30% of cases of TB infection, depending on geographical regions [48].

The demographic characteristics of our study population showed a slight predominance of males in both groups, which is consistent with the global epidemiology of TB and COVID-19 but not of extraPTB [49,50]. Still, epidemiological reports regarding sex-based differences in extraPTB are inconclusive. A large study in Mali, which included 1012 subjects with confirmed extraPTB, reported a male-to-female ratio of 1.59:1 [51]. This study also found differences regarding the affected organ: males are more likely to present pleural TB (OR = 1.51), and women are more likely to present lymph node (OR = 0.57) and abdominal TB (OR = 0.59) [51]. In contrast, a large Korean study places females aged 40 to 60 years at a greater risk of presenting with extraPTB than men [52]. A study from Madrid also showed that women are more likely than men to develop extraPTB. They also associated female sex with an increased likelihood of presenting lymphatic and pleural TB, while males were more likely to present genitourinary and abdominal TB [11]. Furthermore, Pang et al. examined the epidemiology of extrapulmonary TB among inpatients in China, concluding that the most common forms of extrapulmonary TB were osteoarticular and pleural. Most of these diagnoses were based on clinical symptoms, indicating a high risk of diagnostic delays and misdiagnoses in extrapulmonary TB cases [53]. In our study, the subjects presented different types of extraTB infections: a total of thirteen subjects (56%) presented TB pleural effusion, five subjects (22%) presented TB lymphadenitis, two subjects (9%) presented TB meningitis, two subjects (9%) presented bone TB, and one subject (4%) presented gastrointestinal TB. Only four of all cases of extraTB had previously undergone immunosuppressive therapies: one with pleural effusion and two with lymphadenitis. Only four of all cases of extraTB had previously undergone immunosuppressive therapies, one with pleural effusion and two with lymphadenitis. When analyzing sex-based differences regarding the proportion of extraPTB cases, in women, TB pleural effusion and TB lymphadenitis were the most predominant types of TB infections, with equal proportions of 40%, while in men, 69% of cases were of TB pleural effusion, followed by 15% TB meningitis.

The logistic regression analysis revealed that younger age, employment status, and comorbidities such as COPD and type 2 diabetes were significant predictors of extraPTB–SARS-CoV-2 coinfection.

The observation that the extraPTB and SARS-CoV-2 coinfection group in this study was younger than the SARS-CoV-2-only group raises intriguing questions about the role of age in immune responses and clinical outcomes. The negative correlation between age and coinfection may reflect the fact that younger individuals are more likely to develop extraPTB due to their more robust immune responses, while older adults are more prone to pulmonary forms of TB [54]. Young adults, especially those with strong cell-mediated immunity, are more likely to contain the infection in specific sites outside the lungs, leading to localized extrapulmonary manifestations, such as lymph node, pleural, or bone TB. Elders, on the other hand, may experience more disseminated disease, but their overall risk for extraPTB tends to be lower compared to younger adults [55]. Hence, while pulmonary TB is more common in older populations due to the reactivation of latent infections, extraPTB tends to be more prevalent in younger individuals, especially in areas with a high burden of TB [10]. When considering the coinfection with SARS-CoV-2, younger individuals also seem to exhibit better pulmonary outcomes despite the heightened systemic inflammation associated with extraPTB. The improved respiratory outcomes in younger populations with SARS-CoV-2 infection can be attributed to stronger adaptive immune responses. Studies show that younger individuals have higher baseline T cell activity, including cytotoxic CD8+ T cells and helper CD4+ T cells, which play a crucial role in clearing viral infections [56]. This enhanced immune function allows for faster resolution of viral replication and better control of inflammation, limiting pulmonary damage despite the systemic inflammatory milieu associated with extraPTB. Moreover, younger individuals generally have a more robust production of type I and III interferons, which are critical in the early antiviral response [57]. These interferons not only limit viral spread but also modulate the inflammatory response, preventing excessive cytokine release that can lead to acute respiratory distress syndrome in severe COVID-19 cases. This balance between effective immune activation and controlled inflammation likely contributes to the less severe pulmonary involvement observed in the younger coinfected group.

This may be the explanation for the difference in median age between the two groups in our study, with the coinfection group including significantly younger subjects than the SARS-CoV-2 group. Being employed was also associated with a higher probability of having extraPTB, but we associate this result with the younger median age of the group.

This study suggests an association between COPD and type 2 diabetes mellitus and extraPTB coinfection. Individuals with COPD presented 6.5 times higher odds of having the coinfection, while those with type 2 DM had four times higher odds of having the coinfection. Although several previous studies have highlighted the role of these comorbidities in increasing the risk of tuberculous infection and in exacerbating the clinical course of COVID-19 [58–61], those studies have focused on either PTB or on tuberculous infection of either etiology combined. Data are scarce on the implications of these pathologies in extraPTB and SARS-CoV-2 coinfection, and our coinfection group is too small to draw definitive conclusions.

It is clear that COPD is primarily associated with pulmonary complications, leading to worse outcomes in PTB patients. Studies have shown that COPD patients are three times more likely to develop active TB, and when coinfected with SARS-CoV-2, the mortality and hospitalization rates increase significantly. The lung damage caused by COPD makes it easier for Mycobacterium tuberculosis to bypass immune defenses, leading to the development of active TB [58]. TB often leads to post-tubercular airway disease or TB-associated COPD, with COPD being a common comorbidity, second only to diabetes. Smoking accelerates COPD progression, increases TB risk by 3–5 fold, and exacerbates lung damage through inflammatory and proteolytic pathways. Patients with a TB history develop COPD earlier, face more hospitalizations, and have a shorter life expectancy [62]. Moreover, the immune dysregulation in COPD patients, exacerbated by smoking and environmental exposures, often leads to poorer control of both bacterial and viral infections. When these patients develop COVID-19, they are more likely to experience severe respiratory complications [59].

On the other hand, type 2 DM is another key comorbidity associated with adverse outcomes in both TB and COVID-19. Diabetic patients often exhibit impaired immune responses, making them vulnerable to both TB reactivation and severe manifestations of SARS-CoV-2 infection. In PTB and SARS-CoV-2 coinfections, DM exacerbates the clinical course, often leading to prolonged hospitalization and an increased risk for complications, including multi-organ failure and poor prognosis. Studies emphasize the importance of tight glycemic control during hospitalization to mitigate these risks [60,61].

These comorbidities may contribute to the complexity of managing extraPTB–SARS-CoV-2 coinfection. We highlight the need for targeted treatment protocols and further research to develop comprehensive management guidelines for these high-risk populations.

4.3. Hospitalization and Outcomes

This study also found that coinfected patients had significantly longer hospitalization periods compared to those with SARS-CoV-2 infection alone. This aligns with previous studies, which have reported longer recovery times in TB patients coinfected with COVID-19, likely due to the dual burden of managing both infections simultaneously. A recent meta-analysis reported that individuals with TB–COVID-19 coinfection are at heightened risk of hospitalization and protracted recovery periods [55]. Moreover, in patients with concurrent TB and COVID-19 infections, increased mortality rates and extended recovery times have been reported [63].

However, it is notable that mortality was significantly higher in the SARS-CoV-2-alone group compared to the coinfection group in our study. Coinfection was not a significant predictor of fatality, but the lowest value of SpO2 registered and IL-6 levels were. The severity of symptoms increases the probability of a fatal outcome by three-fold. This finding could be explained by the younger age and relatively better respiratory function in the extraPTB cohort, despite the systemic inflammation. It may also indicate that, while extraPTB exacerbates the inflammatory response, it does not necessarily lead to worse pulmonary outcomes compared to COVID-19 infection alone [64].

4.4. Limitations and Future Directions

While this study offers important insights into the interplay between extraPTB and SARS-CoV-2, certain limitations must be acknowledged. Firstly, the relatively small sample size of the coinfected group may limit the generalizability of the findings. Our pre-statistical estimations, however, showed that the cohorts were sufficiently large to provide statistical significance. To this point, we mention the large distribution of data in the cases of coinfected subjects who associated COPD or type 2 DM, which makes us cautiously interpret the higher odds of patients with COPD or type 2 DM to present coinfection. Secondly, the retrospective nature of this study precludes a direct assessment of causality between coinfection and specific outcomes.

Future research should focus on larger, prospective cohort studies to further investigate the mechanisms driving the immune response in coinfected patients. Additionally, longitudinal studies could provide insight into the long-term outcomes of patients with extraPTB and COVID-19, particularly regarding the persistence of inflammatory markers and the risk of relapse or complications as well as of long COVID.

This is the first study to comprehensively investigate the unique clinical and paraclinical parameters associated specifically with coinfected patients with extrapulmonary tuberculosis and COVID-19. While numerous studies have examined pulmonary TB or combined pulmonary and extrapulmonary TB in the context of COVID-19, very few have specifically focused on extraPTB alone. This distinct approach allows for a more detailed understanding of the interplay between extraPTB and COVID-19, which has been largely unexplored.

This study provides valuable insights into a unique patient population, potentially paving the way for more targeted clinical strategies and management guidelines for coinfections involving extraPTB and COVID-19.

Furthermore, these findings emphasize the need for integrated TB–COVID-19 management strategies, particularly in resource-limited settings where dual-burden diseases are prevalent. Clinicians should prioritize monitoring IL-6 and PCT levels for early detection of systemic inflammation and prolonged hospitalization risks. Tailored protocols, including targeted anti-inflammatory therapy and vigilant respiratory support, are critical.

Public health policies should incorporate coinfection screening protocols, especially for younger populations presenting with systemic inflammation. Further, the findings underscore the importance of maintaining uninterrupted TB care services.

5. Conclusions

This study highlights important clinical and paraclinical differences between patients with extraPTB and SARS-CoV-2 coinfection and those with SARS-CoV-2 infection alone.

The susceptibility of younger individuals to extraPTB underscores the complexity of their immune response. While their heightened immune activity may localize Mycobacterium tuberculosis to extrapulmonary sites, coinfection with SARS-CoV-2 seems to amplify systemic inflammation without severely compromising pulmonary function. This duality highlights the need for targeted management strategies in younger coinfected patients, focusing on controlling systemic inflammation without dampening the antiviral response.

Coinfected patients displayed lower CT involvement scores and higher SpO2 levels, indicating less pulmonary compromise but heightened systemic inflammation, evidenced by elevated IL-6, PCT, and inflammatory ratios. This pattern suggests that extraPTB primarily exacerbates systemic inflammatory responses without worsening pulmonary outcomes compared to SARS-CoV-2 infection alone.

Coinfected patients experienced significantly longer hospital stays, but mortality rates were notably lower compared to the SARS-CoV-2-only group. The lower mortality among coinfected patients might be attributed to their younger age and better-preserved respiratory function despite high systemic inflammation levels. For all patients, lower SpO2 and higher IL-6 levels emerged as independent predictors of mortality, emphasizing the importance of monitoring these parameters closely to identify high-risk cases.

Coinfection with SARS-CoV-2 and extraPTB presents distinct clinical characteristics that differ from SARS-CoV-2 alone, primarily due to heightened systemic inflammation rather than increased pulmonary severity. These insights highlight the need for tailored management protocols that address both inflammatory and respiratory factors, especially for younger and at-risk patients.

These findings underscore the need for tailored treatment and monitoring strategies in coinfected patients to address both the inflammatory and infectious aspects of their disease.

Author Contributions: Conceptualization, C.O. and C.M.; methodology, C.O., C.M. and A.S.; software, M.S.M.; validation, C.O. and A.S.; formal analysis, C.M. and A.S.; investigation, C.M. and A.S.; resources, A.S. and C.O.; data curation, M.S.M., P.H. and E.T.; writing—original draft preparation, C.M.; writing—review and editing, A.S. and C.O.; visualization, M.S.M., P.H. and E.T.; supervision, C.O.; project administration, A.S. and C.O. All authors have read and agreed to the published version of the manuscript.

Funding: We would like to acknowledge Victor Babes University of Medicine And Pharmacy Timisoara for their support in covering the costs of publication for this research paper.

Institutional Review Board Statement: This study was conducted in accordance with the Declaration of Helsinki and approved by the Ethics Council for Scientific Research at the Victor Babeș University of Medicine and Pharmacy Timisoara, No. 04/19 January 2021.

Informed Consent Statement: Informed consent was obtained from all subjects involved in this study. Written informed consent has been obtained from the patients to publish this paper.

Data Availability Statement: The findings of this study are supported by data available upon request from the corresponding author, though ethical restrictions prevent public access to the data.

Acknowledgments: We extend our heartfelt gratitude to all the patients who participated in this study. We also acknowledge the valuable contributions of each author and the support from our affiliated institutions, which made this research and its publication possible.

Conflicts of Interest: The authors declare no conflicts of interest.

Abbreviations

ALT	Alanine aminotransferase
AST	Aspartate aminotransferase
AUC	Area under the receiver operating characteristic curve
BMI	Body mass index
COPD	Chronic obstructive pulmonary disease
CRP	C-reactive protein
CT	Computer tomography
DM	Diabetes mellitus
HIV	Human Deficiency Virus
IL-6	Interleukin 6
LDH	Lactate dehydrogenase
n	Number of subjects
NK cells	Natural killer cells
MTB	Mycobacterium tuberculosis
OR	Odds ratio
p	*p*-value
PCT	Procalcitonin
PTB	Pulmonary tuberculosis
ROC	Receiver operating characteristic
RT-PCR	Reverse transcription polymerase chain reaction
SpO2	Saturation of peripheral oxygen
TB	Tuberculosis
WHO	World Health Organization

References

1. World Health Organization. *Global Tuberculosis Report 2023*; World Health Organization: Geneva, Switzerland; Available online: https://www.who.int/teams/global-tuberculosis-programme/tb-reports/global-tuberculosis-report-2023 (accessed on 28 June 2024).
2. Rothan, H.A.; Byrareddy, S.N. The epidemiology and pathogenesis of coronavirus disease (COVID-19) outbreak. *J. Autoimmun.* **2020**, *109*, 102433. [CrossRef] [PubMed]
3. World Health Organization. *COVID-19 Epidemiological Update—15 March 2024*; World Health Organization: Geneva, Switzerland, 2024; Available online: https://www.who.int/publications/m/item/covid-19-epidemiological-update-15-march-2024 (accessed on 28 June 2024).
4. Chan, K.P.; Kwok, W.C.; Ma, T.F.; Hui, C.H.; Tam, T.C.; Wang, J.K.; Ho, J.C.; Lam, D.C.; Sau-Man Ip, M.; Ho, P.L. Territory-Wide Study on Hospital Admissions for Asthma Exacerbations in COVID-19 Pandemic. *Ann. Am. Thorac. Soc.* **2021**, *18*, 1624–1633. [CrossRef] [PubMed]
5. Chan, K.P.F.; Ting-Fung, M.; Sridhar, S.; Lui, M.M.S.; Ho, J.C.M.; Lam, D.C.L.; Ip, M.S.M.; Ho, P.L. Changes in the incidence, clinical features and outcomes of tuberculosis during COVID-19 pandemic. *J. Infect. Public Health* **2024**, *17*, 102511. [CrossRef] [PubMed]
6. Gerstein, S.; Khatri, A.; Roth, N.; Wallach, F. Coronavirus disease 2019 and extrapulmonary tuberculosis co-infection—A case report and review of literature. *J. Clin. Tuberc. Other Mycobact. Dis.* **2021**, *22*, 100213. [CrossRef] [PubMed]
7. Mousquer, G.T.; Peres, A.; Fiegenbaum, M. Pathology of TB/COVID-19 co-infection: The phantom menace. *Tuberculosis* **2020**, *126*, 102020. [CrossRef] [PubMed]
8. Lee, J.Y. Diagnosis and treatment of extrapulmonary tuberculosis. *Tuberc. Respir. Dis.* **2015**, *78*, 47–55. [CrossRef]
9. Lerner, T.R.; Borel, S.; Gutierrez, M.G. The innate immune response in human tuberculosis. *Cell Microbiol.* **2015**, *17*, 1277–1285. [CrossRef]

10. Petro, B.; Katalin, A.W.; Dylan, S. Immune interaction between SARS-CoV-2 and Mycobacterium tuberculosis. *Front. Immunol.* **2023**, *14*, 1254206. [CrossRef]
11. Ramírez-Lapausa, M.; Menéndez-Saldaña, A.; Noguerado-Asensio, A. Extrapulmonary Tuberculosis: An Overview. *Rev. Esp. Sanid. Penit.* **2015**, *17*, 3–11. [CrossRef] [PubMed]
12. Ruiz-Bastián, M.; Díaz-Pollán, B.; Falces-Romero, I.; Toro-Rueda, C.; García-Rodríguez, J.; SARS-CoV-2 Working Group. Impact on tuberculosis diagnostic during COVID-19 pandemic in a tertiary care hospital. *Enferm. Infecc. Microbiol. Clin.* **2024**, *42*, 135–139. [CrossRef]
13. Rodriguez-Takeuchi, S.Y.; Renjifo, M.E.; Medina, F.J. Extrapulmonary tuberculosis: Pathophysiology and imaging findings. *Radiographics* **2019**, *39*, 2023–2037. [CrossRef] [PubMed]
14. Bandyopadhyay, A.; Palepu, S.; Bandyopadhyay, K.; Handu, S. COVID-19 and tuberculosis co-infection: A neglected paradigm. *Monaldi Arch. Chest Dis.* **2020**, *90*, 518–522. [CrossRef] [PubMed]
15. Mihuta, C.; Socaci, A.; Hogea, P.; Tudorache, E.; Mihuta, M.S.; Oancea, C. Colliding Challenges: An Analysis of SARS-CoV-2 Infection in Patients with Pulmonary Tuberculosis versus SARS-CoV-2 Infection Alone. *Medicina* **2024**, *60*, 823. [CrossRef]
16. Prakash, A.K.; Datta, B.; Goyal, P.; Chatterjee, P.; Gupta, G. GENE-XPERT gives early diagnosis in early tuberculosis. *Eur. Respir. J.* **2016**, *48* (Suppl. S60), PA2775.
17. COVID-19 Treatment Guidelines Panel. Coronavirus Disease 2019 (COVID-19) Treatment Guidelines. National Institutes of Health. Available online: https://covid19.nih.gov/treatments-and-vaccines (accessed on 1 June 2024).
18. Gounden, V.; Bhatt, H.; Jialal, I. Renal Function Tests. In *StatPearls*; Updated 17 July 2023; StatPearls Publishing: Treasure Island, FL, USA, 2024. Available online: https://www.ncbi.nlm.nih.gov/books/NBK507821/ (accessed on 13 June 2024).
19. World Health Organization. BCG vaccines: WHO position paper—February 2018. *Wkly. Epidemiol. Rec.* **2018**, *93*, 73–96.
20. Purnell, J.Q. Definitions, Classification, and Epidemiology of Obesity. In *Endotext*; Updated 4 May 2023; Feingold, K.R., Anawalt, B., Blackman, M.R., Boyce, A., Chrousos, G., Corpas, E., de Herder, W.W., Dhatariya, K., Dungan, K., Hofland, J., Eds.; MDText.com, Inc.: South Dartmouth, MA, USA, 2000. Available online: https://www.ncbi.nlm.nih.gov/books/NBK279167/ (accessed on 13 June 2024).
21. Akpek, M. Does COVID-19 Cause Hypertension? *Angiology* **2022**, *73*, 682–687. [CrossRef] [PubMed]
22. Metra, M.; Dinatolo, E.; Dasseni, N. The New Heart Failure Association Definition of Advanced Heart Failure. *Card. Fail. Rev.* **2019**, *5*, 5–8. [CrossRef] [PubMed]
23. Parker, C.S.; Siracuse, C.G.; Litle, V.R. Identifying lung cancer in patients with active pulmonary tuberculosis. *JTD* **2018**, *10* (Suppl. S28), S3392–S3397. [CrossRef]
24. Ramamoorthy, S.; Srinivas, B.H.; Badhe, B.A.; Jinkala, S.; Ganesh, R.N. Coexistence of malignancy and tuberculosis: Is it double disease or double hit related to COVID-19?—Experience from a tertiary care center. *Int. J. Clin. Exp. Pathol.* **2023**, *16*, 1–7.
25. Sanyaolu, A.; Okorie, C.; Marinkovic, A.; Patidar, R.; Younis, K.; Desai, P.; Hosein, Z.; Mangat, J.; Altaf, M. Comorbidity and Its Impact on Patients with COVID-19. SN Compr. *Clin. Med.* **2020**, *2*, 1069–1076. [CrossRef]
26. NHLBI Obesity Education Initiative Expert Panel on the Identification E and T of O in A (US). Clinical Guidelines on the Identification, Evaluation, and Treatment of Overweight and Obesity in Adults: The Evidence Report. In *Obesity Prevention and Management*; National Heart, Lung, and Blood Institute, Ed.; NHLBI Obesity Education Initiative Expert Panel on the Identification, Evaluation, and Treatment of Obesity in Adults (US): Bethesda, MD, USA, 1998.
27. Seifi, S.; Khatony, A.; Moradi, G.; Abdi, A.; Najafi, F. Accuracy of pulse oximetry in detection of oxygen saturation in patients admitted to the intensive care unit of heart surgery: Comparison of finger, toe, forehead, and earlobe probes. *BMC Nurs.* **2018**, *17*, 15. [CrossRef] [PubMed]
28. Fukui, S.; Ikeda, K.; Kobayashi, M.; Nishida, K.; Yamada, K.; Horie, S.; Shimada, Y.; Miki, H.; Goto, H.; Hayashi, K.; et al. Predictive prognostic biomarkers in patients with COVID 19 infection. *Mol. Med. Rep.* **2023**, *27*, 15. [CrossRef]
29. Ali, E.T.; Jabbar, A.S.; Al Ali, H.S.; Hamadi, S.S.; Jabir, M.S.; Albukhaty, S. Extensive Study on Hematological, Immunological, Inflammatory Markers, and Biochemical Profile to Identify the Risk Factors in COVID-19 Patients. *Int. J. Inflamm.* **2022**, *2022*, 5735546. [CrossRef] [PubMed]
30. Ravindra, R.; Ramamurthy, P.; Aslam, S.S.M.; Kulkarni, A.; Suhail, K.; Ramamurthy, P.S. Platelet Indices and Platelet to Lymphocyte Ratio (PLR) as Markers for Predicting COVID-19 Infection Severity. *Cureus* **2022**, *14*, e28206. [CrossRef] [PubMed]
31. Mangoni, A.A.; Zinellu, A. Systemic inflammation index, disease severity, and mortality in patients with COVID-19: A systematic review and meta-analysis. *Front. Immunol.* **2023**, *14*, 1212998. [CrossRef]
32. Hansell, D.M.; Bankier, A.A.; MacMahon, H.; McLoud, T.C.; Müller, N.L.; Remy, J. Fleischner society: Glossary of terms for thoracic imaging. *Radiology* **2008**, *246*, 697–722. [CrossRef]
33. Hernandez-Romieu, A.C.; Little, B.P.; Bernheim, A.; Schechter, M.C.; Ray, S.M.; Bizune, D.; Kempker, R. Increasing Number and Volume of Cavitary Lesions on Chest Computed Tomography Are Associated With Prolonged Time to Culture Conversion in Pulmonary Tuberculosis. *Open Forum Infect. Dis.* **2019**, *6*, ofz232. [CrossRef]
34. Chang, Y.-C.; Yu, C.-J.; Chang, S.-C.; Galvin, J.R.; Liu, H.-M.; Hsiao, C.-H.; Kuo, P.-H.; Chen, K.-Y.; Franks, T.J.; Huang, K.-M.; et al. Pulmonary sequelae in convalescent patients after severe acute respiratory syndrome: Evaluation with thin-section CT. *Radiology* **2005**, *236*, 1067–1075. [CrossRef] [PubMed]

35. Yazdi, N.A.; Ghadery, A.H.; SeyedAlinaghi, S.; Jafari, F.; Jafari, S.; Hasannezad, M.; Koochak, H.E.; Salehi, M.; Manshadi, S.A.D.; Meidani, M.; et al. Predictors of the chest CT score in COVID-19 patients: A cross-sectional study. *Virol. J.* **2021**, *18*, 225, Erratum in *Virol. J.* **2021**, *18*, 241. [CrossRef] [PubMed]
36. Gupta, N.; Ish, P.; Gupta, A.; Malhotra, N.; Caminero, J.A.; Singla, R.; Kumar, R.; Yadav, S.R.; Dev, N.; Agrawal, S.; et al. A Profile of a Retrospective Cohort of 22 Patients with COVID-19 and Active/Treated Tuberculosis. *Eur. Respir. J.* **2020**, *56*, 2003408. [CrossRef] [PubMed]
37. Tan, L.; Wang, Q.; Zhang, D.; Ding, J.; Huang, Q.; Tang, Y.Q.; Wang, Q.; Miao, H. Lymphopenia predicts disease severity of COVID-19: A descriptive and predictive study. *Signal Transduct. Target Ther.* **2020**, *5*, 33. [CrossRef] [PubMed]
38. Ndhlovu, L.C.; Loo, C.P.; Spotts, G.; Nixon, D.F.; Hecht, F.M. FOXP3 expressing CD127lo CD4+ T cells inversely correlate with CD38+ CD8+ T cell activation levels in primary HIV-1 infection. *J. Leukoc. Biol.* **2008**, *83*, 254–262. [CrossRef] [PubMed]
39. Gavin, M.; Rudensky, A. Control of immune homeostasis by naturally arising regulatory $CD4^+$ T cells. *Curr. Opin. Immunol.* **2003**, *15*, 690–696. [CrossRef] [PubMed]
40. Wood, K.J.; Sakaguchi, S. Regulatory T cells in transplantation tolerance. *Nat. Rev. Immunol.* **2003**, *3*, 199–210. [CrossRef] [PubMed]
41. Cardona, P.; Cardona, P.-J. Regulatory T Cells in Mycobacterium Tuberculosis Infection. *Front. Immunol.* **2019**, *10*, 2139. [CrossRef]
42. de Almeida, A.S.; Fiske, C.T.; Sterling, T.R.; Kalams, S.A. Increased frequency of regulatory T cells and T lymphocyte activation in persons with previously treated extrapulmonary tuberculosis. *Clin Vaccine Immunol.* **2012**, *19*, 45–52. [CrossRef]
43. Dhawan, M.; Rabaan, A.A.; Fawarah, M.M.A.; Almuthree, S.A.; Alsubki, R.A.; Alfaraj, A.H.; Mashraqi, M.M.; Alshamrani, S.A.; Abduljabbar, W.A.; Alwashmi, A.S.S.; et al. Updated Insights into the T Cell-Mediated Immune Response against SARS-CoV-2: A Step towards Efficient and Reliable Vaccines. *Vaccines* **2023**, *11*, 101. [CrossRef]
44. Wang, H.; Wang, Z.; Cao, W.; Wu, Q.; Yuan, Y.; Zhang, X. Regulatory T Cells in COVID-19. *Aging Dis.* **2021**, *12*, 1545. [CrossRef] [PubMed]
45. Galván-Peña, S.; Leon, J.; Chowdhary, K.; Michelson, D.A.; Vijaykumar, B.; Yang, L.; Magnuson, A.M.; Chen, F.; Manickas-Hill, Z.; Piechocka-Trocha, A.; et al. Profound Treg Perturbations Correlate with COVID-19 Severity. *Proc. Natl. Acad. Sci. USA.* **2021**, *118*, e2111315118. [CrossRef] [PubMed]
46. Wang, Y.; Zheng, J.; Islam, M.S.; Yang, Y.; Hu, Y.; Chen, X. The Role of $CD4^+FoxP3^+$ Regulatory T Cells in the Immunopathogenesis of COVID-19: Implications for Treatment. *Int. J. Biol. Sci.* **2021**, *17*, 1507–1520. [CrossRef] [PubMed]
47. Yang, Z.; Kong, Y.; Wilson, F.; Foxman, B.; Fowler, A.H.; Marrs, C.F.; Cave, M.D.; Bates, J.H. Identification of Risk Factors for Extrapulmonary Tuberculosis. *Clin. Infect. Dis.* **2004**, *38*, 199–205. [CrossRef]
48. Kulchavenya, E.; Naber, K.G.; Johansen, T.E.B. Epidemiology of Extrapulmonary Tuberculosis. In *Extrapulmonary Tuberculosis*; Sener, A., Erdem, H., Eds.; Springer: Cham, Germany, 2019. [CrossRef]
49. Marçôa, R.; Ribeiro, A.I.; Zão, I.; Duarte, R. Tuberculosis and Gender—Factors Influencing the Risk of Tuberculosis among Men and Women by Age Group. *Pulmonology* **2018**, *24*, 199–202. [CrossRef] [PubMed]
50. Dabitao, D.; Bishai, W.R. Sex and Gender Differences in Tuberculosis Pathogenesis and Treatment Outcomes. In *Sex and Gender Differences in Infection and Treatments for Infectious Diseases*; Klein, S.L., Roberts, C.W., Eds.; Springer: Cham, Germany, 2023; Volume 441. [CrossRef]
51. Baya, B.; Sanogo, I.; Kone, M.; Soumare, D.; Ouattara, K.; Somboro, A.; Wague, M.; Coulibaly, N.; Koloma, I.; Coulibaly, M.; et al. Relationship between patient sex and anatomical sites of extrapulmonary tuberculosis in Mali. *J. Clin. Tuberc. Other Mycobact. Dis.* **2023**, *33*, 100389. [CrossRef] [PubMed]
52. Min, J.; Lee, J.H.; Kim, S.Y.; Park, J.S.; Cho, Y.J.; Yoon, H.I.; Lee, C.T.; Lee, J.H. Differential effects of sex on tuberculosis location and severity across the lifespan. *Sci. Rep.* **2023**, *13*, 33245. [CrossRef]
53. Pang, Y.; An, J.; Shu, W.; Huo, F.; Chu, N.; Gao, M.; Qin, S.; Huang, H.; Chen, X.; Xu, S. Epidemiology of Extrapulmonary Tuberculosis among Inpatients, China, 2008–2017. *Emerg. Infect. Dis.* **2019**, *25*, 457–464. [CrossRef]
54. Ayed, H.B.; Koubaa, M.; Marrakchi, C.; Rekik, K.; Hammami, F.; Smaoui, F.; Ben Hmida, M.; Yaich, S.; Maaloul, I.; Damak, J.; et al. Extrapulmonary Tuberculosis: Update on the Epidemiology, Risk Factors and Prevention Strategies. *Int. J. Trop. Dis.* **2018**, *1*, 006. [CrossRef]
55. Wang, Q.; Cao, Y.; Liu, X.; Fu, Y.; Zhang, J.; Zhang, Y.; Zhang, L.; Wei, X.; Yang, L. Systematic Review and Meta-Analysis of Tuberculosis and COVID-19 Co-Infection: Prevalence, Fatality, and Treatment Considerations. *PLoS Negl. Trop. Dis.* **2024**, *18*, e0012136. [CrossRef] [PubMed]
56. Agrawal, S.; Tran, M.T.; Jennings, T.S.K.; Soliman, M.M.H.; Heo, S.; Sasson, B.; Rahmatpanah, F.; Agrawal, A. Changes in the innate immune response to SARS-CoV-2 with advancing age in humans. *Immun. Ageing.* **2024**, *21*, 21. [CrossRef] [PubMed]
57. Costagliola, G.; Spada, E.; Consolini, R. Age-related differences in the immune response could contribute to determine the spectrum of severity of COVID-19. *Immun. Inflamm. Dis.* **2021**, *9*, 331–339. [CrossRef]
58. Inghammar, M.; Ekbom, A.; Engström, G.; Ljungberg, B.; Romanus, V.; Löfdahl, C.G.; Egesten, A. COPD and the Risk of Tuberculosis—A Population-Based Cohort Study. *PLoS ONE* **2010**, *5*, e10138. [CrossRef] [PubMed]
59. Sershen, C.L.; Salim, T.; May, E.E. Investigating the Comorbidity of COPD and Tuberculosis, a Computational Study. *Front. Syst. Biol.* **2023**, *3*, 940097. [CrossRef]
60. Wilkinson, R.J. Tuberculosis and Type 2 Diabetes Mellitus: An Inflammatory Danger Signal in the Time of Coronavirus Disease 2019. *Clin. Infect. Dis.* **2021**, *72*, 79–81. [CrossRef] [PubMed]

61. Czupryniak, L.; Dicker, D.; Lehmann, R.; Prázný, M.; Schernthaner, G. The Management of Type 2 Diabetes before, during and after COVID-19 Infection: What is the Evidence? *Cardiovasc. Diabetol.* **2021**, *20*, 198. [CrossRef]
62. Jain, N.K. Chronic Obstructive Pulmonary Disease and Tuberculosis. *Lung India* **2017**, *34*, 468–469. [CrossRef] [PubMed]
63. Bostanghadiri, N.; Jazi, F.M.; Razavi, S.; Fattorini, L.; Darban-Sarokhalil, D. Mycobacterium tuberculosis and SARS-CoV-2 Coinfections: A Review. *Front. Microbiol.* **2022**, *12*, 747827. [CrossRef] [PubMed]
64. Cook, T.; Noland, D.K.; Almalouf, P. Extrapulmonary Tuberculosis and COVID-19 Co-Infection as a Complication of TNF-α Inhibitor Therapy. *Chest* **2023**, *164*, A1302–A1303. [CrossRef]

medicina

MDPI

Article

Elevated Cardiac Troponin I as a Mortality Predictor in Hospitalised COVID-19 Patients

Ieva Kubiliute [1,*], Jurgita Urboniene [2], Fausta Majauskaite [1], Edgar Bobkov [3], Linas Svetikas [1] and Ligita Jancoriene [1]

1 Clinic of Infectious Diseases and Dermatovenerology, Institute of Clinical Medicine, Faculty of Medicine, Vilnius University, 03101 Vilnius, Lithuania; fausta.majauskaite@santa.lt (F.M.); linas.svetikas@santa.lt (L.S.); ligita.jancoriene@santa.lt (L.J.)
2 Centre of Infectious Diseases, Vilnius University Hospital Santaros Klinikos, 08661 Vilnius, Lithuania; jurgita.urboniene@santa.lt
3 Faculty of Medicine, Vilnius University, 03101 Vilnius, Lithuania; edgar.bobkov@santa.lt
* Correspondence: ieva.kubiliute@santa.lt

Abstract: *Background and Objectives:* SARS-CoV-2 affects multiple organ systems, including the cardiovascular system, leading to immediate and long-term cardiovascular complications. Acute myocardial injury is one of the earliest and most common cardiac issues in the acute phase of COVID-19. This study aimed to evaluate the prognostic value of cardiac troponin I (cTnI) levels in predicting in-hospital mortality among hospitalised COVID-19 patients. *Materials and Methods:* A retrospective observational cohort study included 2019 adult patients hospitalised with a confirmed COVID-19 infection stratified by cTnI levels on admission into three groups: <19 ng/L (1416 patients), 19–100 ng/L (431 patients), and >100 ng/L (172 patients). Myocardial injury was defined as blood serum cTnI levels increased above the 99th percentile upper reference limit. Depersonalised datasets were extracted from digital health records. Statistical analysis included multivariable binary logistic and Cox proportional hazards regressions. *Results:* Overall, 29.87% of patients experienced acute myocardial injury, which development was associated with age, male sex, chronic heart failure, arterial hypertension, obesity, and chronic kidney disease. Among patients with cTnI levels of 19–100 ng/L, the odds ratio for requiring invasive mechanical ventilation was 3.18 (95% CI 2.11–4.79) and, for those with cTnI > 100 ng/L, 5.38 (95% CI 3.26–8.88). The hazard ratio for in-hospital mortality for patients with cTnI levels of 19–100 ng/L was 2.58 (95% CI 1.83–3.62) and, for those with cTnI > 100 ng/L, 2.97 (95% CI 2.01–4.39) compared to patients with normal cTnI levels. *Conclusions:* Increased cardiac troponin I, indicating myocardial injury, on admission is associated with a more adverse clinical disease course, including a higher likelihood of requiring invasive mechanical ventilation and increased risk of in-hospital mortality. This indicates cardiac troponin I to be a beneficial biomarker for clinicians trying to identify high-risk COVID-19 patients, choosing the optimal monitoring and treatment strategy for these patients.

Keywords: COVID-19; in-hospital mortality; cardiac troponin I; SARS-CoV-2

1. Introduction

The COVID-19 pandemic, caused by severe acute respiratory syndrome coronavirus 2 (SARS-CoV-2), has emerged as a major global public health crisis. It appears that SARS-CoV-2 affects multiple organ systems, including the cardiovascular system, leading to both immediate and long-term cardiovascular complications. During the acute phase of infection, SARS-CoV-2 can cause direct cardiac injury by interacting with the angiotensin-converting enzyme 2 (ACE-2) receptor on various cardiac cells, such as cardiomyocytes, pericytes, macrophages, fibroblasts, and endothelial cells [1,2]. Autopsy studies of COVID-19 patients have confirmed the presence of the SARS-CoV-2 genome in cardiac tissues [3,4]. Furthermore, the immune response to SARS-CoV-2, resulting in a cytokine storm, may also cause direct cardiac damage. Indirect pathways of cardiac injury may involve myocardial ischemia, which could be precipitated by conditions like tachycardia, shock, severe respiratory distress (resembling type 2 myocardial infarction), or acute atherothrombotic incidents (resembling type 1 myocardial infarction). Clinical manifestations of cardiac injury include myocarditis, pericarditis, arrhythmia, myocardial infarction, heart failure, right ventricular dysfunction, and Takotsubo cardiomyopathy [5–8]. Acute myocardial injury, characterised by elevated serum cardiac troponin without the typical signs of acute ischemia on electrocardiograms or echocardiograms, is identified as one of the earliest and most common cardiac issues in the acute phase of COVID-19 [5].

This study aimed to evaluate the prognostic value of cardiac troponin I (cTnI) levels in predicting in-hospital mortality among hospitalised COVID-19 patients.

2. Materials and Methods

A retrospective observational cohort study was conducted at Vilnius University Hospital Santaros Klinikos in Lithuania from March 2020 to May 2021 [9].

The study included adult patients, 18 years and older, who were admitted to the hospital with confirmed COVID-19 infection and treated in various units, including standard care, high dependency, or intensive care units. The confirmation of the infection was based on a positive result on either a SARS-CoV-2 reverse transcriptase polymerase chain reaction or a rapid SARS-CoV-2 antigen test conducted on a nasopharyngeal sample. For symptomatic patients, the rapid antigen test was utilised within the first five days of the onset of COVID-19 symptoms. Initially, 2179 patients, who underwent cTnI testing upon admission, were considered for the study. Exclusion criteria included individuals with end-stage chronic kidney disease, defined by an estimated glomerular filtration rate (eGFR) less than 15 mL/min/1.73 m^2, and those who developed myocardial infarction subsequent to admission. After applying these exclusions, the study population was finalised at 2019 patients. These individuals were stratified by cTnI levels on admission into three groups: 1416 patients exhibited cTnI levels below 19 ng/L, 431 patients had cTnI levels within the 19–100 ng/L range, and 172 patients presented with cTnI levels above 100 ng/L (Figure 1). Myocardial injury was defined as blood serum cTnI levels increased above the 99th percentile upper reference limit [10]. The concentration of cTnI was measured using the Snibe MAGLUMI 2000 Chemoluminescence Immunoassay System, Shenzhen New Industries Biomedical Engineering Co., Ltd., Shenzhen, China.

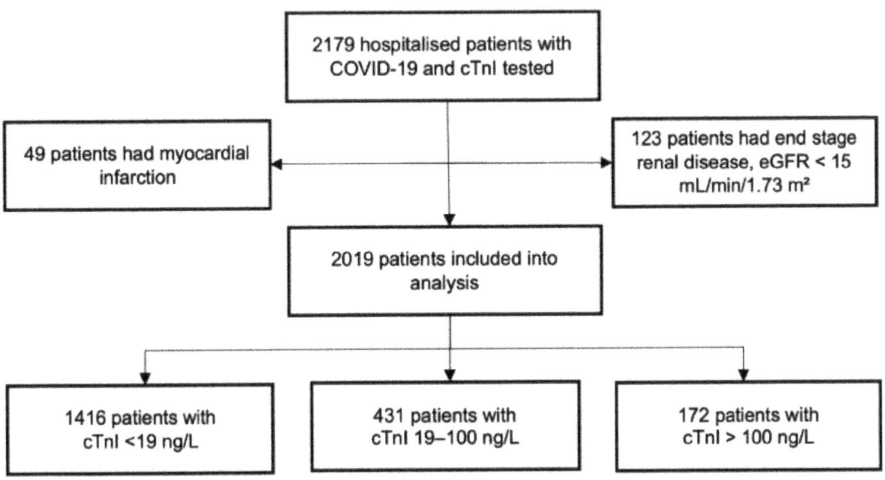

Figure 1. Distribution of patients hospitalised with COVID-19 infection.

Depersonalised datasets were extracted from digital health records, facilitated by the Centre for Informatics and Development, in compliance with the procedures authorised by Vilnius University Hospital Santaros Klinikos. The demographic parameters encompassed sex and age. Comorbid conditions included arterial hypertension (AH), coronary artery disease (CAD), congestive heart failure (CHF), atrial fibrillation (AF), diabetes mellitus, obesity, chronic obstructive pulmonary disease (COPD), chronic kidney disease (CKD), and a history of cerebrovascular accidents. These conditions were identified within the electronic medical records using the corresponding International Classification of Diseases, Tenth Revision (ICD-10) codes. If a medical condition was not documented in the electronic medical records related to the hospitalisation due to COVID-19, the individual was classified as not having that specific comorbidity.

Initial laboratory test results, including a complete blood count, creatinine, urea, eGFR, sodium, potassium, alanine aminotransferase (ALT), aspartate aminotransferase (AST), lactate dehydrogenase (LDH), C-reactive protein (CRP), ferritin, interleukin 6 (IL-6), D-dimer, and cTnI levels, were extracted from electronic medical records and analysed. Additionally, information regarding the duration of hospitalisation and patient outcomes was gathered from depersonalised medical records.

Statistical analysis was performed using IBM SPSS version 20.0. Continuous and categorical variables were presented as the median (interquartile range (IQR)) and numbers (percentages), respectively. Mann–Whitney *U* test was used to compare continuous variables, and χ^2 test or Fisher's exact test was used to compare categorical variables. Multivariable binary logistic regression was used to determine the association of myocardial injury development with age, sex, and comorbid conditions. Another multivariable binary logistic regression model was created to determine the association of cTnI levels with the need for invasive mechanical ventilation (IMV). The model included the need for IMV as the dependent variable and age; sex; and comorbid conditions (AH, CAD, CHF, AF, diabetes, obesity, COPD, CKD, and previous stroke) as predictors. We conducted a survival analysis to assess the effects of cTnI levels on outcomes within 30 days of hospitalisation. Patients were considered to be right-censored if they were discharged from the hospital alive or remained in the hospital. Cox proportional hazards regression models were created with in-hospital mortality as the dependent variable and age; comorbid conditions (AH, CAD, CHF, AF, diabetes, obesity, COPD, CKD, and previous stroke); treatment with remdesivir; systemic steroids; and antibiotics as predictors. Survival curves were plotted to illustrate the survival rates stratified by the cTnI groups. A two-sided *p*-value <0.05 was considered significant.

3. Results

Among 2019 adults, 56% were men. The median age was 60 years (IQR 50–69). Table 1 presents the demographic details, clinical features, and initial laboratory findings of the patients included in the analysis.

Table 1. Demographic, clinical, and initial laboratory characteristics of hospitalised COVID-19 patients.

Demographic and Clinical Characteristic (N = 2019)	N (%)	Laboratory Characteristics	N	Median (IQR)
Age, years, median (IQR)	60 (50–69)	Haemoglobin, g/L	2019	140.0 (127.0–150.0)
Male	1130 (55.97)	WBC, $\times 10^9$/L	2019	6.34 (4.76–8.61)
Female	889 (44.03)	Neutrophils, $\times 10^9$/L	2019	4.66 (3.28–6.69)
Any comorbid condition	1000 (49.53)	Lymphocytes, $\times 10^9$/L	2019	1.0 (0.71–1.40)
Arterial hypertension	802 (39.72)	Platelets, $\times 10^9$/L	2019	195.0 (153.0–253.0)
Coronary artery disease	79 (3.91)	cTnI	2019	9.70 (5.0–23.0)

Table 1. *Cont.*

Demographic and Clinical Characteristic (N = 2019)	N (%)	Laboratory Characteristics	N	Median (IQR)
Congestive heart failure	160 (7.92)	Glucose, mmol/L	1984	6.22 (5.54–7.30)
Atrial fibrillation	203 (10.05)	Creatinine, μmol/L	2019	81.0 (67.0–100.0)
Diabetes mellitus	277 (13.72)	eGFR, mL/min/1.73 m^2	2019	84.0 (64.0–96.0)
Obesity	106 (5.25)	Urea, mmol/L	1883	5.50 (4.07–7.91)
COPD	34 (1.68)	Sodium, mmol/L	2019	140.0 (137.0–143.0)
Chronic kidney disease	109 (5.40)	Potassium, mmol/L	2019	4.20 (3.87–4.50)
Previous stroke	23 (1.14)	ALT, U/L	1993	33.0 (21.0–53.0)
Invasive mechanical ventilation	170 (8.42)	AST, U/L	1986	37.0 (26.98–57.0)
Treatment with antibiotics	1514 (74.99)	LDH, U/L	1910	308.0 (243.0–410.0)
Treatment with antivirals (Remdesivir)	711 (35.22)	CRP, mg/L	2018	63.25 (25.45–125.53)
Treatment with systemic steroids	1371 (67.90)	Ferritin, μg/L	1939	471.0 (235.00–1 002.0)
In-hospital mortality	247 (12.23)	IL-6, ng/L	1892	30.40 (15.01–57.30)
Length of hospital stay, days, median (IQR)	11 (8–16)	D-dimer, μg/L	1972	490.0 (295.0–910.0)

ALT: alanine aminotransferase; AST: aspartate aminotransferase; COPD: chronic obstructive pulmonary disease; CRP: C-reactive protein; cTnI: cardiac troponin I; eGFR: estimated glomerular filtration rate; IL-6: interleukin 6; IQR: interquartile range; LDH: lactate dehydrogenase; N: number; WBC: white blood cell count. Reference values: haemoglobin: 128–160 g/L (for males), 117–145 g/L (for females); WBC: 4.0–9.8 $\times 10^9$/L; neutrophils: 1.5–6.0 $\times 10^9$/L; lymphocytes: 1.0–4.0 $\times 10^9$/L; NLR: 1–2; platelets: 140–450 $\times 10^9$/L; glucose: 4.2–6.1 mmol/L; creatinine: 64–104 μmol/L (for males), 49–90 μmol/L (for females); urea: 2.5–7.5 mmol/L; sodium: 134–145 mmol/L; potassium: 3.8–5.3 mmol/L; ALT: ≤40 U/L; AST: ≤40 U/L; LDH: 125–243 U/L; CRP: <5 mg/L; ferritin: 25–350 μg/L (for men), 13–232 μg/L (for women); IL-6: 0–7 ng/L; D-dimer: <250 μg/L.

Out of 2019 patients, 603 (29.87%) experienced acute myocardial injury, characterised by elevated levels of cTnI. Multivariable regression analysis revealed that age, male sex, the presence of CHF, AF, obesity, and CKD were associated with the development of acute myocardial injury (Figure 2).

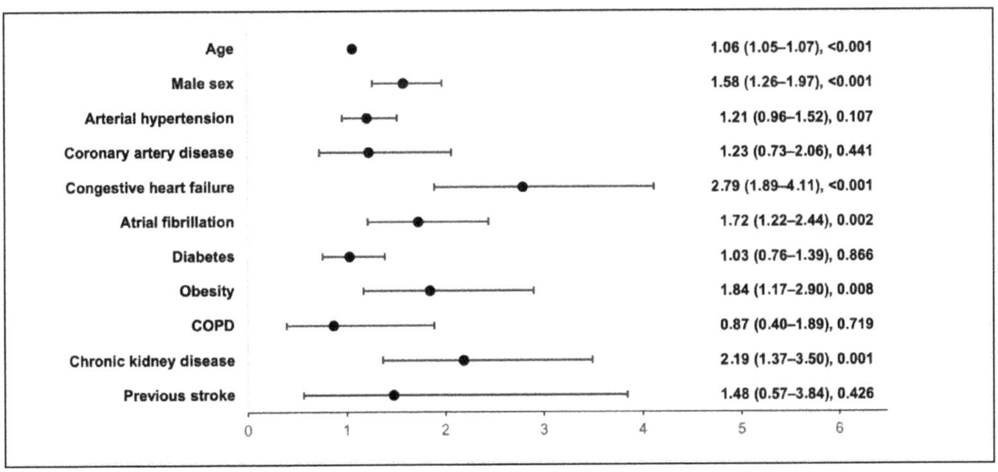

Figure 2. Risk factors and odds ratio (OR) associated with acute myocardial injury in COVID-19 patients.

Out of the 603 patients with elevated cTnI levels, 431 (71.48%) had cTnI levels between 19 and 100 ng/L, and 172 (28.52%) had cTnI levels above 100 ng/L. Patients with elevated cTnI levels were, on average, older than those presenting with normal cTnI levels upon admission. The prevalence of any comorbid condition, including AH, CAD, CHF, AF, diabetes, COPD, CKD, and previous stroke, was higher among patients with cTnI levels of 19–100 ng/L and in those with cTnI levels above 100 ng/L compared to patients with normal cTnI levels. The prevalence of CAD and AF was greater in patients with cTnI levels of 19–100 ng/L than in those with cTnI levels above 100 ng/L (Table 2).

Table 2. Baseline characteristics of hospitalised patients stratified by cardiac troponin I concentration.

Characteristic	cTnI < 19 ng/L (N = 1416), *n* (%)	19 ≤ cTnI ≤ 100 ng/L (N = 431), *n* (%)	cTnI > 100 ng/L (N = 172), *n* (%)	*p*-Value [1]	*p*-Value [2]	*p*-Value [3]
Age in years, median (IQR)	57 (47–65)	67 (58–77)	74 (62–81)	<0.001	<0.001	<0.001
Male	771 (54.45)	253 (58.70)	106 (61.63)	0.120	0.074	0.508
Any underlying condition	584 (41.24)	287 (66.59)	129 (75.00)	<0.001	<0.001	0.044
Hypertension	481 (33.97)	220 (51.04)	101 (58.72)	<0.001	<0.001	0.088
Coronary artery disease	33 (2.33)	27 (6.26)	19 (11.05)	<0.001	<0.001	0.046
Congestive heart failure	50 (3.53)	72 (16.71)	38 (22.09)	<0.001	<0.001	0.122
Atrial fibrillation	74 (5.23)	81 (18.79)	48 (27.91)	<0.001	<0.001	0.014
Diabetes	160 (11.30)	82 (19.03)	35 (20.35)	<0.001	0.001	0.711
Obesity	63 (4.45)	29 (6.73)	14 (8.14)	0.057	0.033	0.543
COPD	17 (1.20)	11 (2.55)	6 (3.49)	0.044	0.031	0.587
Chronic kidney disease	37 (2.61)	46 (10.67)	26 (15.12)	<0.001	<0.001	0.129
Previous stroke	7 (0.49)	10 (2.32)	6 (3.49)	0.002	0.001	0.410
Complications						
Pulmonary embolism	20 (1.41)	17 (3.94)	16 (9.30)	0.001	<0.001	0.009
Stroke	12 (0.85)	15 (3.48)	3 (1.74)	<0.001	0.216	0.258
Remdesivir	513 (36.23)	162 (37.59)	36 (20.93)	0.608	<0.001	<0.001
Systemic steroids	961 (67.87)	315 (73.09)	95 (55.23)	0.040	0.001	<0.001
Antibiotics use	1066 (75.28)	336 (77.96)	112 (65.12)	0.255	0.004	0.001
Invasive ventilation	61 (4.31)	66 (15.31)	43 (25.00)	<0.001	<0.001	0.005
Length of hospital stay, days	11 (7–15)	12 (8–19)	13 (8–21)	<0.001	0.001	0.579
In-hospital mortality	76 (5.37)	106 (24.59)	65 (37.79)	<0.001	<0.001	0.001

(1) *p*-value comparing patients with cTnI < 19 ng/L vs. patients with 19 ≤ cTnI ≤ 100 ng/L. (2) *p*-value comparing patients with cTnI < 19 ng/L vs. patients with cTnI > 100 ng/L. (3) *p*-value comparing patients with 19 ≤ cTnI ≤ 100 ng/L vs. patients with cTnI > 100 ng/L. cTnI: cardiac troponin I; IQR: interquartile range; N or n: number.

Patients with cTnI levels of 19–100 ng/L exhibited statistically significantly higher levels of WBC, neutrophil count, glucose, creatinine, urea, AST, LDH, CRP, ferritin, IL-6, and D-dimer compared to patients with normal cTnI levels. Conversely, their lymphocyte count, eGFR, and sodium concentration were significantly lower (Table 3).

Patients with cTnI levels above 100 ng/L showed higher levels of WBC, neutrophil count, glucose, creatinine, urea, AST, LDH, and D-dimer compared to both patients with normal cTnI levels and those with cTnI levels of 19–100 ng/L. CRP, ferritin, and IL-6 concentrations were higher in patients with cTnI levels above 100 ng/L than in those with normal cTnI levels; however, there was no statistically significant difference in CRP, ferritin, and IL-6 concentrations between patients with cTnI levels above 100 ng/L and those with levels of 19–100 ng/L. Lymphocyte count, eGFR, and sodium concentration were significantly lower in patients with cTnI levels above 100 ng/L compared to those with normal cTnI levels (Table 3).

Table 3. Laboratory tests of hospitalised COVID-19 patients stratified by cardiac troponin I concentration.

Variable	cTnI < 19 ng/L (N = 1416), Median (IQR)	19 ≤ cTnI ≤ 100 ng/L (N = 431), Median (IQR)	cTnI > 100 ng/L (N = 172), Median (IQR)	*p*-Value [1]	*p*-Value [2]	*p*-Value [3]
Haemoglobin, g/L	142.00 (130.00–151.00)	135.00 (121.00–147.00)	133.00 (116.00–145.75)	<0.001	<0.001	0.164
WBC, $\times 10^9$/L	6.15 (4.65–8.06)	6.72 (5.02–9.41)	8.83 (6.08–12.38)	<0.001	<0.001	<0.001
Neutrophils, $\times 10^9$/L	4.42 (3.14–6.15)	4.95 (3.50–7.53)	7.10 (4.38–10.23)	<0.001	<0.001	<0.001
Lymphocytes, $\times 10^9$/L	1.04 (0.77–1.40)	0.90 (0.60–1.39)	0.80 (0.53–1.30)	<0.001	<0.001	0.071
Platelets, $\times 10^9$/L	195.00 (154.00–252.00)	192.00 (151.00–245.00)	207.00 (150.25–261.25)	0.202	0.495	0.195
Glucose, mmol/L	6.07 (5.46–6.92)	6.67 (5.82–8.23)	7.64 (6.02–9.76)	<0.001	<0.001	0.003
Creatinine, µmol/L	78.00 (65.00–91.00)	92.00 (72.00–125.00)	103.50 (77.00–148.75)	<0.001	<0.001	0.018
eGFR, mL/min/1.73 m^2	88.00 (73.08–98.30)	68.40 (43.60–89.00)	57.20 (34.00–82.00)	<0.001	<0.001	0.002
Urea, mmol/L	4.91 (3.74–6.48)	7.37 (5.24–11.14)	10.17 (6.68–16.25)	<0.001	<0.001	<0.001
Sodium, mmol/L	140.75 (137.88–143.00)	140.00 (136.10–143.00)	139.00 (135.00–142.00)	0.001	0.002	0.386
Potassium, mmol/L	4.15 (3.90–4.50)	4.20 (3.80–4.60)	4.20 (3.85–4.60)	0.468	0.075	0.314
ALT, U/L	33.00 (21.00–53.00)	31.00 (19.35–50.00)	32.50 (19.00–59.75)	0.066	0.676	0.552
AST, U/L	35.00 (25.72–53.00)	40.00 (29.08–61.07)	50.00 (31.00–78.75)	<0.001	<0.001	0.004
LDH, U/L	295.00 (236.00–388.00)	335.00 (264.00–487.00)	385.50 (280.75–564.75)	<0.001	<0.001	0.031
CRP, mg/L	59.00 (24.43–108.90)	85.60 (32.60–157.60)	92.08 (19.88–146.30)	<0.001	0.003	0.486
Ferritin, µg/L	441.00 (225.50–952.55)	543.00 (252.50–1115.50)	543.29 (239.70–1286.73)	0.011	0.046	0.739
IL-6, ng/L	27.70 (13.90–51.05)	42.50 (19.85–71.05)	34.15 (16.85–87.73)	<0.001	0.001	0.739
D-dimer, µg/L	430.00 (270.00–720.00)	677.50 (410.00–1330.00)	1 255.00 (587.50–2360.00)	<0.001	<0.001	<0.001

ALT: alanine aminotransferase; AST: aspartate aminotransferase; CRP: C-reactive protein; cTnI: cardiac troponin I; eGFR: estimated glomerular filtration rate; IL-6: interleukin 6; IQR: interquartile range; LDH: lactate dehydrogenase; N: number; WBC: white blood cell count. (1) *p*-value comparing cTnI < 19 ng/L vs. 19 ≤ cTnI ≤ 100 ng/L. (2) *p*-value comparing cTnI < 19 ng/L vs. cTnI > 100 ng/L. (3) *p*-value comparing 19 ≤ cTnI ≤ 100 ng/L vs. cTnI > 100 ng/L. Reference values: haemoglobin: 128–160 g/L (for males), 117–145 g/L (for females); WBC: 4.0–9.8 $\times 10^9$/L; neutrophils: 1.5–6.0 $\times 10^9$/L; lymphocytes: 1.0–4.0 $\times 10^9$/L; platelets: 140–450 $\times 10^9$/L; glucose: 4.2–6.1 mmol/L; creatinine: 64–104 µmol/L (for males), 49–90 µmol/L (for females); eGFR: >90 mL/min/1.73 m^2; urea: 2.5–7.5 mmol/L; sodium: 134–145 mmol/L; potassium: 3.8–5.3 mmol/L; ALT: ≤40 U/L; AST: ≤40 U/L; LDH: 125–243 U/L; CRP: <5 mg/L; ferritin: 25–350 µg/L (for men), 13–232 µg/L (for women); IL-6: 0–7 ng/L; D-dimer: <250 µg/L.

Remdesivir was administered to 711 (35.22%) patients upon admission or the following day for a standard 5-day course (IQR 5 days). Patients with normal cTnI levels and those with cTnI levels of 19–100 ng/L were more likely to receive remdesivir than those with cTnI levels above 100 ng/L at 36.23% and 37.59%, respectively, compared to 20.93% ($p < 0.001$ for both comparisons).

Systemic steroids were administered to 1371 (67.90%) patients, with the majority (97.67%) being treated with dexamethasone for a median duration of 9 days (IQR 6–10 days).

Fewer patients with cTnI levels greater than 100 ng/L received steroids compared to those with cTnI levels of 19–100 ng/L (55.23% vs. 73.09%, $p < 0.001$) and those with normal cTnI levels (55.23% vs. 67.87%, $p = 0.001$).

A total of 1514 (74.99%) patients received antibiotics. The most commonly administered antibiotics were amoxicillin and clavulanic acid, which were used in 1269 of the 1514 cases (83.82%). Other antibiotics were prescribed less frequently—piperacillin and tazobactam—in 454 cases (29.99%) and azithromycin in 120 cases (7.93%). Antibiotic use was less frequent in patients with cTnI levels greater than 100 ng/L compared to those with cTnI levels of 19–100 ng/L (65.12% vs. 77.96%, $p = 0.001$) and also compared to patients with normal cTnI levels (65.12% vs. 77.96%, $p = 0.004$).

The need for IMV was highest in patients with cTnI levels above 100 ng/L at 25% compared to 15.31% in those with cTnI levels between 19 and 100 ng/L, and 4.31% in patients with normal cTnI levels (Table 2). Among patients with cTnI 19–100 ng/L, the odds ratio (OR) for IMV was 3.18 (95% CI 2.11–4.79, $p < 0.001$); in those with cTnI levels above 100 ng/L, the OR was 5.38 (95% CI 3.26–8.88, $p < 0.001$) compared to patients presenting normal cTnI levels on admission. Other risk factors for IMV were male sex (OR 1.49, 95% CI 1.04–2.12, $p = 0.029$) and CHF (OR 2.85, 95% CI 1.82–4.45, $p < 0.001$).

The in-hospital mortality rate was highest among patients with cTnI levels above 100 ng/L at 37.79% compared to 24.59% in those with cTnI levels of 19–100 ng/L and 5.37% in patients with normal cTnI levels.

Cox regression analysis revealed that the hazard ratio (HR) for 30-day in-hospital mortality for patients with cTnI levels of 19–100 ng/L upon admission was 2.58 (95% CI 1.83–3.62, $p < 0.001$), and for those with cTnI levels above 100 ng/L, the HR was 2.97 (95% CI 2.01–4.39, $p < 0.001$) compared to those with normal cTnI levels (Figure 3).

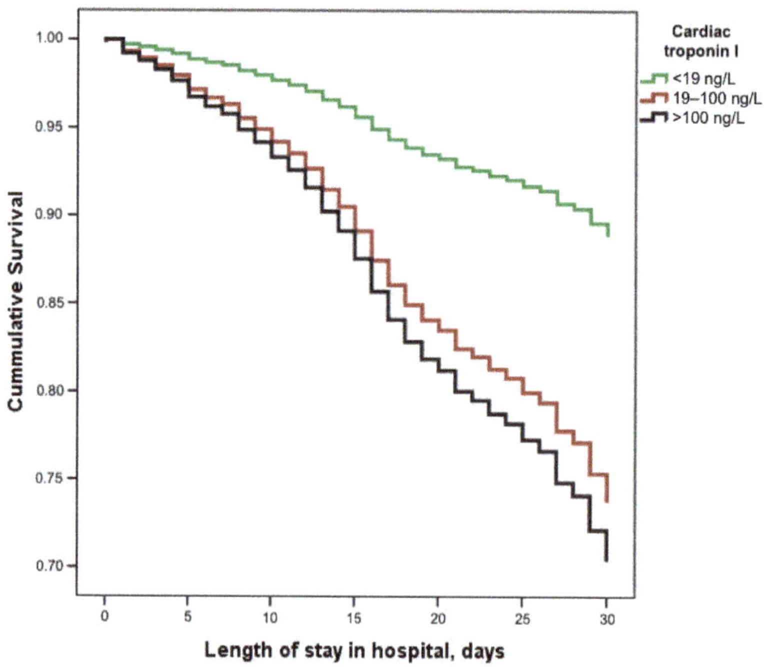

Figure 3. Survival of hospitalised COVID-19 patients stratified by cardiac troponin I concentration.

Other risk factors associated with an increased HR for 30-day in-hospital mortality included age, CHF, obesity, and previous stroke. Treatment with remdesivir was associated with a reduced HR for 30-day in-hospital mortality: HR 0.61 (95% CI 0.43–0.86, $p = 0.005$) (Table 4).

Table 4. Hazards ratio for 30 days in-hospital mortality in hospitalised COVID-19 patients.

Characteristic	In-Hospital Mortality	
	HR (95% CI)	***p*-Value**
TnI < 19 ng/L	Reference	
19 ≤ TnI ≤ 100 ng/L	2.58 (1.83–3.62)	<0.001
TnI > 100 ng/L	2.97 (2.01–4.39)	<0.001
Age in years	1.05 (1.03–1.06)	<0.001
Arterial hypertension	0.71 (0.53–0.95)	0.019
Coronary artery disease	1.03 (0.63–1.67)	0.906
Congestive heart failure	1.81 (1.33–2.46)	<0.001
Atrial fibrillation	1.45 (1.06–1.98)	0.021
Diabetes	0.92 (0.66–1.29)	0.636
Obesity	2.40 (1.50–3.84)	<0.001
COPD	1.75 (0.96–3.18)	0.068
Chronic kidney disease	0.70 (0.46–1.05)	0.083
Previous stroke	1.67 (0.88–3.16)	0.114
Treatment with remdesivir	0.61 (0.43–0.86)	0.005
Treatment with systemic steroids	1.40 (1.00–1.96)	0.051
Antibiotics	0.85 (0.59–1.24)	0.413

COPD: chronic obstructive pulmonary disease; cTnI: cardiac troponin I; HR: hazard ratio.

4. Discussion

Several viral infections are identified as potential causes of heart damage. These include enteroviruses (Coxsackie B viruses, echoviruses, and poliovirus), herpesviruses (human herpes virus 6, Epstein–Barr virus, cytomegalovirus, and varicella zoster virus); parvoviruses (such as parvovirus B19); adenoviruses; influenza viruses; retroviruses (human immunodeficiency virus (HIV)); and coronaviruses [11,12]. In addition, accumulating data suggest that hepatitis C virus may also contribute to heart diseases [13]. Viruses can damage the heart through various mechanisms, including direct virus-mediated damage to cardiomyocytes (Coxsackievirus B, Epstein–Barr virus, cytomegalovirus, and HIV); endothelial cells (human herpes virus 6, parvovirus B19, and cytomegalovirus); and fibroblasts (cytomegalovirus). During the acute phase of infection, SARS-CoV-2 can cause direct cardiac injury by interacting with the ACE-2 receptor on cardiomyocytes, pericytes, macrophages, fibroblasts, and endothelial cells [1,2]. Moreover, viruses can cause heart damage through an immune response, which may result from the development of autoimmune myocarditis or excessive cytokine production [11]. In our research, we focused on myocardial injury caused by SARS-CoV-2 and analysed the data of one of the largest hospitals in Lithuania from March 2020, when the first COVID-19 patient was admitted to the hospital, until May 2021. In the initial stages of the pandemic, until the autumn of 2020, no single SARS-CoV-2 lineage clearly dominated in Lithuania. By the end of 2020, the B.1.177.60 lineage began to spread. Subsequently, this lineage was overtaken by the B.1.1.7 (alpha variant) and its localised version Q.1., which dominated until June 2021 [14].

In our single-centre retrospective cohort study of 2019 hospitalised COVID-19 patients, several key observations were made: (1) myocardial injury was quite common among patients hospitalised with COVID-19, affecting nearly 30% of patients, but in the majority of cases, it was associated with low-level elevations in cTnI concentrations; (2) age, male sex, the presence of CHF, AF, obesity, and CKD were associated with the development of acute myocardial injury; (3) patients with acute myocardial injury exhibited higher levels of inflammatory biomarkers; and (4) more significant myocardial injury was associated with a five-fold higher risk of requiring invasive mechanical ventilation and nearly a three-fold higher risk of in-hospital mortality.

The detection of elevated myocardial injury markers, particularly cTnI, has garnered considerable scientific interest due to its widespread measurement in various healthcare settings and its clinical significance [15–18]. Numerous studies have reported myocardial injury, defining it as troponin elevation above the 99th percentile of the upper reference limit, with varying prevalence rates based on the population studied. For instance, Lala et al., in a study involving 2736 hospitalised COVID-19 patients, found a 36% prevalence of myocardial injury [16]. De Marzo et al. reported a myocardial injury prevalence of 25.7% among individuals exceeding 60 years of age [17], while Shi et al. documented myocardial injury in 19.7% of their study cohort [18]. In alignment with these findings, our research demonstrated that 29.87% of patients admitted to hospital for COVID-19 infection presented with increased cTnI levels. Despite varying prevalence rates of myocardial injury reported across studies, there is a consensus that myocardial injury occurs more frequently in severe or critically ill COVID-19 patients and non-survivors [19–21].

Furthermore, myocardial injury has been found to occur more frequently among older patients with a greater number of comorbidities, particularly chronic cardiovascular conditions [16,18,22,23]. Lala et al. highlighted that patients with more severe myocardial injury had a higher prevalence of cardiovascular diseases, such as coronary artery disease, atrial fibrillation, and heart failure, compared to those with mildly elevated or normal troponin levels [16]. Our research further quantified this risk, showing that age increased the odds ratio for myocardial injury by 1.06 times, male sex by 1.58 times, the presence of CHF by 2.79 times, AF by 1.72 times, obesity by 1.84 times, and CKD by 2.19 times. Similarly, Papageorgiou et al. identified that age (OR 1.68), hypertension (OR 1.81), and moderate CKD (OR 9.12) were independent predictors of myocardial injury [23]. Additionally, Lombardi and colleagues found significant associations between myocardial injury with heart failure (OR 2.01) and a history of coronary artery disease (OR 2.04) [22]. The existence of numerous comorbidities can exacerbate the severity of COVID-19, resulting in more severe myocardial injury.

Our study revealed that patients with myocardial injury presented with elevated levels of WBC, neutrophil count, glucose, creatinine, urea, AST, LDH, CRP, ferritin, IL-6, and D-dimer in comparison to those with normal cTnI levels. This correlation between myocardial injury and an increase in inflammatory and prothrombotic markers is consistent with findings from other researchers. Specifically, myocardial injury patients demonstrated significant rises in inflammatory biomarkers such as CRP [18,22,24] and thrombotic indicators like D-dimer [22–24]. Moreover, Li et al. identified correlations between high sensitivity cTnI levels and IL-6 ($r = 0.59$ to 0.66, $p < 0.001$), CRP ($r = 0.54$ to 0.62, $p < 0.001$), and D-dimer ($r = 0.54$ to 0.65, $p < 0.001$) at various stages: upon admission, within the first week, and after the first week of hospitalisation, further underscoring the link between cardiac injury and systemic inflammation and thrombosis in this patient population [20].

In our study, 35% of patients received treatment with remdesivir, and this treatment was associated with a 1.64-fold reduction in HR for 30-day in-hospital mortality. These findings are consistent with prior research, indicating that remdesivir administration is linked to improved time to recovery and potentially reduced mortality rates [25]. However, this finding should be approached with caution, as remdesivir was more frequently administered to patients with less severe COVID-19 and less severe acute myocardial injury, taking into consideration the reported potential cardiac effects associated with its use, such as hypotension, bradycardia, and prolonged QTc interval, that are more frequently observed in patients with COVID-19 and concomitant cardiovascular diseases [7,26,27]. Randomised controlled trials have provided strong evidence supporting the beneficial therapeutic effect of corticosteroids in COVID-19 patients requiring oxygen therapy, with no impact on cardiovascular events [28,29]. Our study demonstrated that patients with more severe acute myocardial injury were less frequently administered systemic steroids and that treatment with systemic steroids had no effect on the HR for 30-day mortality.

Our study revealed a 3.18-fold increase in the odds ratio for IMV and a 2.58-fold increase in the hazard ratio for 30-day in-hospital mortality among patients with cTnI levels between 19 and 100 ng/L. Higher cTnI levels correlated with even greater increases, up to 5.38 times for the OR for IMV and up to 2.97 times for the HR for in-hospital mortality. These findings are in close agreement with those of Lala et al., who observed a 3.03-fold increase in the HR for mortality (95% CI 2.42–3.80) in patients with troponin levels more than three times the upper reference limit, although in an older study population with higher incidences of coronary artery disease (CAD) and heart failure at 16.6% and 10.1%, respectively [16]. Similarly, Shi et al. noted a higher mortality risk in patients with myocardial injury, with a HR of 3.41 [18]. Papageorgiou et al. identified that patients with elevated troponin levels were significantly more likely to require non-invasive and IMV (with ORs of 2.40 and 6.81, respectively) to develop acute kidney injury (with 6.76-times higher odds), to necessitate urgent renal replacement therapy (with 4.14-times higher odds), to experience thromboembolic events (with 11.99-times higher odds), and to die (with 2.40-times higher odds) compared to patients with normal troponin levels [23].

The role of elevated cTnI levels as a critical prognostic marker for severe outcomes in COVID-19, including the necessity for IMV and higher mortality rates, has sparked discussions on its potential integration into routine diagnostics and its implications for tailoring treatment approaches for patients with myocardial injury [30,31]. Sandoval et al. proposed a structured method for leveraging cTnI in risk stratification. An initial cTnI measurement could be instrumental in the early classification of COVID-19 patients, aiding in their preliminary assessment. Patients deemed clinically stable or marginally stable yet presenting with significant laboratory anomalies such as elevated cTnI levels are categorised at an intermediate risk level. Conversely, patients who are clinically unstable with notable laboratory abnormalities fall into the high-risk category and necessitate hospital admission. For hospitalised patients, repeated cTnI monitoring is recommended. Individuals whose cTnI levels remain stable and do not exhibit significant increases might not require further interventions. On the other hand, patients exhibiting escalating cTnI levels should be subjected to more in-depth evaluations and potentially more intensive therapeutic interventions [19].

We acknowledge that our study has several limitations. Firstly, the identification of comorbidities relied on ICD-10-AM codes encoded in medical records, which might not have captured all relevant conditions. Another issue was the absence of data regarding the duration of COVID-19 symptoms prior to hospitalisation, which prevented the specification of the time of myocardial injury and the more precise evaluation of the potential mechanism of the myocardial injury in regard to its relation to virus-mediated or immune-mediated damage and evolution over time. The dataset did not include the dates of hospitalisation, which did not allow for the analysis of acute myocardial damage across various COVID-19 pandemic waves. Conducted in the largest hospital of the capital of Lithuania, the single-centre nature of this study may lead to selection bias and limit the applicability of the results to wider populations. The specific healthcare practices, patient demographics, and treatment approaches of this hospital may not accurately reflect those of the broader population. Furthermore, our retrospective study's design did not allow for the assessment of the long-term effects of acute myocardial injury in COVID-19 patients, as it focused on short-term outcomes during the hospital stay and not addressing the potential prolonged impact of acute myocardial injury beyond the acute phase of the infection.

5. Conclusions

Cardiac troponin I serves as an effective biomarker for risk stratification in COVID-19 patients upon admission. Increased levels of cardiac troponin I, indicating myocardial injury, on admission are associated with a more adverse clinical disease course, including a higher likelihood of the need for invasive mechanical ventilation and increased risk of in-hospital mortality. This indicates cardiac troponin I to be a beneficial biomarker for clinicians trying to identify high-risk COVID-19 patients, choosing the optimal monitoring and treatment strategy for these patients.

Author Contributions: I.K., Conceptualisation, Writing—original draft preparation, Methodology, and Writing—review and editing; J.U., Conceptualisation, Formal analysis, Writing—original draft preparation, and Writing—review and editing; E.B., Writing—original draft preparation and Visualisation; F.M., Writing—review and editing; L.S., Writing—review and editing; L.J., Writing—review and editing and Supervision. All authors participated in manuscript writing. All authors have read and agreed to the published version of the manuscript.

Funding: This research received no external funding.

Institutional Review Board Statement: Ethical review and approval were waived for this study, as the research involved the use of depersonalised and pseudonymised clinical data.

Informed Consent Statement: The use of depersonalised and pseudonymised clinical data made it unnecessary to obtain patient informed consent, as the data processing ensured privacy and confidentiality, eliminating potential ethical concerns related to personal data identification.

Data Availability Statement: The data presented in this study are available on request from the corresponding author.

Conflicts of Interest: The authors declare no conflicts of interest.

References

1. Fairweather, D.; Beetler, D.J.; Di Florio, D.N.; Musigk, N.; Heidecker, B.; Cooper, L.T. COVID-19, Myocarditis and Pericarditis. *Circ. Res.* **2023**, *132*, 1302–1319. [CrossRef] [PubMed]
2. Devaux, C.A.; Camoin-Jau, L. An update on angiotensin-converting enzyme 2 structure/functions, polymorphism, and duplicitous nature in the pathophysiology of coronavirus disease 2019: Implications for vascular and coagulation disease associated with severe acute respiratory syndrome coronavirus infection. *Front. Microbiol.* **2022**, *13*, 1042200. [CrossRef] [PubMed]
3. Lindner, D.; Fitzek, A.; Bräuninger, H.; Aleshcheva, G.; Edler, C.; Meissner, K.; Scherschel, K.; Kirchhof, P.; Escher, F.; Schultheiss, H.-P.; et al. Association of Cardiac Infection with SARS-CoV-2 in Confirmed COVID-19 Autopsy Cases. *JAMA Cardiol.* **2020**, *5*, 1281. [CrossRef] [PubMed]
4. Bearse, M.; Hung, Y.P.; Krauson, A.J.; Bonanno, L.; Boyraz, B.; Harris, C.K.; Helland, T.L.; Hilburn, C.F.; Hutchison, B.; Jobbagy, S.; et al. Factors associated with myocardial SARS-CoV-2 infection, myocarditis, and cardiac inflammation in patients with COVID-19. *Mod. Pathol.* **2021**, *34*, 1345–1357. [CrossRef] [PubMed]
5. Terzic, C.M.; Medina-Inojosa, B.J. Cardiovascular Complications of Coronavirus Disease-2019. *Phys. Med. Rehabil. Clin. North Am.* **2023**, *34*, 551–561. [CrossRef] [PubMed]
6. Liu, F.; Liu, F.; Wang, L. COVID-19 and cardiovascular diseases. *J. Mol. Cell Biol.* **2021**, *13*, 161–167. [CrossRef] [PubMed]
7. Vosko, I.; Zirlik, A.; Bugger, H. Impact of COVID-19 on Cardiovascular Disease. *Viruses* **2023**, *15*, 508. [CrossRef] [PubMed]
8. Nandy, S.; Wan, S.-H.; Brenes-Salazar, J. Cardiovascular Manifestations of COVID-19. *CCR* **2021**, *17*, e230421187503. [CrossRef] [PubMed]
9. Kubiliute, I.; Vitkauskaite, M.; Urboniene, J.; Svetikas, L.; Zablockiene, B.; Jancoriene, L. Clinical characteristics and predictors for in-hospital mortality in adult COVID-19 patients: A retrospective single center cohort study in Vilnius, Lithuania. *PLoS ONE* **2023**, *18*, e0290656. [CrossRef]
10. Thygesen, K.; Alpert, J.S.; Jaffe, A.S.; Chaitman, B.R.; Bax, J.J.; Morrow, D.A.; White, H.D.; Executive Group on behalf of the Joint European Society of Cardiology (ESC)/American College of Cardiology (ACC)/American Heart Association (AHA)/World Heart Federation (WHF) Task Force for the Universal Definition of Myocardial Infarction. Fourth Universal Definition of Myocardial Infarction (2018). *J. Am. Coll. Cardiol.* **2018**, *72*, 2231–2264. [CrossRef]
11. Martens, C.R.; Accornero, F. Viruses in the Heart: Direct and Indirect Routes to Myocarditis and Heart Failure. *Viruses* **2021**, *13*, 1924. [CrossRef] [PubMed]
12. Schultheiss, H.P.; Baumeier, C.; Pietsch, H.; Bock, C.T.; Poller, W.; Escher, F. Cardiovascular consequences of viral infections: From COVID to other viral diseases. *Cardiovasc. Res.* **2021**, *117*, 2610–2623. [CrossRef] [PubMed]
13. Ilyas, S.Z.; Tabassum, R.; Hamed, H.; Rehman, S.U.; Qadri, I. Hepatitis C Virus-Associated Extrahepatic Manifestations in Lung and Heart and Antiviral Therapy-Related Cardiopulmonary Toxicity. *Viral Immunol.* **2017**, *30*, 633–641. [CrossRef] [PubMed]
14. Zemaitis, L.; Alzbutas, G.; Gecyte, E.; Gecys, D.; Lesauskaite, V. SARS-CoV-2: Two Years in the Pandemic: What Have We Observed from Genome Sequencing Results in Lithuania? *Microorganisms* **2022**, *10*, 1229. [CrossRef]
15. Battaglini, D.; Lopes-Pacheco, M.; Castro-Faria-Neto, H.C.; Pelosi, P.; Rocco, P.R.M. Laboratory Biomarkers for Diagnosis and Prognosis in COVID-19. *Front. Immunol.* **2022**, *13*, 857573. [CrossRef]

16. Lala, A.; Johnson, K.W.; Januzzi, J.L.; Russak, A.J.; Paranjpe, I.; Richter, F.; Zhao, S.; Somani, S.; Van Vleck, T.; Vaid, A.; et al. Prevalence and Impact of Myocardial Injury in Patients Hospitalized with COVID-19 Infection. *J. Am. Coll. Cardiol.* **2020**, *76*, 533–546. [CrossRef] [PubMed]
17. De Marzo, V.; Di Biagio, A.; Della Bona, R.; Vena, A.; Arboscello, E.; Emirjona, H.; Mora, S.; Giacomini, M.; Da Rin, G.; Pelosi, P.; et al. Prevalence and prognostic value of cardiac troponin in elderly patients hospitalized for COVID-19. *J. Geriatr. Cardiol.* **2021**, *18*, 338–345. [CrossRef] [PubMed]
18. Shi, S.; Qin, M.; Shen, B.; Cai, Y.; Liu, T.; Yang, F.; Gong, W.; Liu, X.; Liang, J.; Zhao, Q.; et al. Association of Cardiac Injury with Mortality in Hospitalized Patients with COVID-19 in Wuhan, China. *JAMA Cardiol.* **2020**, *5*, 802. [CrossRef] [PubMed]
19. Sandoval, Y.; Januzzi, J.L.; Jaffe, A.S. Cardiac Troponin for Assessment of Myocardial Injury in COVID-19. *J. Am. Coll. Cardiol.* **2020**, *76*, 1244–1258. [CrossRef]
20. Li, C.; Jiang, J.; Wang, F.; Zhou, N.; Veronese, G.; Moslehi, J.J.; Ammirati, E.; Wang, D.W. Longitudinal correlation of biomarkers of cardiac injury, inflammation, and coagulation to outcome in hospitalized COVID-19 patients. *J. Mol. Cell. Cardiol.* **2020**, *147*, 74–87. [CrossRef]
21. Metkus, T.S.; Sokoll, L.J.; Barth, A.S.; Czarny, M.J.; Hays, A.G.; Lowenstein, C.J.; Michos, E.D.; Nolley, E.P.; Post, W.S.; Resar, J.R.; et al. Myocardial Injury in Severe COVID-19 Compared with Non–COVID-19 Acute Respiratory Distress Syndrome. *Circulation* **2021**, *143*, 553–565. [CrossRef]
22. Lombardi, C.M.; Carubelli, V.; Iorio, A.; Inciardi, R.M.; Bellasi, A.; Canale, C.; Camporotondo, R.; Catagnano, F.; Dalla Vecchia, L.A.; Giovinazzo, S.; et al. Association of Troponin Levels with Mortality in Italian Patients Hospitalized with Coronavirus Disease 2019: Results of a Multicenter Study. *JAMA Cardiol.* **2020**, *5*, 1274. [CrossRef] [PubMed]
23. Papageorgiou, N.; Sohrabi, C.; Merino, D.P.; Tyrlis, A.; Atieh, A.E.; Saberwal, B.; Lim, W.-Y.; Creta, A.; Khanji, M.; Rusinova, R.; et al. High sensitivity troponin and COVID-19 outcomes. *Acta Cardiol.* **2022**, *77*, 81–88. [CrossRef] [PubMed]
24. Guo, T.; Fan, Y.; Chen, M.; Wu, X.; Zhang, L.; He, T.; Wang, H.; Wan, J.; Wang, X.; Lu, Z. Cardiovascular Implications of Fatal Outcomes of Patients with Coronavirus Disease 2019 (COVID-19). *JAMA Cardiol.* **2020**, *5*, 811. [CrossRef] [PubMed]
25. Davies, M.; Osborne, V.; Lane, S.; Roy, D.; Dhanda, S.; Evans, A.; Shakir, S. Remdesivir in Treatment of COVID-19: A Systematic Benefit-Risk Assessment. *Drug Saf.* **2020**, *43*, 645–656. [CrossRef] [PubMed]
26. Nabati, M.; Parsaee, H. Potential Cardiotoxic Effects of Remdesivir on Cardiovascular System: A Literature Review. *Cardiovasc. Toxicol.* **2022**, *22*, 268–272. [CrossRef] [PubMed]
27. Rafaniello, C.; Ferrajolo, C.; Sullo, M.G.; Gaio, M.; Zinzi, A.; Scavone, C.; Gargano, F.; Coscioni, E.; Rossi, F.; Capuano, A. Cardiac Events Potentially Associated to Remdesivir: An Analysis from the European Spontaneous Adverse Event Reporting System. *Pharmaceuticals* **2021**, *14*, 611. [CrossRef] [PubMed]
28. RECOVERY Collaborative Group; Horby, P.; Lim, W.S.; Emberson, J.R.; Mafham, M.; Bell, J.L.; Linsell, L.; Staplin, N.; Brightling, C.; Ustianowski, A.; et al. Dexamethasone in Hospitalized Patients with COVID-19. *N. Engl. J. Med.* **2021**, *384*, 693–704. [CrossRef] [PubMed]
29. Caiazzo, E.; Rezig, A.O.M.; Bruzzese, D.; Ialenti, A.; Cicala, C.; Cleland, J.G.F.; Guzik, T.J.; Maffia, P.; Pellicori, P. Systemic administration of glucocorticoids, cardiovascular complications and mortality in patients hospitalised with COVID-19, SARS, MERS or influenza: A systematic review and meta-analysis of randomised trials. *Pharmacol. Res.* **2022**, *176*, 106053. [CrossRef]
30. Chapman, A.R.; Bularga, A.; Mills, N.L. High-Sensitivity Cardiac Troponin Can Be an Ally in the Fight against COVID-19. *Circulation* **2020**, *141*, 1733–1735. [CrossRef]
31. De Michieli, L.; Jaffe, A.S.; Sandoval, Y. Use and Prognostic Implications of Cardiac Troponin in COVID-19. *Cardiol. Clin.* **2022**, *40*, 287–300. [CrossRef] [PubMed]

medicina

MDPI

Article

Lung Ultrasound Efficacy in Monitoring Post-SARS-CoV-2 Pneumonia and Inflammatory Biomarkers in Pediatric Patients

Ramona Chelcea [1], Mihaela Dediu [2], Diana Dabica [1], Sorina Maria Denisa Laitin [3,*] and Ioana Mihaiela Ciuca [2]

1 Doctoral School, "Victor Babes" University of Medicine and Pharmacy, Eftimie Murgu Square 2, 300041 Timisoara, Romania; ramona.chelcea@umft.ro (R.C.); diana.popin@umft.ro (D.D.)
2 Department of Pediatrics, "Victor Babes" University of Medicine and Pharmacy, Eftimie Murgu Square 2, 300041 Timisoara, Romania; dediu.mihaela@umft.ro (M.D.); ciuca.ioana@umft.ro (I.M.C.)
3 Discipline of Epidemiology, Victor Babes University of Medicine and Pharmacy, 300041 Timisoara, Romania
* Correspondence: laitin.sorina@umft.ro

Abstract: *Background and Objectives*: Recognizing the crucial gaps in our understanding of pediatric pneumonia post-SARS-CoV-2 infection, this study aimed to assess the relationship between Pediatric Pneumonia Ultrasound Scores (PedPne) and inflammatory biomarkers. The primary objective of this study is to evaluate the predictive value of PedPne in comparison with inflammatory biomarkers (IL-6 and dNLR) for the development of pneumonia in pediatric patients following SARS-CoV-2 infection. *Materials and Methods*: This longitudinal observational study collected data from pediatric patients diagnosed with pneumonia after an acute SARS-CoV2 infection. The study focused on analyzing changes in PedPne scores and inflammatory markers such as IL-6 and dNLR from initial admission to follow-up at 7 days. Statistical analysis involved calculating the sensitivity, specificity, and Area Under the Curve (AUC) for each biomarker, alongside regression analysis to determine their hazard ratios for predicting pneumonia development. *Results*: The analysis identified significant cutoff values for dNLR at 1.88 (sensitivity 77.0%, specificity 85.7%, AUC 0.802, $p < 0.001$), IL-6 at 6.1 pg/mL (sensitivity 70.3%, specificity 92.9%, AUC 0.869, $p < 0.001$), and PedPne score at 3.3 (sensitivity 75.7%, specificity 78.6%, AUC 0.794, $p < 0.001$). Conversely, NLR showed lower diagnostic performance (AUC 0.485, $p = 0.327$). Regression analysis further highlighted the strong predictive power of these markers, with IL-6 showing a fourfold increase in pneumonia risk (HR = 4.25, CI: 2.07–9.53, $p < 0.001$), dNLR indicating more than a twofold increase (HR = 2.53, CI: 1.19–6.97, $p = 0.006$), and PedPne score associated with more than a doubling of the risk (HR = 2.60, CI: 1.33–5.18, $p < 0.001$). *Conclusions*: The study conclusively demonstrated that both PedPne ultrasound scores and specific inflammatory biomarkers such as dNLR and IL-6 are significant predictors of pneumonia development in pediatric patients post-COVID-19 infection. These findings advocate for the integration of these biomarkers in routine clinical assessments to enhance the diagnostic accuracy and management of pneumonia in children following SARS-CoV-2 infection.

Keywords: pediatrics; pediatric disease; SARS-CoV-2

1. Introduction

Recent studies have underscored the heightened risk of developing secondary bacterial pneumonia after a primary viral infection such as SARS-CoV-2 [1,2]. This type of pneumonia, often severe, necessitates a better understanding of its pathogenesis and diagnostic markers. Reports indicate that approximately 15% of hospitalized COVID-19 patients develop secondary pneumonia, characterized by persistent fever, worsening respiratory symptoms, and new infiltrates on chest imaging, which complicates the clinical course and can significantly extend hospital stay and increase mortality [3–5].

Chest ultrasound has emerged as a vital tool in pediatric pneumonia, offering a radiation-free alternative to traditional imaging techniques like chest X-rays and CT scans [6,7]. Its application has proven particularly valuable in assessing lung involvement and guiding treatment decisions in real time. The Pediatric Pneumonia Ultrasound Score (PedPne) is a quantifiable measure that has been correlated with clinical outcomes, allowing clinicians to monitor disease progression and response to treatment with greater precision [8].

Inflammatory biomarkers also play a crucial role in the diagnosis and management of infectious diseases, including pneumonia. Markers such as C-reactive protein (CRP), procalcitonin, and interleukin-6 (IL-6) have been widely studied for their ability to indicate the presence and severity of infection, where elevated levels have been associated with worse outcomes in respiratory infections, reflecting the intensity of the inflammatory response triggered by pathogens [9–11].

Despite the established roles of ultrasound scoring and inflammatory markers, there is a notable gap in longitudinal studies that integrate these parameters in the context of post-SARS-CoV-2 pneumonia [12,13]. Furthermore, there is an important focus in examining the correlation between ultrasound findings and inflammatory markers over the course of the illness and during recovery [14,15]. As such, an integrated approach utilizing both PedPne ultrasound scores and inflammatory biomarkers could provide a comprehensive assessment of pneumonia's impact and progression, potentially leading to more tailored and effective treatment strategies.

Given the critical gaps in our understanding and the potential of ultrasound and biomarker integration, this study hypothesizes that a significant correlation exists between PedPne ultrasound scores and inflammatory biomarkers in pediatric patients developing pneumonia post-SARS-CoV-2 infection. The objectives of this study are to analyze the changes in PedPne scores and inflammatory markers from the initial presentation to the subsequent follow-up at 7 days of treatment, and to evaluate how these measurements correlate with pneumonia development. Pediatric pneumonia post-SARS-CoV-2 infection poses unique diagnostic challenges due to its variable symptoms and overlap with other respiratory infections, often leading to delayed treatment [16–18]. This study addresses these challenges by assessing the utility of PedPne and inflammatory biomarkers, aiming to enhance early diagnosis and management. Integrating these tools into clinical practice can improve diagnostic accuracy, enable timely interventions, and ultimately reduce morbidity and healthcare burdens associated with pediatric respiratory infections.

2. Materials and Methods

2.1. Study Design and Ethics

This longitudinal observational study evaluates the correlation between PedPne and inflammatory biomarkers in pediatric patients who developed pneumonia following SARS-CoV-2 infection. The study cohort comprises patients evaluated in outpatient settings at Pediatric Pulmonology Ward of the Pediatric Clinic, Clinical County Hospital Timisoara, between September 2022 and April 2024, presenting pneumonia signs, who had previously been diagnosed with SARS-CoV2 infection. The research protocol involved collecting data at initial presentation for hospital admission and during follow-up visits at 7–10 days of treatment. Data collection was carried out through both electronic health records and direct clinical assessments.

This study has received approval from the institutional Ethic Committee (number 461/18.04.2024), of Clinical County Hospital Timisoara adhering to the ethical standards set by the Declaration of Helsinki and the EU Good Clinical Practice Directive (2005/28/EC). All patient information was anonymized prior to analysis to ensure confidentiality. Additionally, written informed consent was obtained from the legal guardians of all participants, confirming compliance with ethical requirements.

2.2. Inclusion and Exclusion Criteria

Inclusion criteria for the study required participants to have a confirmed diagnosis of SARS-CoV-2 infection, established through RT-PCR testing, and subsequent development of pneumonia, identified through clinical and ultrasound findings. All participants were pediatric patients admitted to the outpatient or inpatient services of the pediatric clinic during the specified study period. Eligibility also depended on the availability of comprehensive medical records, including detailed ultrasound evaluations, inflammatory biomarker levels (e.g., CRP, procalcitonin), and clinical outcomes.

Exclusion criteria included patients who did not develop pneumonia following SARS-CoV-2 infection, those who had pre-existing lung diseases that could confound the ultrasound and biomarker results, and patients whose legal guardians did not provide written consent for participation in the study. Additionally, patients with incomplete data sets, such as missing follow-up ultrasound scores or biomarker results, were excluded to maintain the integrity of the research findings.

2.3. Data Collection and Variables

For our study, we systematically collected and analyzed variables from pediatric patients hospitalized with COVID-19, focusing on differences between those with and without pneumonia. The primary demographic variable was age, categorized into three groups: 1–6 years, 7–12 years, and 13–18 years. Additionally, body mass index (BMI) and vitamin D levels were measured to explore their potential influence on the disease severity. We included clinical and laboratory data, assessing initial and subsequent changes at 7 days post-hospitalization. Key inflammatory markers were evaluated, including C-reactive protein (CRP), procalcitonin, interleukin-6 (IL-6), white blood cell (WBC) count, percentages of neutrophils, and erythrocyte sedimentation rate (ESR). Ferritin levels and derived neutrophil-to-lymphocyte ratio (dNLR) were also calculated to provide insights into the systemic inflammatory response. Additionally, previously data on SARS-CoV2-specific immunoglobulins M and G were collected from patients' data. General immunoglobulin levels (IgG, IgM, IgA, IgE) were measured in patients with pneumonia. Pediatric pneumonia severity was quantitatively assessed using the Pediatric Pneumonia Ultrasound Score (PedPne US) at first evaluation and after 7 to 10 days to monitor progression or resolution of pneumonia.

In the study protocol, lung ultrasound was performed at admission by a pediatric pulmonologist proficient in LUS techniques, using a Venue Go™ by GE HealthCare (Chicago, Illinois, USA) ultrasound system with both linear (7–12 MHz) and convex (3.5–5 MHz) probes. The ultrasound examination involved scanning through longitudinal and transversal sections across various anatomical lines and included a transabdominal approach for deeper insights. The lung was sectioned into six areas for detailed analysis, and specific ultrasound artifacts like the presence of consolidation and pleural effusion were quantified. The diagnostic criteria included hypoechoic images erasing A-lines, dynamic bronchograms, and B-line patterns with specified points assigned based on the severity and nature of the findings in the PedPne score.

The PedPne score, a systematic tool for assessing pediatric pneumonia severity using lung ultrasound, is quantified based on specific ultrasound findings reflecting lung pathology [19]. The score incorporates several diagnostic features: perilesional B-lines (more than three B-lines per intercostal space score 1 point and coalescent B-lines score 2 points), varying sizes of lung consolidations (non-translobar consolidations smaller than 2 cm score 3 points, larger than 2 cm score 4 points, and translobar consolidations score 5 points), and pleural effusions (simple pleural effusion scores 6 points, complicated nonseptated pleural effusion scores 7 points, complex septate pleural effusion scores 8 points, and homogenous hyperechoic effusion or empyema scores 9 points). Each of these elements is assessed during a detailed lung ultrasound, where each hemithorax was divided into six areas, and each lung feature was scored according to its severity and diagnostic impact on pediatric pneumonia.

2.4. Statistics

Data management and analysis were carried out using the statistical software R version 4.0.3. A sample size of minimum 62 patients was calculated as being sufficient for the current study. Continuous variables were presented as means ± standard deviation (SD), while categorical variables were summarized using frequencies and percentages. To compare the means of continuous data across groups, the study employed Student's *t*-test, whereas categorical data comparisons were made using the Chi-square test. For the key laboratory markers under study, the optimal cutoff values were determined using receiver operating characteristic (ROC) curves, from which the sensitivity, specificity, and Area Under the Curve (AUC) were calculated to evaluate their predictive power. Additionally, regression analysis was conducted to ascertain the hazard ratios for pneumonia development based on the biomarkers crossing their respective cutoff values. The significance level was set at a *p*-value of less than 0.05.

3. Results

The study retrospectively analyzed the background characteristics of children hospitalized with and without pneumonia following SARS-CoV-2 infection. Age and vitamin D levels were compared between the two groups, with children having pneumonia tending to be older (mean ± SD: 6.67 ± 5.01 years) than those without pneumonia (mean ± SD: 5.04 ± 3.95 years), although this difference was not statistically significant ($p = 0.121$). The distribution of children across age categories also did not significantly differ between the groups ($p = 0.372$), with a higher percentage of older children (13–18 years) in the pneumonia group (19.4%) compared to those without pneumonia (7.7%). Similarly, no significant differences were observed in the body mass index (BMI) ($p = 0.742$) and vitamin D levels ($p = 0.110$) between the groups.

Significantly higher Pediatric Pneumonia Ultrasound (PedPne US) scores were observed in children with pneumonia both at initial assessment and after 7 days of hospitalization. Initially, the mean PedPne US score was substantially higher in the pneumonia group (3.89 ± 1.08) compared to the no pneumonia group (1.93 ± 0.27), with this difference reaching statistical significance ($p < 0.001$). Similarly, after 7 days, children with pneumonia showed a significant increase in the mean PedPne US score (0.99 ± 0.74) compared to those without pneumonia (0.21 ± 0.43), again demonstrating a significant association ($p < 0.001$), as presented in Table 1.

Table 1. Background characteristics of children with and without pneumonia during COVID-19 hospitalization.

Variables	No Pneumonia (*n* = 28)	Pneumonia (*n* = 38)	*p*-Value
Age, years (mean ± SD)	5.04 ± 3.95	6.67 ± 5.01	0.121
Age category			0.372
1–6 years	15 (53.8%)	17 (47.2%)	
7–12 years	11 (38.5%)	12 (33.3%)	
13–18 years	2 (7.7%)	7 (19.4%)	
BMI (mean ± SD)	17.01 ± 1.94	16.63 ± 3.05	0.742
Vitamin D (mean ± SD)	19.65 ± 6.11	20.52 ± 6.64	0.110
PedPne US initial score (mean ± SD)	1.93 ± 0.27	3.89 ± 1.08	<0.001
PedPne US 7-day score (mean ± SD)	0.21 ± 0.43	0.99 ± 0.74	<0.001

SD—standard deviation; BMI—body mass index; PedPne—pediatric pneumonia; US—ultrasound.

Significant elevations were observed in CRP levels (44.2 ± 51.4 mg/L vs. 18.1 ± 18.1 mg/L, $p = 0.006$), procalcitonin (2.47 ± 1.51 ng/mL vs. 0.69 ± 0.70 ng/mL, $p < 0.001$), interleukin-6 (IL-6) (6.75 ± 6.59 pg/mL vs. 1.43 ± 1.77 pg/mL, $p < 0.001$), and ferritin (80.85 ± 73.51 ng/mL vs. 51.44 ± 33.54 ng/mL, $p = 0.020$). White blood cell (WBC) count, neutrophil percentage, neutrophil-to-lymphocyte ratio (NLR), and derived

NLR (dNLR) also showed significant increases in the pneumonia group. The erythrocyte sedimentation rate (ESR) was notably higher in the pneumonia group (22.4 ± 13.4 mm/h) compared to those without pneumonia (11.1 ± 5.4 mm/h), with a p-value less than 0.001.

COVID-19-specific immunoglobulin M (IgM) levels were considerably higher in children with pneumonia (147.6 ± 75.8 IU/mL) compared to those without (10.9 ± 52.1 IU/mL, $p < 0.001$), indicating a more recent infection; the levels of COVID-19-specific immunoglobulin G (IgG) did not differ significantly ($p = 0.255$). Additionally, significant differences were noted in the levels of IgA ($p = 0.028$) and IgE ($p = 0.002$) (Table 2).

Table 2. Comparison of laboratory findings of children with and without pneumonia during COVID-19 hospitalization (initial measurements).

Variables (Mean ± SD)	Normal Range	No Pneumonia ($n = 28$)	Pneumonia ($n = 38$)	p-Value
Inflammatory markers				
ESR	0–20 mm/h	11.1 ± 5.4	22.4 ± 13.4	<0.001
C-reactive protein	<10 mg/L	18.1 ± 18.1	44.2 ± 51.4	0.006
WBC	4.0–10.0 × 10^9/L	12.5 ± 5.0	14.8 ± 5.9	0.004
Neutrophil %	40–60%	51.0 ± 24.4	62.0 ± 22.3	0.048
Lymphocyte %	20–40%	17.6 ± 17.0	23.0 ± 20.2	0.363
Procalcitonin	<0.5 ng/mL	0.69 ± 0.70	2.47 ± 1.51	<0.001
IL-6	<7 pg/mL	1.43 ± 1.77	6.75 ± 6.59	<0.001
Ferritin	30–400 ng/mL	51.44 ± 33.54	80.85 ± 73.51	0.020
NLR	-	5.36 ± 9.33	8.80 ± 11.17	0.008
dNLR	-	0.73 ± 1.65	1.49 ± 2.63	0.006
Antibody count				
COVID-19-specific Immunoglobulin G	-	115.1 ± 81.7	154.4 ± 127.0	0.255
COVID-19-specific Immunoglobulin M	-	10.9 ± 52.1	147.6 ± 75.8	<0.001
IgG	-	551.7 ± 199.1	795.6 ± 297.7	0.238
IgM	-	123.2 ± 64.3	207.9 ± 53.1	<0.001
IgA	-	86.6 ± 29.0	100.3 ± 96.4	0.028
IgE	-	169.3 ± 284.0	82.2 ± 161.0	0.002

SD—standard deviation; WBC—white blood cell; dNLR—derived neutrophil-to-lymphocyte ratio; IL-6—interleukin 6; ESR—erythrocyte sedimentation rate.

CRP showed a significant increase in patients with post-COVID-19 pneumonia (9.57 ± 9.02 mg/L vs. 4.85 ± 2.80 mg/L, $p = 0.046$) as well as interleukin-6 (IL-6) levels that were substantially elevated in the pneumonia group (6.75 ± 6.59 pg/mL vs. 1.43 ± 1.77 pg/mL, $p < 0.001$). The erythrocyte sedimentation rate significantly increased in patients with pneumonia (12.92 ± 6.90 mm/h) compared to those without (8.43 ± 3.41 mm/h), with a p-value of less than 0.001.

COVID-19-specific immunoglobulin G and M showed a significant increase ($p < 0.001$ for both). This pattern was echoed in the general IgG levels, which were significantly higher in children with pneumonia (810.9 ± 290.6 mg/dL vs. 760.5 ± 200.3 mg/dL, $p < 0.001$), whereas IgM levels did not differ significantly ($p < 0.001$). Additionally, dNLR—an indicator of systemic inflammation—was higher in those with pneumonia (1.09 ± 2.63 vs. 0.73 ± 1.65, $p = 0.003$). Conversely, there was an increase in ferritin levels (80.85 ± 73.31 ng/mL vs. 51.44 ± 33.54 ng/mL, $p = 0.002$) and a significant change in IgE levels ($p = 0.029$) (Table 3).

Table 3. Comparison of laboratory findings of children with and without pneumonia during COVID-19 hospitalization (7-day measurements).

Variables (Mean ± SD)	Normal Range	No Pneumonia (n = 28)	Pneumonia (n = 38)	p-Value
Inflammatory markers				
ESR	0–20 mm/h	8.43 ± 3.41	12.92 ± 6.90	<0.001
C-reactive protein	<10 mg/L	4.85 ± 2.80	9.57 ± 9.02	0.046
WBC	4.0–10.0 × 10^9/L	12.51 ± 5.02	14.77 ± 5.89	0.058
Neutrophil %	40–60%	56.01 ± 24.44	61.97 ± 22.27	0.027
Lymphocyte %	20–40%	17.61 ± 17.08	23.04 ± 20.21	0.530
Procalcitonin	<0.5 ng/mL	0.69 ± 0.70	2.47 ± 11.51	0.408
IL-6	<7 pg/mL	1.43 ± 1.77	6.75 ± 6.59	<0.001
Ferritin	30–400 ng/mL	51.44 ± 33.54	80.85 ± 73.31	0.002
NLR	-	8.36 ± 9.33	8.80 ± 11.17	0.628
dNLR	-	0.73 ± 1.65	1.09 ± 2.63	0.003
Antibody count				
COVID-19-specific Immunoglobulin G	-	130.1 ± 80.5	266.3 ± 120.7	<0.001
COVID-19-specific Immunoglobulin M	-	45.2 ± 30.1	150.7 ± 75.4	<0.001
IgG	-	760.5 ± 200.3	810.9 ± 290.6	<0.001
IgM	-	120.4 ± 65.1	115.3 ± 55.2	<0.001
IgA	-	88.2 ± 30.5	102.7 ± 98.2	0.564
IgE	-	170.2 ± 285.0	85.3 ± 162.5	0.029

SD—standard deviation; WBC—white blood cell; dNLR—derived neutrophil-to-lymphocyte ratio; IL-6—interleukin 6; ESR—erythrocyte sedimentation rate.

The subgroup analysis in Table 4 of children with pneumonia reveals significant differences in certain inflammatory markers across age categories. Notably, while the initial PedPne scores did not show significant differences (p = 0.084), the analysis highlighted a substantial variation in the white blood cell (WBC) counts (p = 0.002) and ferritin levels (p = 0.001), suggesting age-related differences in the immune response to pneumonia. Specifically, WBC counts were highest in the 7–13 year age group. Ferritin also showed significant variation, which may reflect different inflammatory or infection processes in pediatric pneumonia across different age groups.

Table 4. Subgroup analysis of PedPne scores and inflammatory markers by age categories of children with pneumonia.

Variables (Mean ± SD)	1–6 Years (n = 32)	7–13 Years (n = 23)	13–18 Years (n = 9)	p-Value
Initial PedPne score	3.58 ± 0.32	3.46 ± 0.16	3.72 ± 0.37	0.084
7-day PedPne score	0.94 ± 0.36	0.87 ± 0.38	0.74 ± 0.32	0.293
ESR	11.14 ± 6.19	10.98 ± 6.47	11.57 ± 5.40	0.365
C-reactive protein	9.87 ± 9.43	9.16 ± 7.37	8.74 ± 8.17	0.093
WBC	14.28 ± 6.39	15.52 ± 5.18	13.67 ± 5.35	0.002
Neutrophil %	68.21 ± 22.26	62.67 ± 20.18	67.89 ± 21.28	0.297
Lymphocyte %	21.74 ± 21.37	23.39 ± 20.21	22.26 ± 20.39	0.831
Procalcitonin	3.23 ± 6.17	2.12 ± 10.46	2.07 ± 8.30	0.007
IL-6	1.52 ± 5.31	1.68 ± 7.44	1.83 ± 6.22	0.067
Ferritin	80.47 ± 70.19	73.89 ± 73.23	77.32 ± 71.21	0.001
NLR	8.21 ± 9.31	7.89 ± 8.43	8.53 ± 10.37	0.144
dNLR	1.92 ± 2.16	1.63 ± 1.44	1.29 ± 2.50	0.758

SD—standard deviation; WBC—white blood cell; dNLR—derived neutrophil-to-lymphocyte ratio; IL-6—interleukin 6; ESR—erythrocyte sedimentation rate.

In the evaluation of best cutoff values for predicting pneumonia development post-SARS-CoV-2 infection, significant findings were observed for several laboratory parameters, which were analyzed for their diagnostic efficacy. The dNLR, IL-6, and PedPne scores demonstrated high diagnostic accuracy. Specifically, dNLR exhibited a cutoff value of 1.88, with a sensitivity of 77.0% and specificity of 85.7%, achieving an AUC of 0.802 with a statistically significant *p*-value of less than 0.001. Similarly, IL-6 was identified as a robust biomarker with a cutoff of 6.1 pg/mL, which achieved a sensitivity of 70.3% and a specificity of 92.9%, with an AUC of 0.869, also showing a *p*-value of less than 0.001.

Furthermore, the PedPne ultrasound score, which directly assessed pneumonia severity, was set at a cutoff of 3.3, yielding a sensitivity of 75.7% and a specificity of 78.6%, with an AUC of 0.794, indicating high predictive power ($p < 0.001$). In contrast, the neutrophil-to-lymphocyte ratio (NLR) displayed a lower predictive capability with a cutoff of 3.84, sensitivity of 52.7%, specificity of 57.1%, and an AUC of 0.485, coupled with a non-significant *p*-value of 0.327, as presented in Table 5 and Figure 1.

Table 5. Best cutoff values for pneumonia development.

Laboratory Parameter	Best Cutoff Value	Sensitivity	Specificity	AUC	*p*-Value
NLR	3.84	52.7%	57.1%	0.485	0.327
dNLR	1.88	77.0%	85.7%	0.802	<0.001
IL-6	6.1 pg/mL	70.3%	92.9%	0.869	<0.001
PedPne Score	3.3	75.7%	78.6%	0.794	<0.001

dNLR—derived neutrophil-to-lymphocyte ratio; AUC—Area Under Curve.

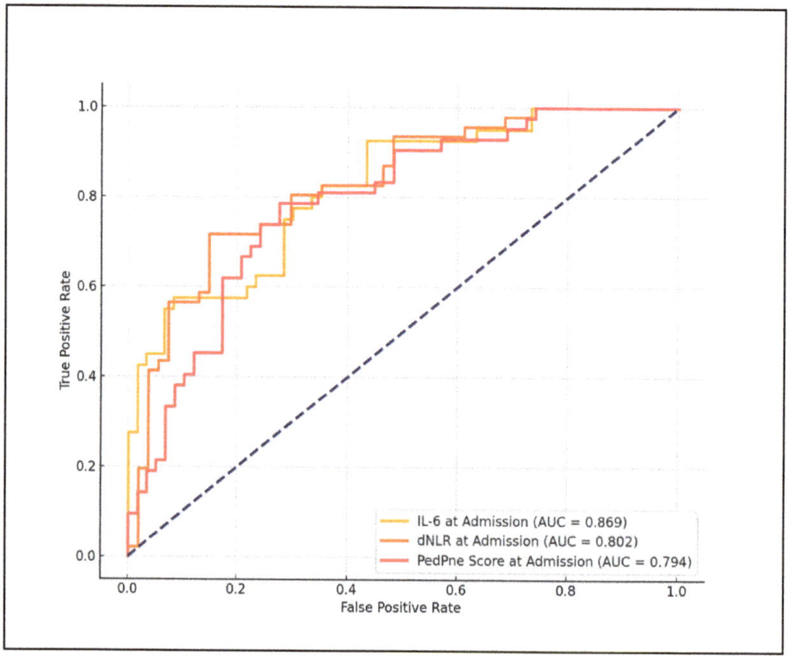

Figure 1. ROC analysis for pneumonia development among children admitted with COVID-19.

dNLR showed a hazard ratio (HR) of 2.53 with a confidence interval (CI) ranging from 1.19 to 6.97 and a *p*-value of 0.006, indicating a more than a twofold increase in the risk of pneumonia when dNLR values were above the cutoff. Similarly, IL-6 emerged as a strong predictor, with a hazard ratio of 4.25 (CI: 2.07–9.53) and a p-value of less than 0.001, suggesting a fourfold increase in pneumonia risk. Additionally, the PedPne score, which evaluates the ultrasound findings indicative of pneumonia, had a hazard ratio of 2.60 (CI: 1.33–5.18) with a p-value of less than 0.001, reinforcing its utility in predicting pneumonia development. In contrast, the neutrophil-to-lymphocyte ratio (NLR) displayed a hazard ratio of 1.16 (CI: 0.95–2.61) with a p-value of 0.118, indicating that while there was an observed increase in risk, it was not statistically significant, as described in Table 6 and Figure 2.

Table 6. Regression analysis for pneumonia development among children admitted for COVID-19.

Factors above the Best Cutoff	Hazard Ratio	95% CI	p-Value
NLR	1.16	0.95–2.61	0.118
dNLR	2.53	1.19–6.97	0.006
IL-6	4.25	2.07–9.53	<0.001
PedPne Score	2.60	1.33–5.18	<0.001

dNLR—derived neutrophil-to-lymphocyte ratio; CI—confidence interval.

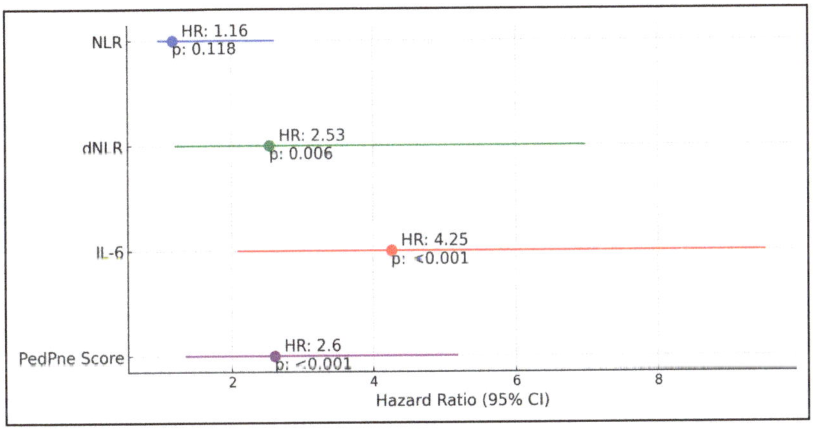

Figure 2. Regression analysis for pneumonia development among children admitted for COVID-19.

4. Discussion

4.1. Analysis of Findings

This study delineated the prognostic utility of Pediatric Pneumonia Ultrasound Scores (PedPne) and specific inflammatory biomarkers like dNLR and IL-6 in pediatric patients developing pneumonia post-SARS-CoV-2 infection. The significant correlation found between high PedPne scores and the progression of pneumonia underscores the importance of ultrasound evaluations in clinical settings for early detection and management. Notably, the study's findings indicate that elevations in dNLR and IL-6 not only signify an active inflammatory response but are also predictive of pneumonia outcomes, aligning with emerging literature that supports their roles as critical markers of systemic inflammation and disease severity in viral infections.

The derivation of optimal cutoff values for these markers provided objective criteria to aid in the clinical decision-making process. For instance, dNLR showed a high specificity and sensitivity (85.7% and 77.0%, respectively), suggesting that it can reliably distinguish between pediatric patients at higher risk for pneumonia from those with less severe manifestations. Similarly, IL-6's cutoff value at 6.1 pg/mL, demonstrating an AUC of 0.869, highlighted its strong predictive power, consistent with its recognized role in orchestrating prolonged inflammatory responses in viral pneumonias.

Regression analysis further substantiated the predictive strength of these biomarkers, with IL-6 showing substantial hazard ratios, indicating a significant increase in the likelihood of pneumonia development as these marker levels rise. PedPne score correlated with inflammation, and insights into the inflammatory dynamics allow for a more nuanced understanding and anticipation of disease progression, potentially guiding targeted therapeutic interventions and monitoring strategies.

In the development and application of a lung ultrasound score, Ciuca et al. [8] first introduced this novel diagnostic tool, finding a very strong positive correlation between the PedPne score and inflammatory markers such as C-reactive protein and erythrocyte sedimentation rate among 64 patients diagnosed from 217 that were screened. A median lung ultrasound score of 8.02 aligned closely with radiographic findings, confirming its reliability. Subsequently, in 2022, the same group published an extensive exhaustive score, named the PedPne score, and expanded the utility across a larger cohort of 321 screened patients with 81 confirmed cases of pneumonia, demonstrating its consistent application over the disease course with strong correlations noted between the US score and CRP, procalcitonin, and leukocyte counts across multiple evaluations [20]. These findings underscore the clinical relevance of the PedPne score as a robust, non-invasive measure for both the diagnosis and ongoing monitoring of pediatric pneumonia.

In a randomized clinical trial by Guitart et al. [20], the integration of a lung ultrasound and procalcitonin markedly improved the management of pediatric bacterial pneumonia by guiding antibiotic use and reducing unnecessary radiation exposure, demonstrating that when LUS and PCT values were below a set threshold, antibiotic use could be safely reduced, evidenced by a 77% decrease in chest X-rays and no significant cost increase. This method contrasts with findings from Bazdyrev et al. [21], who explored the long-term management of post-COVID-19 organizing pneumonia (PCOP), noting that up to 25% of patients required extended treatment with corticosteroids, fraught with potential relapses and severe side effects. The juxtaposition of these studies highlights the evolving understanding and management strategies in pediatric pneumonia—from acute care optimizations to addressing chronic post-viral effects—underscoring the critical need for precise diagnostic and therapeutic approaches in diverse clinical scenarios.

Indolfi et al. [22] and Ciuca et al. [23] provided significant insights into the utility of lung ultrasound in pediatric respiratory conditions post-COVID-19 and pneumonia, respectively. Indolfi et al. focused on the long-term respiratory complications associated with COVID-19 in children, finding that 27.0% of the 104 children evaluated showed positive LUS findings, indicating persistent pulmonary abnormalities. This study, which noted a significant association of a higher body mass index with worse COVID-19 symptoms and LUS scores ($p < 0.05$), highlights the potential of LUS in monitoring long COVID effects in pediatric patients. On the other hand, Ciuca et al. demonstrated the effectiveness of LUS over chest X-ray in diagnosing consolidated pneumonia in children, with LUS showing superior sensitivity. They reported an almost perfect agreement between LUS and CXR with a Cohen's kappa coefficient of $K = 0.89 \pm 0.04$ SD, $p = 0.000$. Both studies underline LUS as a valuable diagnostic tool, with Indolfi et al. emphasizing its role in long-term management of post-COVID-19 complications and Ciuca et al. confirming its higher diagnostic accuracy for acute pneumonia, suggesting a shift towards more widespread use of LUS in pediatric respiratory assessments.

The findings of this study introduce novel insights into the clinical utility of combining PedPne with inflammatory biomarkers such as dNLR and IL-6 for diagnosing and managing pneumonia in pediatric patients post-SARS-CoV-2 infection. This approach offers a robust predictive framework, enhancing early diagnostic capabilities and potentially guiding tailored therapeutic strategies. The demonstrated sensitivity and specificity of these biomarkers, especially in a pediatric population, signify a significant advancement in our ability to not only detect but also prognosticate the course of pneumonia following COVID-19, providing a valuable tool in the clinical arsenal against the variable presentations of the SARS-CoV-2 infection in children.

In understanding the linkage between PedPne scores and inflammatory biomarkers with pneumonia progression, it becomes evident that these metrics can provide critical insights into disease severity and trajectory. Elevated WBC counts and ferritin levels, as noted in specific age groups, could signify more intense inflammatory responses, which correlate with increased disease severity. Clinically, incorporating these biomarkers into routine diagnostic protocols could enhance the early detection and stratification of pneumonia severity, guiding more tailored treatment approaches. For instance, higher PedPne scores alongside elevated ferritin might prompt earlier initiation of anti-inflammatory treatments. By integrating such biomarkers systematically, clinicians can better predict patient outcomes, optimize resource allocation, and potentially reduce hospital stay durations through more precise management strategies.

4.2. Study Limitations and Future Perspectives

The sample size, though sufficient to achieve statistical significance, was relatively small, which might limit the generalizability of the findings. The observational nature of the study also restricts the ability to infer causality between the biomarkers and pneumonia development. Furthermore, the study relied on data from a single pediatric center, which might introduce center-specific biases in patient management and diagnostic criteria that could affect the study's outcomes. The study's limitations include potential biases from sample size and demographic homogeneity, which may impact the generalizability of the findings. Future research should focus on including a broader range of biomarkers and expanding to multi-center studies to enhance the robustness and applicability of the results.

5. Conclusions

In conclusion, this study validated the significant predictive value of PedPne scores, dNLR, and IL-6 in identifying and managing pediatric pneumonia post-COVID-19, with these tools demonstrating high specificity and sensitivity in clinical assessments. The integration of these biomarkers into routine clinical protocols could potentially enhance the diagnostic accuracy and therapeutic management of pediatric pneumonia, leading to improved patient outcomes. Future studies with larger, multi-center cohorts are recommended to further substantiate these findings and refine the predictive models for broader clinical application.

Author Contributions: Conceptualization, R.C. and M.D.; methodology, R.C. and M.D.; software, R.C. and M.D.; validation, D.D.; formal analysis, D.D.; investigation, D.D.; resources, D.D.; data curation, S.M.D.L. and I.M.C.; writing—original draft preparation, R.C.; writing—review and editing, S.M.D.L. and I.M.C.; visualization, S.M.D.L. and I.M.C.; project administration, S.M.D.L. and I.M.C. All authors have read and agreed to the published version of the manuscript.

Funding: The article processing charge was paid by the Victor Babes University of Medicine and Pharmacy Timisoara.

Institutional Review Board Statement: Ethic Committee Name: Ethic Committee of Clinical County Hospital Timisoara (Approval Code: 461; Approval Date: 18 April 2021). The Local Commission of Ethics for Scientific Research from the Timis County Emergency Clinical Hospital "Pius Brinzeu" from Timisoara, Romania, operates under article 167 provisions of Law no. 95/2006, art. 28, chapter VIII of order 904/2006; with EU GCP Directives 2005/28/EC, International Conference of Harmonisation of Technical Requirements for Registration of Pharmaceuticals for Human Use (ICH); and with the Declaration of Helsinki—Recommendations Guiding Medical Doctors in Biomedical Research Involving Human Subjects.

Informed Consent Statement: Informed consent was obtained from all subjects involved in the study.

Data Availability Statement: The data presented in this study are available on request from the corresponding author.

Acknowledgments: We would like to acknowledge VICTOR BABES UNIVERSITY OF MEDICINE AND PHARMACY TIMISOARA for their support in covering the costs of publication for this research paper.

Conflicts of Interest: The authors declare no conflicts of interest.

References

1. Wu, G.; Lu, J.; Liu, D.; He, Y. Characteristics and risk factors of secondary bacterial infections in COVID-19 patients. *Antimicrob Steward. Healthc. Epidemiol.* **2023**, *3*, e156. [CrossRef] [PubMed]
2. Manohar, P.; Loh, B.; Nachimuthu, R.; Hua, X.; Welburn, S.C.; Leptihn, S. Secondary Bacterial Infections in Patients with Viral Pneumonia. *Front. Med.* **2020**, *7*, 420. [CrossRef] [PubMed]
3. Chong, W.H.; Saha, B.K.; Chopra, A. Does COVID-19 pneumonia signify secondary organizing pneumonia? A narrative review comparing the similarities between these two distinct entities. *Heart Lung* **2021**, *50*, 667–674. [CrossRef] [PubMed]
4. Naranje, P.; Bhalla, A.S.; Jana, M.; Garg, M.; Nair, A.D.; Singh, S.K.; Banday, I. Imaging of Pulmonary Superinfections and Co-Infections in COVID-19. *Curr. Probl. Diagn. Radiol.* **2022**, *51*, 768–778. [CrossRef] [PubMed]
5. Bhat, K.A.; Madi, D.; Bhat, S.; Mary, T.; Shenoy Mulki, S.; Kotian, H. Profile of Secondary Bacterial and Fungal Infections in Hospitalized COVID-19 Patients in a Tertiary Care Centre. *Infect. Drug. Resist.* **2022**, *15*, 5705–5714. [CrossRef] [PubMed]
6. Dong, Z.; Shen, C.; Tang, J.; Wang, B.; Liao, H. Accuracy of Thoracic Ultrasonography for the Diagnosis of Pediatric Pneumonia: A Systematic Review and Meta-Analysis. *Diagnostics* **2023**, *13*, 3457. [CrossRef] [PubMed]
7. Elabbas, A.; Choudhary, R.; Gullapalli, D.; Mistry, S.; MH, F.; Mallick, A.H.; Kevu, E.P.; Asif, J.; Mostafa, J.A. Lung Ultrasonography Beyond the Diagnosis of Pediatrics Pneumonia. *Cureus* **2022**, *14*, e22460. [CrossRef] [PubMed]
8. Ciuca, I.M.; Marc, M.S.; Dediu, M.; Popin, D.; Liviu, P. Lung Ultrasound Score for Pediatric Pneumonia Surveillance. *Eur. Respir. J.* **2022**, *60*, 3205. [CrossRef]
9. Carbonell, R.; Moreno, G.; Martín-Loeches, I.; Bodí, M.; Rodríguez, A. The Role of Biomarkers in Influenza and COVID-19 Community-Acquired Pneumonia in Adults. *Antibiotics* **2023**, *12*, 161. [CrossRef]
10. Cioboata, D.M.; Boia, M.; Manea, A.M.; Costescu, O.C.; Costescu, S.; Doandes, F.M.; Popa, Z.L.; Sandesc, D. Predictive Value of Neutrophil-to-Monocyte Ratio, Lymphocyte-to-Monocyte Ratio, C-Reactive Protein, Procalcitonin, and Tumor Necrosis Factor Alpha for Neurological Complications in Mechanically Ventilated Neonates Born after 35 Weeks of Gestation. *Pediatr. Rep.* **2024**, *16*, 313–326. [CrossRef]
11. Capraru, I.D.; Vulcanescu, D.D.; Bagiu, I.C.; Horhat, F.G.; Popescu, I.M.; Baditoiu, L.M.; Muntean, D.; Licker, M.; Radulescu, M.; Mot, I.C.; et al. COVID-19 Biomarkers Comparison: Children, Adults and Elders. *Medicina* **2023**, *59*, 877. [CrossRef]
12. Lugarà, M.; Tamburrini, S.; Coppola, M.G.; Oliva, G.; Fiorini, V.; Catalano, M.; Carbone, R.; Saturnino, P.P.; Rosano, N.; Pesce, A.; et al. The Role of Lung Ultrasound in SARS-CoV-19 Pneumonia Management. *Diagnostics* **2022**, *12*, 1856. [CrossRef]
13. Zeng, Z.; Yu, H.; Chen, H.; Qi, W.; Chen, L.; Chen, G.; Yan, W.; Chen, T.; Ning, Q.; Han, M.; et al. Longitudinal changes of inflammatory parameters and their correlation with disease severity and outcomes in patients with COVID-19 from Wuhan, China. *Crit. Care* **2020**, *24*, 525. [CrossRef]
14. Wolszczak-Biedrzycka, B.; Dorf, J.; Milewska, A.; Łukaszyk, M.; Naumnik, W.; Kosidło, J.W.; Dymicka-Piekarska, V. The Diagnostic Value of Inflammatory Markers (CRP, IL6, CRP/IL6, CRP/L, LCR) for Assessing the Severity of COVID-19 Symptoms Based on the MEWS and Predicting the Risk of Mortality. *J. Inflamm. Res.* **2023**, *16*, 2173–2188. [CrossRef]
15. Stoicescu, E.R.; Iacob, R.; Ilie, A.C.; Iacob, E.R.; Susa, S.R.; Ghenciu, L.A.; Constantinescu, A.; Cocolea, D.M.; Oancea, C.; Manolescu, D.L. Differentiating Viral from Bacterial Pneumonia in Children: The Diagnostic Role of Lung Ultrasound-A Prospective Observational Study. *Diagnostics* **2024**, *14*, 480. [CrossRef] [PubMed]
16. Sansone, F.; Attanasi, M.; Di Filippo, P.; Sferrazza Papa, G.F.; Di Pillo, S.; Chiarelli, F. Usefulness of Lung Ultrasound in Paediatric Respiratory Diseases. *Diagnostics* **2021**, *11*, 1783. [CrossRef] [PubMed]
17. Tomczonek-Moruś, J.; Krysiak, N.; Blomberg, A.; Depczyk-Bukała, M.; Tkaczyk, M.; Zeman, K. Role of Lung Ultrasonography (LUS) as a Tool for Evaluating Children with Pediatric Inflammatory Multisystem Syndrome Temporally Associated with SARS-CoV-2 (PIMS-TS). *J. Clin. Med.* **2023**, *12*, 2850. [CrossRef] [PubMed]
18. Ansar, W.; Ghosh, S. Inflammation and Inflammatory Diseases, Markers, and Mediators: Role of CRP in Some Inflammatory Diseases. *Biol. C React. Protein Health Disease* **2016**, 67–107. [CrossRef]
19. Ciuca, I.M.; Dediu, M.; Pop, L.L. Pediatric pneumonia (PedPne) lung ultrasound score and inflammatory markers: A pilot study. *Pediatr. Pulmonol.* **2022**, *57*, 576–582. [CrossRef]
20. Guitart, C.; Bobillo-Perez, S.; Rodríguez-Fanjul, J.; Carrasco, J.L.; Brotons, P.; López-Ramos, M.G.; Cambra, F.J.; Balaguer, M.; Jordan, I. Lung ultrasound and procalcitonin, improving antibiotic management and avoiding radiation exposure in pediatric critical patients with bacterial pneumonia: A randomized clinical trial. *Eur. J. Med. Res.* **2024**, *29*, 222. [CrossRef]
21. Bazdyrev, E.; Panova, M.; Zherebtsova, V.; Burdenkova, A.; Grishagin, I.; Novikov, F.; Nebolsin, V. The Hidden Pandemic of COVID-19-Induced Organizing Pneumonia. *Pharmaceuticals* **2022**, *15*, 1574. [CrossRef] [PubMed]

22. Indolfi, C.; Klain, A.; Dinardo, G.; D'Addio, E.; Ferrara, S.; Decimo, F.; Ciprandi, G.; Tosca, M.A.; Miraglia del Giudice, M. COVID-19 Pediatric Follow-Up: Respiratory Long COVID-Associated Comorbidities and Lung Ultrasound Alterations in a Cohort of Italian Children. *Children* **2024**, *11*, 166. [CrossRef] [PubMed]
23. Ciuca, I.M.; Dediu, M.; Marc, M.S.; Lukic, M.; Horhat, D.I.; Pop, L.L. Lung Ultrasound Is More Sensitive for Hospitalized Consolidated Pneumonia Diagnosis Compared to CXR in Children. *Children* **2021**, *8*, 659. [CrossRef]

medicina

MDPI

Article

Antiretroviral Therapy Switch in HIV-Infected Adults from a Regional HIV/AIDS Center in NE Romania

Isabela Ioana Loghin [1,2], Șerban Alin Rusu [2], Andrei Vâţă [1,2,*], Mihaela Cobaschi [3,4,*], Ion Cecan [2], Carmen Manciuc [1,2] and Carmen Mihaela Dorobăţ [2]

1 Department of Infectious Diseases, "Grigore T. Popa" University of Medicine and Pharmacy, 700115 Iasi, Romania; isabelabegezsan@yahoo.com (I.I.L.); dmanciuc@yahoo.com (C.M.)
2 Department of Infectious Diseases, "St. Parascheva" Clinical Hospital of Infectious Diseases, 700116 Iasi, Romania; rususerbanalin@yahoo.com (Ș.A.R.); ion11cecan@gmail.com (I.C.); carmendorobat@yahoo.com (C.M.D.)
3 Faculty of Medicine/Clinical II Department, "Carol Davila" University of Medicine and Pharmacy, 050474 Bucharest, Romania
4 National Institute for Infectious Diseases "Prof. Dr. Matei Balș", 021105 Bucharest, Romania
* Correspondence: andreiandrei@yahoo.com (A.V.); cobaschimihaela@gmail.com (M.C.)

Abstract: *Background and Objectives*: Antiretroviral therapy (ART) has revolutionized the management of HIV infection, transforming it from a once-debilitating disease to a chronic, manageable condition. However, challenges such as treatment resistance, medication side effects, and long-term tolerability persist, prompting the exploration of novel therapeutic approaches. We aimed to highlight the characteristics and related comorbidities of HIV/AIDS cases in which the antiretroviral therapy was modified. *Material and Methods*: A cross-sectional clinical investigation was conducted on adults diagnosed with HIV/AIDS who were hospitalized at the "St. Parascheva" Clinical Hospital of Infectious Diseases in Iasi in the Northeastern region of Romania. The timeframe under investigation was 1 January 2023 to 30 June 2023. *Results*: In the Northeastern part of Romania, from a total of 1692 patients in the active records, there were a total of 148 recorded cases of antiretroviral therapy switch in HIV-infected patients. The main reason for the ART switch was the simplification of the ART regimen (82 cases, 55.40%), viro-immunological failure (16 cases, 10.66%), other disturbances correlated to the ART regimen, dyslipidemia (34 cases 22.97%), depression (3 cases, 2.02%), suicide attempt (1 case, 0.67%), new situations, including the appearance of pregnancy (3 cases 2.02%), and tuberculosis (9 cases, 6.08%). ART before the switch was represented by protease inhibitors that accounted for 84 cases (56.75%) of the ART switch. Following the therapy switch, integrase inhibitor-based ART single-tablet regimens accounted for 43.91% (65 cases) of all changeovers, with non-nucleoside reverse transcriptase inhibitor regimens coming in second, in 63 cases, 42.66%. *Conclusions*: ART switch as an experimental therapy offers a promising approach to optimizing HIV treatment outcomes. By focusing on viral suppression and immune reconstitution, addressing treatment challenges, and exploring novel ARV agents, ART switch strategies aim to improve the overall health and well-being of individuals living with HIV.

Keywords: HIV infection; ART switch; HIV-AIDS; treatment-experienced patients

1. Introduction

Antiretroviral therapy (ART) has revolutionized the management of HIV infection, transforming it from a once-debilitating disease to a chronic, manageable condition. However, challenges such as treatment resistance, medication side effects, and long-term tolerability persist, prompting the exploration of novel therapeutic approaches. In recent years, deliberate antiretroviral (ART) regimen switching has emerged as an intriguing strategy to optimize treatment outcomes for individuals living with HIV [1,2].

One of the primary goals of ART switch strategies is to optimize viral suppression, which is crucial for controlling HIV replication and preventing disease progression. Studies have demonstrated that a strategic switch from one ART regimen to another can lead to a significant reduction in viral load, thereby enhancing treatment efficacy. By targeting distinct mechanisms of action and overcoming resistance pathways, ART switches offer a renewed opportunity to achieve and maintain the durable suppression of the virus [3,4].

In addition to viral suppression, ART switch interventions have been associated with improvements in immune reconstitution. Research has indicated that switching ART regimens can result in notable increases in CD4 cell counts, reflecting a restoration of immune function and resilience against opportunistic infections. This immune recovery is essential for halting disease progression and improving the overall health outcomes in individuals living with HIV [5,6].

ART switch strategies also provide solutions to challenges related to treatment adherence and medication tolerability. Some patients may experience adverse effects or difficulties adhering to their current regimen, leading to suboptimal treatment outcomes. By switching to alternative ARV drugs, patients may experience reduced side effects, improved adherence, and an enhanced quality of life [7,8].

The requirement of adjusting HIV treatment according to the needs of each patient has been highlighted by the era of customized medicine. In order to determine the best regimens depending on variables like the virus subtype, treatment history, and comorbidities, comparative efficacy studies have assessed a variety of ART switch techniques. These studies have provided valuable insights into the efficacy and safety profiles of different switch options, enabling clinicians to make informed and personalized treatment decisions [9,10].

Safety considerations are paramount when implementing ART switch strategies. Research has focused on evaluating the safety profiles of different ART regimens, including potential risks such as drug interactions, metabolic disturbances, and cardiovascular events. Clinicians must carefully assess the benefits and risks of ART switch interventions to ensure the long-term success of treatment while minimizing adverse effects [5]. An important aspect is pre-conception counseling in couples with prospective ART modification. In this situation, the guidelines for treatment-naïve pregnant patients recommend regimens that include ritonavir-boosted atazanavir (ATV/r), darunavir (DRV/r), or raltegravir (RAL), in combination with one of the following NRTI backbones: abacavir (ABC)/lamivudine (3TC), tenofovir disoproxil fumarate (TDF)/emtricitabine (FTC), TDF/3TC, or AZT/3TC [1,11,12].

Emerging research has highlighted the potential use of novel ARV agents in ART switch strategies. Investigational drugs such as long-acting injectable formulations and novel classes of ARVs offer the promise of improved treatment adherence and a reduced pill burden [13,14].

Furthermore, the creation of medications with distinct modes of action opens up new possibilities for treating HIV patients and overcoming treatment resistance [14,15].

Effective patient education and support programs play a vital role in the success of ART switch strategies. Studies have shown that comprehensive patient counseling, adherence support, and regular follow-ups significantly enhance treatment outcomes and patient satisfaction. Empowering patients with knowledge about their treatment options and the potential side effects can lead to improved treatment adherence and overall well-being.

ART switch, as an experimental therapy, offers a promising approach to optimizing HIV treatment outcomes. By focusing on viral suppression and immune reconstitution, addressing treatment challenges, and exploring novel ARV agents, we aim to observe the evolution of the study group after the ART switch so that we can improve the overall health and well-being of individuals living with HIV.

2. Materials and Methods

2.1. Database Description

To highlight the characteristics and related comorbidities of HIV/AIDS cases in which the antiretroviral therapy was modified, we conducted a cross-sectional clinical investigation of patients diagnosed with HIV/AIDS who were hospitalized at the "Sf. Parascheva" Clinical Hospital of Infectious Diseases in Iasi in the Northeastern region of Romania. The timeframe under investigation was 1 January 2023 to 30 June 2023.

The study included 148 patients who were admitted to our Regional HIV/AIDS Center of Northeastern Romania, were diagnosed with HIV/AIDS, had a positive test for HIV using the enzyme-linked immunosorbent assay (ELISA) and had the disease confirmed by western blot (WB), were under different antiretroviral regimens and were evaluated for switching therapy. In addition, the patients' CD4+ T cell counts and HIV plasma viral load were evaluated.

2.2. Ethical Approval

Ethical approval was obtained from the "St. Parascheva" Clinical Hospital of Infectious Diseases in Iasi, Romania, according to the Ethical Committee in March/2024; Approval No. 5/21. At admission, every person signed the informed consent form.

2.3. Study Design

Data on demographics specific to age and gender, individual pathological histories, clinical characteristics, blood tests (viro-immunological testing), assessments of possible opportunistic infections, patient staging, the initiation of antiretroviral therapy, and the course and prognosis of HIV/AIDS were all collected. Because of this type of design, this study is classified as a cross-sectional study.

The HIV infection stage was identified using an age-specific CD4+ T-lymphocyte count or the CD4+ T-lymphocyte percentage of the total CD4 T-lymphocyte cell level, according to the Centers for Disease Control and Prevention (CDC) in Atlanta. Three phases are distinguished between HIV infection and AIDS: stage 1, characterized by CD4+ T-lymphocyte levels greater than 500 cells/mL; stage 2, characterized by levels between 200 and 499 cells/mL; and stage 3, characterized by levels less than 200 cells/mL. Stages 1 and 2 depict HIV infection, whereas Stage 3 represents AIDS (https://www.cdc.gov/hiv/library/reports/hiv-surveillance/vol-26-no-2/content/technical-notes.html (accessed on 15 January 2023)). ART switch was made according to the Liverpool drug–drug interaction checker, to avoid drug–drug interactions if the patient was taking other co-medication (https://www.hiv-druginteractions.org/checker (accessed on 1 February 2023)).

The adherence and therapeutic compliance were monitored in order to establish the necessity of switching the ART.

2.4. Study Setting and Data Collection

The "St. Parascheva" Clinical Hospital of Infectious Disease in Iasi is a primary referral medical facility for the Moldova region of Romania, with a capacity of 300 beds. It is divided into six pavilions. This includes a compartment for Infectious Diseases and the HIV/AIDS Regional Center. The Regional Center has a capacity of 12 beds, where the patients are periodically evaluated based on CDC and EACS recommendations.

All blood tests were performed by the hospital's central laboratory, and the patient's HIV plasmatic viral load (RT-PCR HIV 1 using Cepheid's GeneXpert® (Cepheid, CA, USA)) and CD4+ T cell count were assessed by the molecular biology lab. The viral load was classified as low if undetectable or with less than 40 copies/mL, and high if detectable with more than 40 copies/mL.

Periodically, the clinical and biological status of every newly diagnosed PLWH (people living with HIV) was assessed for metabolic syndrome and liver enzymes. The laboratory reference values were within 5–31 UI/L for AST (aspartate trans-aminase) and for ALT (alanine transaminase), within 7–32 UI/L for GGT (gamma-glutamyl transferase), within 122–200 mg/dL for COL (cholesterol), within 30–159 mg/dL for LDL-COL (low-density lipoprotein cholesterol), within 40–66 mg/dL for HDL-COL (high-density lipoprotein cholesterol), and within 30–150 mg/dL for TG (triglycerides), with no differences between sexes.

There are 1710 patients in total on the active register of the Regional HIV/AIDS Center, Iasi. Every six months, they receive a periodic evaluation to make sure they are adhering to and complying with the antiretroviral treatment. Every patient has a medical file that includes information on their related conditions, blood test results, CD4 T cell count, HIV viral load, and ART regimens. The paper charts kept by our center's patients provided the data for our investigation.

2.5. Statistical Analysis

The analysis included the patients' demographic data, medical history, clinical and laboratory results, treatment administered, and evolution.

The Chi square test in the XLSTAT version 2019 program was used to determine the correlation between demographic characteristics and clinical and laboratory data. Statistical Software for Excel (XLSTAT) version 2019 was used to conduct the statistical analysis. T-test statistics were used to quantify the difference between two data samples selected. *p*-value test statistics were performed, obtaining significant values under 0.05. All the data were analyzed, and on this basis, the statistic was made. No data were omitted.

3. Results

3.1. General Characteristics

From the 1710 patients in the active records of the Regional HIV/AIDS Department in the Northeastern part of Romania, there were a total of 148 recorded cases of antiretroviral therapy switch. Men were the ones who experienced more antiretroviral therapy switches (96 cases, 64.86%), and the difference in the M/F ratio between those with ART switch and those without was significant (1.23 vs. 1.84, $p = 0.025$). The study group's median age was 35 years old, significantly lower than that of the patients without a therapy switch (40 years, $p = 0.046$). The age distribution was as follows: young adults, aged between 30–39 years old—85 patients (57.43%); 40–49—19 patients (12.83%); 50–59 years—17 patients (11.48%); 20–29 years—20 patients (13.50%); and over 60 years old—7 patients (4.79%) (Table 1).

Table 1. Distribution of the study group by age.

	With Switch		Without Switch		*p*
Age (Years)	n (148)	%	n (1562)	%	
20–29	20	13.5	260	16.6	
30–39	85	57.4	473	30.3	
40–49	19	12.8	387	24.8	$p < 0.00001$
50–59	17	11.5	344	22.0	
Over 60	7	4.8	98	6.3	

At the time of switch, 54 cases (36.48%) had a CD4+ T-lymphocyte level between 1 and 199 cells/µL, 52 cases (35.13%) had a CD4+ T-lymphocyte value between 200 and 499 cells/µL, and 42 cases (28.37%) had a value over 500 cells/µL. The mean CD4+ T-lymphocyte level was 330.95 cells/µL, with a standard deviation of 284.22. Based on both gender and the CD4+ T-lymphocyte levels, men were the most affected, with lower overall CD4+ T-lymphocyte levels. The average HIV viral load was 494.627 copies/mL, with a standard deviation of 109.703.

The following findings were obtained using the CDC (Center for Disease Control and Prevention) phases of HIV/AIDS. According to our data, 28 patients (18.91%) had stage 1 HIV infection, 52 patients (35.13%) had stage 2 HIV infection, and 68 patients (45.94%) had stage 3 HIV infection at the time of switch.

It was discovered that in the study group, abnormal ALT and AST values were present in 35 cases (23.64). Regarding the metabolic profile, 49 cases (33.10%) had abnormal triglyceride levels, which affected both genders almost equally (18.24% men and 14.86% women). Cholesterol blood levels were elevated in 54 cases at baseline (Table 2).

Table 2. Distribution of cases according to sex, metabolic disorder, and liver enzyme levels.

Laboratory Marker	Value	Before Switch		After Switch		
		N (148)	%	N (148)	%	*p*
ALT	normal	113	76.4	135	91.2	0.0005
	elevated	35	23.6	13	8.8	
AST	normal	113	76.4	135	91.2	0.0005
	elevated	35	23.6	13	8.8	
GGT	normal	117	79.1	131	88.5	0.028
	elevated	31	20.9	17	11.5	
Total cholesterol	normal	94	63.5	112	75.7	0.023
	elevated	54	36.5	36	24.3	
HDL-col	normal	101	68.24	112	75.67	0.15
	elevated	47	31.75	36	24.32	
LDL-col	normal	99	66.89	112	75.67	0.095
	elevated	49	33.10	36	24.32	
Triglycerides	normal	97	65.5	121	81.75	0.001
	elevated	51	34.5	27	18.24	

3.2. Antiretroviral Regimens

Some of the study group cases had multiple antiretroviral treatment drug associations (regimens) before the present switch. Almost half of the patients were at their first ARV treatment change—69; 51 cases had between 2 and 4 regimens, 26 cases had between 5 and 9 regimens, and 2 cases had more than 9 antiretroviral therapy regimens (Figure 1).

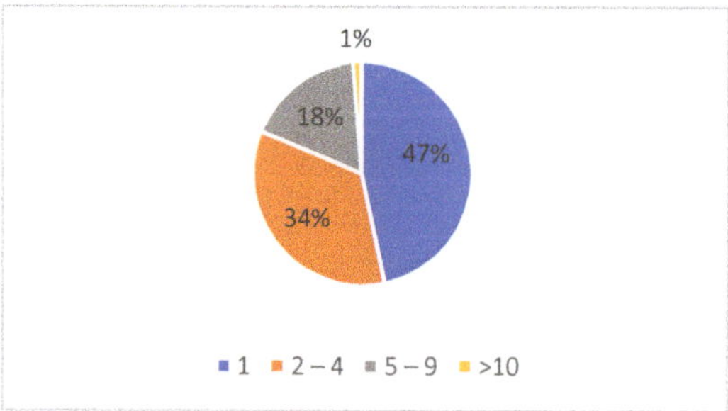

Figure 1. Number of antiretroviral regimens before the present switch.

ART switch was made according to the Liverpool drug–drug interaction checker, to avoid drug–drug interactions if the patient was taking other co-medication.

Before the ART switch, the patients had a cardiological (106 cases, 72%), neurological (82 cases, 55.33%), internal medicine (51 cases, 34.66%), psychiatric (15 cases, 10.13%), and gastroenterological (20 cases, 13.33%) check-up.

3.3. Switching Antiretroviral Therapy Criteria

The main reason for the ART switch was the simplification of the ART regimen (82 cases, 55.40%), viro-immunological failure (16 cases, 10.66%), side effects correlated to the ART regimen, dyslipidemia (34 cases 22.97%), depression (3 cases, 2.02%), suicide attempt (1 case, 0.67%), pregnancy (3 cases 2.02%) and tuberculosis (9 cases, 6.08%) (Figure 2).

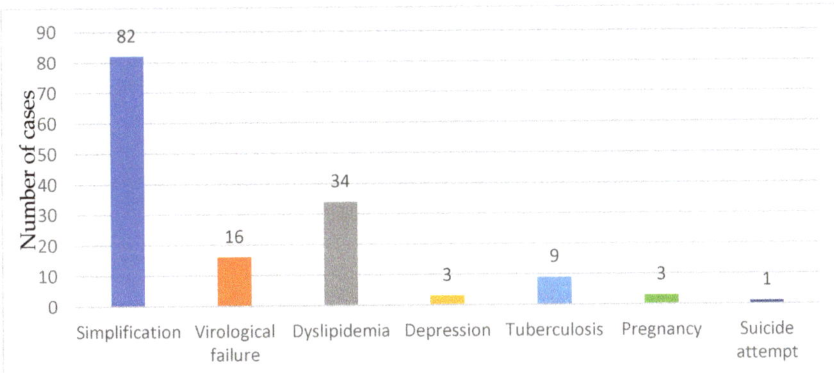

Figure 2. The reasons for ART switch.

ART before the switch was represented by protease inhibitors (PI) that accounted for 84 cases (56.75%) of the ART switch, followed by non-nucleoside reverse transcriptase inhibitor (NNRTI) regimens (37 cases, 25%), integrase inhibitor (INSTI) regimens using more than one pill (13 cases, 8.78%), and other regimens (14 cases, 9.45%) (Table 3).

Table 3. HIV/AIDS cases by ART regimen before the present switch.

ART Regimen	N (148)	%
Protease inhibitors + 2 NRTI (more than one pill)	84	56.7
Non-nucleoside reverse transcriptase inhibitor + 2 NRTI (more than one pill)	37	25
Integrase inhibitors + 2 NRTI (more than one pill)	13	8.7
Other	14	9.45

Following the therapy switch, integrase inhibitor-based ART single-tablet regimens accounted for 65 cases, at 43.91% (from which Bictegravir/Emtricitabine/tenofovir Alafenamide accounted for 38 cases, 25.67%, and Dolutegravir/ Lamivudine 27 cases, 18.24%), with non-nucleoside reverse transcriptase inhibitor single-tablet regimens coming in second, in 63 cases (42.66%), followed by other regimens (integrase inhibitors + 2 NRTI MTR-15 cases, 10.13%, Protease inhibitors+ 2 NRTI MTR, 5 cases, 3.37%) (Figure 3).

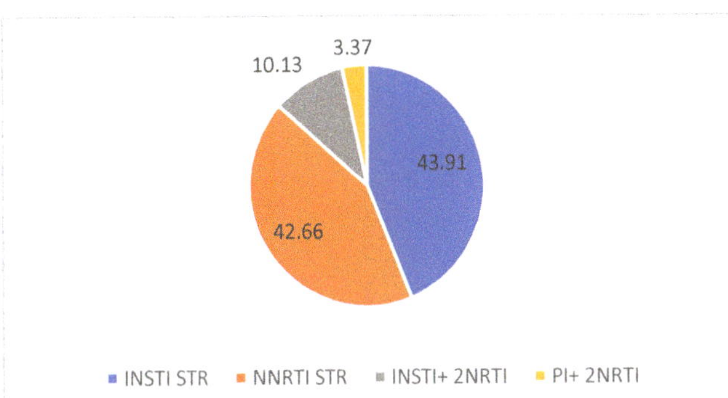

Figure 3. ARV regimens selected after the therapy switch (%).

The patients were evaluated one month after the ART switch, and the viro-immunological condition showed a significant decrease in HIV viremia, with an increased level of CD4+ T cells. As a result, 103 patients (69.59%) had a value between 200 and 499 cells/µL, 26 patients (17.50%) had a value exceeding 500 cells/µL, and 19 patients (12.83%) had a CD4 value below 200 cells/µL. The majority of patients, regardless of gender, exhibited a CD4+ T-lymphocyte count of 200–499 cells/µL or above (Figure 4).

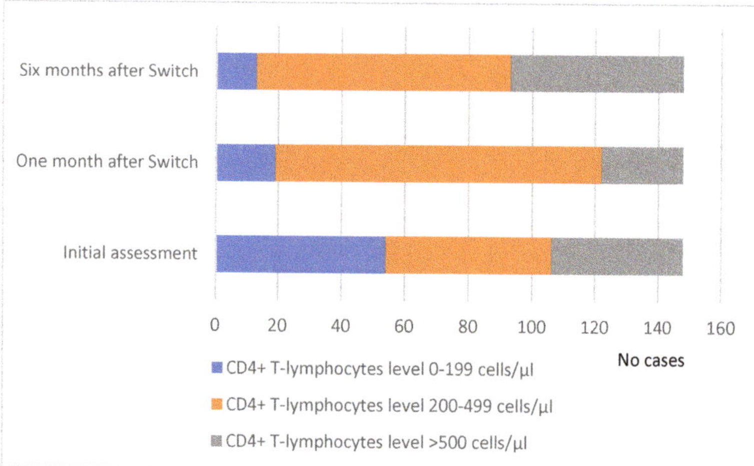

Figure 4. Evolution of the CD4+ T cell number distribution at baseline and one and six months after the ART switch.

The HIV viral load decreased after starting antiretroviral therapy, with viral suppression happening in 55.26% of cases (21 cases). The patients who had undetectable viremia during the first evaluation were either transferred from another regional HIV/AIDS center or had received their diagnosis overseas and had begun antiretroviral therapy (ART) at the time of their initial evaluation at our center (Figure 5).

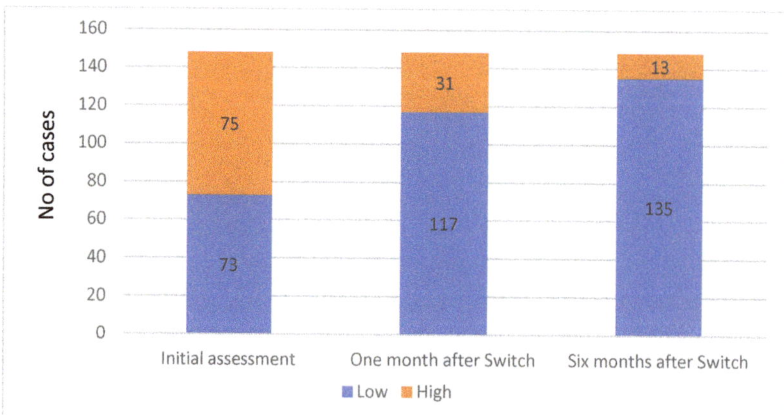

Figure 5. HIV viral load status distribution at baseline and one and six months after the ART switch.

At the six-month evaluation, abnormal ALT and AST values were present in 13 cases (8.78%). Regarding the metabolic profile, 27 cases had abnormal triglyceride levels, which affected both genders almost equally (10.13% men and 8.10% women). Additionally, elevated blood cholesterol levels were found in 36 cases, 24.32%) (Table 2).

4. Discussion

Antiretroviral therapy has revolutionized the management of HIV infection, significantly improving the quality of life and life expectancy of individuals living with this chronic disease.

ART switch with an individualized therapy offers a promising approach to optimizing HIV treatment outcomes. By focusing on viral suppression and immune reconstitution, addressing treatment challenges, and exploring novel ARV agents, we aimed to observe the evolution of the study group after the ART switch so that we can improve the overall health and well-being of individuals living with HIV.

In our cohort, the ART switch occurred more frequently in men, in younger patients, and in the 30–39-year-old group. Similar findings were revealed by a team of authors analyzing the antiretroviral therapy switch rate and switching pattern for people living with HIV from a national database in Japan [3]. Simplification was shown, as switching to a single daily tablet regimen is probably better received by this demographic category, with an active, busy lifestyle.

The CD4 T lymphocytes and HIV viremia load one month after the switch were favorable, obtaining viral suppression in some cases that had detectable viremia before the switch. Furthermore, the adherence and compliance of the patients to the ART were observed because the new switch regimens were mostly single-tablet regimens.

However, challenges such as drug resistance, treatment toxicity, and long-term tolerability remain, necessitating the exploration of innovative treatment strategies. Among these approaches, ART switch—an intentional change from one ARV regimen to another—has emerged as a promising experimental therapy in the field of HIV management [16,17].

The primary goal of ART switch is to optimize viral suppression, enhance immune reconstitution, and minimize treatment-associated complications. Previous studies [18,19] found that ART switch strategies have the potential to significantly reduce the viral load in HIV patients, leading to improved clinical outcomes. This is particularly crucial in cases of virological failure on current regimens, where a switch to alternative ARVs can offer a fresh chance at viral suppression. We agree with this statement. We observed that patients had a significantly improved virological status after the ART switch.

In addition to virological benefits, ART switch has been associated with notable improvements in immunological parameters, including increases in CD4 cell counts following the ART switch, indicating enhanced immune reconstitution. This immune recovery is crucial for bolstering the body's defenses against opportunistic infections and disease progression in HIV patients [20,21]. At the one- and six-month evaluation after the ART switch, many of our patients showed significant increases in their CD4 cell counts.

Despite the potential advantages of ART switch, challenges in treatment adherence often arise. Several studies highlighted the importance of adherence support programs, as many patients reported difficulties in maintaining consistent medication routines post-switch. Adherence remains a cornerstone of successful HIV treatment, emphasizing the need for comprehensive patient education and support services [22,23]. We observed that in our patients, pill burden was the major factor correlated with adherence.

Comparative effectiveness studies have delved into the various ART switch strategies used to identify optimal approaches. Lodi et al. conducted a network meta-analysis comparing the efficacy of different switch regimens, providing valuable insights for clinicians. This research highlighted the importance of tailoring switch strategies to individual patient needs and treatment histories [24]. It is important to ponder the benefits and risks of ART switch. We need more studies regarding the outcome of ART switch.

While ART switch holds promise as an experimental therapy, the consideration of safety profiles is paramount. A study [25] that investigated the safety outcomes of different ART switch regimens shed light on their potential risks, such as cardiovascular events and metabolic disturbances. Clinicians must weigh the benefits against the potential adverse effects when making switch decisions.

Special attention must be given to women of childbearing age, and in this situation, the guidelines offer the right recommendation [26,27]. Dyslipidemia is associated with increased cardiovascular disease and cognitive decline [28,29]. Other studies have shown that PI-based therapy has deleterious effects on lipid metabolism [30,31]. We also observed that protease inhibitors increase metabolic disorders such as dyslipidemia, this being one of the reasons for ART switch. At the six-month evaluation after the switch, patients showed decreased values of triglycerides and cholesterol, and also increased hepatic enzyme levels.

The change in antiretroviral therapy among HIV-infected adults from the Regional HIV/AIDS Center in NE Romania during the COVID-19 pandemic was carried out with the careful supervision of both the clinical-biological and viro-immunological evaluation parameters, and in the context of psychological counseling.

In our country, as a single-tablet regimen, the most affordable is Doravirine/lamivudine/tenofovir disopoxil fumarate, with Bictegravir/emtricitabine/tenofovir alafenamide at the opposite pole. The ART regimens are being supported by the national program currently in Romania, making it easier to access the new ART co-formulated single-tablet regimens.

This study has several limitations regarding the limited area that contains the study group, the northeastern part of Romania. It would be more significant if we could include the other regions of our country. Difficulties related to the quantification of the patient's adherence to treatment could interfere with the interpretation of the reasons that led to the ART switch.

ART switch, as an individualized therapy in people living with HIV, offers a multifaceted approach to treatment optimization. Through optimizing viral suppression, enhancing immune reconstitution, and addressing treatment challenges, ART switch has the potential to improve the long-term outcomes and quality of life for individuals living with HIV. However, it requires careful patient monitoring, adherence support, and the consideration of safety profiles to ensure its effectiveness. In the future, we aim to include the other regions of our country to better understand the impact of ART switches on the lives of people living with HIV. It is crucial to continue routinely monitoring the virologic efficacy and safety parameters to look for any new adverse events connected to ART modification and drug–drug interactions. Many of the newer medicines tested for ART switches allow patients to stay on these regimens for many years without having to switch again because of their decreased pill burden, frequency of administration, and similar if not improved virologic efficacy, safety, and tolerability.

5. Conclusions

In our study group, the ART switch occurred more frequently in young male adults, the most common reason being treatment simplification involving novel ARV agents in order to improve the overall health and well-being of individuals living with HIV. Most responded well to the change in the treatment, with improved CD4 counts, decreased viral loads and a better lipid and hepatic enzyme profile.

ART switch, as an individualized therapy, offers a promising approach to optimizing HIV treatment outcomes. The integration of personalized treatment approaches, safety considerations, patient education, and support programs will be crucial in maximizing the benefits of ART switch therapies.

Author Contributions: Conceptualization, I.I.L. and C.M.D.; data curation, I.I.L. and M.C.; formal analysis, I.C. and Ş.A.R.; investigation, A.V. and I.I.L.; methodology, I.I.L. and C.M.; resources, Ş.A.R. and A.V.; software, I.C. and Ş.A.R.; supervision, C.M.D.; validation, I.I.L. and C.M.D.; visualization, I.I.L., A.V., C.M. and M.C.; writing—original draft, I.I.L. and Ş.A.R.; writing—review and editing, I.I.L., C.M., A.V. and C.M.D. All authors have read and agreed to the published version of the manuscript.

Funding: This research received no external funding.

Institutional Review Board Statement: The study was conducted in accordance with the Declaration of Helsinki and approved by the Ethics Committee of the "St. Parascheva" Clinical Hospital of Infectious Diseases, Iasi, Romania. (Approval No. 5 from 21 March 2024).

Informed Consent Statement: This was a retrospective study, and written informed consent had been obtained from the patients when they were admitted to our hospital, according to the hospital policy.

Data Availability Statement: All data generated or analyzed during this study are included in this published article.

Conflicts of Interest: The authors declare no conflicts of interest.

References

1. The ART-LINC of IeDEA Study Group. Switching to second-line antiretroviral therapy in resource-limited settings: Comparison of programmes with and without viral load monitoring. *AIDS* **2009**, *23*, 1867–1874. [CrossRef] [PubMed]
2. Müller, M.; Wandel, S.; Colebunders, R.; Attia, S.; Furrer, H.; Egger, M.; IeDEA Southern and Central Africa. Immune reconstitution inflammatory syndrome in patients starting antiretroviral therapy for HIV infection: A systematic review and meta-analysis. *Lancet Infect Dis.* **2010**, *10*, 251–261. [CrossRef] [PubMed] [PubMed Central]
3. Naito, T.; Mori, H.; Fujibayashi, K.; Fukushima, S.; Yuda, M.; Fukui, N.; Tsukamoto, S.; Suzuki, M.; Goto-Hirano, K.; Kuwatsuru, R. Analysis of antiretroviral therapy switch rate and switching pattern for people living with HIV from a national database in Japan. *Sci. Rep.* **2022**, *12*, 1732. [CrossRef] [PubMed]
4. Kabarambi, A.; Balinda, S.; Abaasa, A.; Cogill, D.; Orrell, C. Determinants and reasons for switching anti-retroviral regimen among HIV-infected youth in a large township of South Africa (2002–2019). *AIDS Res. Ther.* **2022**, *19*, 32. [CrossRef] [PubMed]
5. Chastain, D.; Badowski, M.; Huesgen, E.; Pandit, N.S.; Pallotta, A.; Michienzi, S. Optimizing Antiretroviral Therapy in Treatment-Experienced Patients Living with HIV: A Critical Review of Switch and Simplification Strategies. An Opinion of the HIV Practice and Research Network of the American College of Clinical Pharmacy. *J. Int. Assoc. Provid. AIDS Care (JIAPAC)* **2019**, *18*, 2325958219867325. [CrossRef] [PubMed] [PubMed Central]
6. Ruzicka, D.J.; Kuroishi, N.; Oshima, N.; Sakuma, R.; Naito, T. Switch rates, time-to-switch, and switch patterns of antiretroviral therapy in people living with human immunodeficiency virus in Japan, in a hospital-claim database. *BMC Infect. Dis.* **2019**, *19*, 505. [CrossRef] [PubMed]
7. Nachega, J.B.; Uthman, O.A.; Anderson, J.; Peltzer, K.; Wampold, S.; Cotton, M.F.; Mills, E.J.; Ho, Y.-S.; Stringer, J.S.; McIntyre, J.A.; et al. Adherence to antiretroviral therapy during and after pregnancy in low-income, middle-income, and high-income countries: A systematic review and meta-analysis. *AIDS* **2012**, *26*, 2039–2052. [CrossRef]
8. Lester, R.T.; Ritvo, P.; Mills, E.J.; Kariri, A.; Karanja, S.; Chung, M.H.; Jack, W.; Habyarimana, J.; Sadatsafavi, M.; Najafzadeh, M.; et al. Effects of a mobile phone short message service on antiretroviral treatment adherence in Kenya (WelTel Kenya1): A randomised trial. *Lancet* **2010**, *376*, 1838–1845. [CrossRef] [PubMed]
9. Papot, E.; Kaplan, R.; Vitoria, M.; Polizzotto, M.N. Optimizing switching strategies to simplify antiretroviral therapy: The future of second-line from a public health perspective. *AIDS* **2021**, *35* (Suppl. S2), S153–S163. [CrossRef]
10. Watt, M.H.; Maman, S.; Golin, C.E.; Earp, J.A.; Eng, E.; Bangdiwala, S.I.; Jacobson, M. Factors associated with self-reported adherence to antiretroviral therapy in a Tanzanian setting. *AIDS Care* **2010**, *22*, 381–389. [CrossRef] [PubMed] [PubMed Central]
11. Li, Y.; Wang, Q.; Liang, S.; Feng, C.; Yang, H.; Yu, H.; Yuan, D.; Yang, S. Effect of Switching Antiretroviral Treatment Regimen in Patients With Drug-Resistant HIV-1 Infection: Retrospective Observational Cohort Study. *JMIR Public Health Surveill.* **2022**, *8*, e33429. [CrossRef] [PubMed]
12. Collaborative Initiative for Paediatric HIV Education and Research (CIPHER) Global Cohort Collaboration. Incidence of switching to second-line antiretroviral therapy and associated factors in children with HIV: An international cohort collaboration. *Lancet HIV* **2019**, *6*, e105–e115; Erratum in *Lancet HIV* **2020**, *7*, e803. [CrossRef] [PubMed] [PubMed Central]
13. Alemu, K.D.; Moges, N.A.; Boneya, D.J.; Asrade, A.A.; Tsega, T.D.; Tewachew, A.S. Time to Switch to Second-Line Anti-Retroviral Treatment and Its Predictors Among HIV Infected Adults with Virological Failure in Northwest Ethiopia: A Retrospective Follow-Up Study. *HIV/AIDS-Res. Palliat. Care* **2022**, *14*, 87–100. [CrossRef] [PubMed]
14. Panel on Clinical Practices for Treatment of HIV Infection. Guidelines for the use of antiretroviral agents in HIV-infected adults and adolescents. *Ann. Intern. Med.* **1998**, *128 Pt 2*, 1079–1100. [CrossRef] [PubMed]
15. Gandhi, R.T.; Bedimo, R.; Hoy, J.F.; Landovitz, R.J.; Smith, D.M.; Eaton, E.F.; Lehmann, C.; Springer, S.A.; Sax, P.E.; Thompson, M.A.; et al. Antiretroviral Drugs for Treatment and Prevention of HIV Infection in Adults: 2022 Recommendations of the International Antiviral Society–USA Panel. *JAMA-J. Am. Med. Assoc.* **2023**, *329*, 63–84. [CrossRef]
16. Rizzardini, G.; Overton, E.T.; Orkin, C.; Swindells, S.; Arasteh, K.; Górgolas Hernández-Mora, M.; Pokrovsky, V.; Girard, P.M.; Oka, S.; Andrade-Villanueva, J.F.; et al. Long-Acting Injectable Cabotegravir + Rilpivirine for HIV Maintenance Therapy: Week 48 Pooled Analysis of Phase 3 ATLAS and FLAIR Trials. *J. Acquir. Immune Defic. Syndr.* **2020**, *85*, 498–506. [CrossRef] [PubMed] [PubMed Central]
17. Margolis, D.A.; Gonzalez-Garcia, J.; Stellbrink, H.-J.; Eron, J.J.; Yazdanpanah, Y.; Podzamczer, D.; Lutz, T.; Angel, J.B.; Richmond, G.J.; Clotet, B.; et al. Long-acting intramuscular cabotegravir and rilpivirine in adults with HIV-1 infection (LATTE-2): 96-week results of a randomised, open-label, phase 2b, non-inferiority trial. *Lancet* **2017**, *390*, 1499–1510. [CrossRef] [PubMed]
18. Achhra, A.C.; Mwasakifwa, G.; Amin, J.; Boyd, M.A. Efficacy and safety of contemporary dual-drug antiretroviral regimens as first-line treatment or as a simplification strategy: A systematic review and meta-analysis. *Lancet HIV* **2016**, *3*, e351–e360. [CrossRef] [PubMed]

19. Plum, P.E.; Maes, N.; Sauvage, A.S.; Frippiat, F.; Meuris, C.; Uurlings, F.; Lecomte, M.; Léonard, P.; Paquot, N.; Fombellida, K.; et al. Impact of switch from tenofovir disoproxil fumarate-based regimens to tenofovir alafenamide-based regimens on lipid profile, weight gain and cardiovascular risk score in people living with HIV. *BMC Infect. Dis.* **2021**, *21*, 910. [CrossRef] [PubMed] [PubMed Central]
20. Cohen, C. Low-level viremia in HIV-1 infection: Consequences and implications for switching to a new regimen. *HIV Clin. Trials* **2009**, *10*, 116–124. [CrossRef] [PubMed]
21. Baril, J.G.; Angel, J.B.; Gill, M.J.; Gathe, J.; Cahn, P.; van Wyk, J.; Walmsley, S. Dual Therapy Treatment Strategies for the Management of Patients Infected with HIV: A Systematic Review of Current Evidence in ARV-Naive or ARV-Experienced, Virologically Suppressed Patients. *PLoS ONE* **2016**, *11*, e0148231. [CrossRef] [PubMed] [PubMed Central]
22. Bronkhorst, E.; Hattingh, S.; Poka, M. Antiretroviral stewardship in a tertiary academic hospital: The need for a clinical pharmacist. *Health SA* **2023**, *28*, 2135. [CrossRef] [PubMed] [PubMed Central]
23. Tuot, S.; Sim, J.W.; Nagashima-Hayashi, M.; Chhoun, P.; Teo, A.K.J.; Prem, K.; Yi, S. What are the determinants of antiretroviral therapy adherence among stable people living with HIV? A cross-sectional study in Cambodia. *AIDS Res. Ther.* **2023**, *20*, 47. [CrossRef] [PubMed]
24. Lodi, S.; Günthard, H.F.; Gill, J.; Phillips, A.N.; Dunn, D.; Vu, Q.; Siemieniuk, R.; Garcia, F.; Logan, R.; Jose, S.; et al. Effectiveness of Transmitted Drug Resistance Testing Before Initiation of Antiretroviral Therapy in HIV-Positive Individuals. *J. Acquir. Immune Defic. Syndr.* **2019**, *82*, 314–320. [CrossRef] [PubMed] [PubMed Central]
25. Iannone, V.; Passerotto, R.A.; Lamanna, F.; Steiner, R.J.; Lombardi, F.; Salvo, P.F.; Dusina, A.; Farinacci, D.; Borghetti, A.; Di Giambenedetto, S.; et al. Changes in Metabolic Profile in PLWHIV Switching to Doravirine-Based Regimen. *Viruses* **2023**, *15*, 1046. [CrossRef] [PubMed] [PubMed Central]
26. Panel on Treatment of HIV-Infected Pregnant Women and Prevention of Perinatal Transmission. Recommendations for Use of Antiretroviral Drugs in Pregnant HIV-1-Infected Women for Maternal Health and Interventions to Reduce Perinatal HIV Transmission in the United States. 2015. Available online: http://aidsinfo.nih.gov/contentfiles/lvguidelines/PerinatalGL.pdf (accessed on 1 April 2024).
27. World Health Organization HIV/AIDS Programme. *Consolidated Guidelines on the Use of Antiretroviral Drugs for Treating and Preventing HIV Infection: Recommendations for a Public Health Approach*; WHO: Geneva, Switzerland, 2013.
28. Collins, S.E.; Grant, P.M.; Shafer, R.W. Modifying Antiretroviral Therapy in Virologically Suppressed HIV-1-Infected Patients. *Drugs* **2015**, *76*, 75–98. [CrossRef] [PubMed] [PubMed Central]
29. Zhang, Y.; Xiao, J.; Zhang, W.; Han, N.; Yang, D.; Liu, W.; Zeng, H.; Han, J.; Zhao, H. Cumulative effects of hypertriglyceridemia in HIV-infected patients switching from NNRTIs to PI-based antiretroviral therapy. *J. Infect. Dev. Ctries.* **2022**, *16*, 528–536. [CrossRef] [PubMed]
30. Mukerji, S.S.; Locascio, J.J.; Misra, V.; Lorenz, D.R.; Holman, A.; Dutta, A.; Penugonda, S.; Wolinsky, S.M.; Gabuzda, D. Lipid profiles and APOE4 allele impact midlife cognitive decline in HIV-infected men on antiretroviral therapy. *Clin. Infect. Dis.* **2016**, *63*, 1130–1139. [CrossRef] [PubMed]
31. Esser, S.; Eisele, L.; Schwarz, B.; Schulze, C.; Holzendorf, V.; Brockmeyer, N.H.; Hower, M.; Kwirant, F.; Rudolph, R.; Neumann, T.; et al. Rates of cardiovascular events and deaths are associated with advanced stages of HIV-infection: Results of the HIV HEART study 7, 5-year follow-up. *J. Int. AIDS Soc.* **2014**, *17*, 19542. [CrossRef]

medicina

MDPI

Article

Antibiotic Utilization and Resistance According to the WHO AWaRe Classification in Intensive Care Units After COVID-19 Third Wave in Pakistan: Findings and Implications

Muhammad Shahid Iqbal [1,*], Mohd Faiyaz Khan [1,*], Sadaf Farooqui [1], Salah-Ud-Din Khan [2], Saeed Vohra [3], Shahzad Rasheed [3], Muhammad Zahid Iqbal [4,5] and Shafqat Qamer [6]

1 Department of Clinical Pharmacy, College of Pharmacy, Prince Sattam bin Abdulaziz University, Al-Kharj 11942, Saudi Arabia
2 Department of Biochemistry, College of Medicine, Imam Mohammad Ibn Saud Islamic University (IMSIU), Riyadh 11432, Saudi Arabia
3 Department of Anatomy and Physiology, College of Medicine, Imam Mohammad Ibn Saud Islamic University (IMSIU), Riyadh 11432, Saudi Arabia
4 Department of Clinical Pharmacy, College of Pharmacy, King Khalid University, Abha 61421, Saudi Arabia
5 Department of Pharmacy Practice, Faculty of Pharmaceutical Sciences, Lahore University of Biological & Applied Sciences, Lahore 53400, Pakistan
6 Department of Basic Medical Sciences, College of Medicine, Prince Sattam bin Abdulaziz University, Al-Kharj 11942, Saudi Arabia
* Correspondence: profdrmsi@gmail.com or m.javed@psau.edu.sa (M.S.I.); moh.khan@psau.edu.sa (M.F.K.)

Abstract: *Background and Objective:* Irrational use and overuse of antibiotics is considered a major cause of antimicrobial resistance (AMR) among patients admitted to hospitals, especially in intensive care units (ICUs). ICUs are the most critical wards in healthcare settings, where the use of antibiotics is much higher compared to other wards. Therefore, the appropriate administration and monitoring of antibiotic usage in these units is a matter of concern. *Materials and Methods:* This retrospective study evaluated the types, utilization patterns, sensitivity, and resistance of various antibiotics used among patients admitted to the ICUs of different hospitals after the third wave of the coronavirus disease in 2019 (COVID-19) in Pakistan. *Results:* It was observed that more than 40% of the patients were given two antibiotics and 54.3% were given at least one antibiotic each day. A total of 768 antibiotics from different groups, based on the World Health Organization (WHO) Access, Watch, and Reserve (AWaRe) classification, were prescribed to 313 patients admitted to ICUs between April and August 2021. Among the types of antibiotics, amoxicillin/clavulanic acid was the most frequently used antibiotic (75 prescriptions). It was also observed that the majority of the bacterial isolates were more sensitive to carbapenems than the other antibiotics. The current study showed that antibiotic usage according to the AWaRe classifications was 31.8% in the Access category, 59.5% in the Watch category, and 8.7% in the Reserve category in ICUs of the studied hospitals after the third wave of COVID-19. *Conclusions:* The findings of the study also highlight the importance and continuous need for the implementation of antibiotic stewardship programs to optimize the appropriate utilization of antibiotics in the ICUs of the studied hospitals.

Keywords: antibiotics; AMR; COVID-19; ICUs; AWaRe; AMS; WHO; Pakistan

1. Introduction

Antimicrobial resistance (AMR) has been partially managed after the introduction of the World Health Organization (WHO) Access, Watch, and Reserve (AWaRe) classification of antibiotic usage [1]. The WHO Expert Committee on Selection and Use of Essential Medicines developed the AWaRe tool to lessen the clinical burden, address the global spread of AMR, and minimize the side effects associated with irrational antibiotic use [1–4]. The three categories of the AWaRe classification are as follows: "Access" (the first- and second-choice antibiotics, such as amoxicillin, ampicillin, and amikacin, with a narrow spectrum and less potential for resistance), "Watch" (broader-spectrum antibiotics such as fluoroquinolones, macrolides, and second- and third-generation cephalosporins, carrying a higher risk of developing resistance), and Reserve (the last-resort choice antibiotics to treat infections, such as linezolid and colistin, resistant to multiple drugs) [4–6]. The WHO AWaRe classification system has two major objectives. The first is reporting antibiotic use according to AWaRe classification worldwide. The second objective is setting targets and assessing and implementing the outcome of antimicrobial stewardship (AMS) initiatives that aim to reduce AMR and maximize apt antibiotic usage [2–6]. AMS, a program that encourages prudent antibiotic use and precise prescribing patterns of antibiotics, also includes the AWaRe tool [7,8]. Various countries like Brazil, the UK, Bangladesh, and Germany have adopted this AWaRe classification tool and found it beneficial in controlling AMR [2,9]. Adoption of the AWaRe classification can also be utilized to track antimicrobial usage trends and encourage sensible prescription patterns among the prescribers [10–12]. By encouraging the sensible use of antibiotics in healthcare settings, AMS initiatives significantly contribute to the reduction of AMR [13].

Recent WHO initiatives have highlighted the necessity of structured AMS approaches to address issues brought on by the Coronavirus disease 2019 (COVID-19) pandemic, which resulted in a rise in antibiotic use (despite fewer bacterial co-infections) in a post-pandemic era [14]. Though its implementations are still lacking, WHO's AWaRe categorization has been progressively included in AMS frames worldwide to help with appropriate antibiotic selection [15]. Furthermore, to implement precise antibiotic usage, AMS programs in low- and middle-income countries often face budget constraints and resource restrictions [16]. This necessitates the need for continuous evaluations of AMS programs all over the world, particularly in low-income countries, to enhance their effectiveness and their alignment with WHO guidelines.

Multidrug-resistant microorganisms have been documented in various parts of Pakistan in the past few years. In Pakistan, Enterobacteriaceae resistance to quinolones has increased over the past 10 years [17,18]. The Salmonella outbreaks in 2016 were resistant to fluoroquinolones [18,19]. According to a prior study, 94% of bloodstream bacteria were resistant to third-generation cephalosporins [19,20]. Several other studies have also reported that various factors contribute enormously to AMR. These include irrational antibiotic prescriptions, incorrect and under-dosing prescribing patterns, antibiotic self-medication, incompetent healthcare staff, insufficient self-training, lack of culture and sensitivity (C&S) testing, and discontinuation of AMS programs [20,21].

In Pakistan, pharmaceutical companies can aggressively market and sell antibiotics without adequate quality control due to the lack of strict monitoring and lenient regulations of the Drug Regulatory Authority of Pakistan (DRAP) [22–24]. Another factor contributing to AMR in Pakistan is overprescription and self-medication among the majority of the public [22–24]. In Pakistan, many prescribers prescribe antibiotics needlessly, while others do so in response to patient requests [23,24]. Furthermore, a lot of people buy antibiotics from drug stores and pharmacies without any legitimate prescription, making self-medication widespread, which is another contributing factor for AMR in Pakistan [24–26]. Furthermore, broad-spectrum antibiotics are frequently prescribed in Pakistan rather than narrow-spectrum antibiotics, which further aids in the development of AMR [24,25]. The general public's lack of awareness and inadequate education regarding the apt usage of antibiotics is another significant factor contributing to AMR in Pakistan [22–24]. Typically, pharmaceutical companies also provide prescribers with hefty incentives to over-prescribe their products, which also results in AMR [24,25]. Some studies have reported that the prescription rate of irrational antibiotics in Pakistan is quite high, i.e., >50% as compared to other developing countries [22,26]. Due to the lack of precise and updated AMS programs in hospitals, abundant irrational antibiotics are being prescribed with less or no effect against most of the microbes [27]. This is concerning because, to enhance WHO AWaRe recommendation adherence and minimize AMR, the susceptibility patterns of microorganisms should be closely observed at primary, secondary, and tertiary care facilities across the entire country [18,19,24].

Intensive care units (ICUs) are the most sensitive areas in hospitals where critically ill patients are kept under intensive care. In ICUs, irrationality and overuse of antibiotics not only result in AMR but can also reduce antibiotic effectiveness [28]. As bacteria become resistant to antibiotics, providing therapy for various life-threatening infections like sepsis, CNS infections, and intra-abdominal infections becomes more challenging in ICUs [27,28]. AMR often leads to longer hospital stays, higher healthcare costs, decreased therapeutic outcomes, and ultimately an increased mortality rate [27–29]. Antibiotic use in ICUs is around ten times higher than in the other wards of the hospitals [28,29].

ICUs are critical settings in hospitals where broad-spectrum antibiotics are frequently prescribed and used due to the high prevalence of severe infections [30]. However, inappropriate and unnecessary antibiotic prescription and utilization often results in AMR, making treatments more complex and prolonged in the ICUs [30,31]. According to a recent study, around 50% of antibiotics prescribed in ICUs are unnecessary and inappropriate [30–32]. Therefore, monitoring antibiotic prescription is crucial to identify concerning signs of misuse or overuse in ICUs [31–33]. Many low and middle-income countries have struggled to implement a robust antimicrobial stewardship program (ASP), especially as recommended by the WHO. Unfortunately, more than half of hospitals in Pakistan do not have any ASP that could help to combat AMR.

In January 2021, the third COVID-19 wave was officially declared by the WHO after a new variant of SARS-CoV-2 (B.1.1.7) from the United Kingdom was detected in more than 70 countries including Pakistan [34–36]. This variant was also associated with an increased risk of casualties compared to previous variants. In Pakistan, an average of more than 100 patient deaths was reported daily due to this variant [35,36]. Major cities in Pakistan like Islamabad, Lahore, Faisalabad, Multan, and Peshawar were affected the most by B.1.1.7 during the third wave of COVID-19. A strict lockdown was imposed by the Government of Pakistan in these cities to control the spread of the third wave of COVID-19 [36].

Various studies reported that during the COVID-19 pandemic, several infected patients were admitted to hospitals for inappropriate antimicrobial therapy, which resulted in increased AMR worldwide [37,38]. Conversely, there were several reasons to prescribe antibiotics during the COVID-19 pandemic, especially to treat COVID-19 and non-COVID-19 patients suffering from different bacterial infections. These infections included pneumonia, co-infections, secondary bacterial infections, and several nosocomial infections [39]. According to another study, a large number of hospitalized patients were given empirical antimicrobial therapies during the COVID-19 pandemic which was not appropriate at all and led to an increase in AMR [38]. Some other studies also reported that during the COVID-19 pandemic, a higher number of patients admitted to ICUs were administered unnecessary antibiotics [37–40]. Overall, the frequency of various infections increased dramatically during the third wave of COVID-19 across the globe [41]. Therefore, this study was designed to determine types, utilization (according to AWaRe classification), sensitivity, and resistance patterns of various antibiotics used in patients admitted to the

ICUs of different hospitals in Pakistan. This was a pioneering study, as no previous research has been conducted in the ICUs of the studied hospitals during or after the COVID-19 third wave.

2. Materials and Methods

2.1. Study Design and Study Period

A retrospective study was conducted between April and August 2021 in the ICUs of four public hospitals in Pakistan. All aspects of the study protocol, including information about participants' identity and background, were strictly confidential and for research purposes only. This study was approved by the Research Ethics Committee, Lahore Pharmacy College, Lahore Medical & Dental College under ETH/LPC/06/01/21.

2.2. Data Management and Confidentiality

All subject names were kept in a password-protected folder and were allocated with study identification numbers. Identification numbers instead of patient names were used in the final dataset of this research. On completion of the study, data from the computer were copied to a USB flash drive, and computer data were deleted permanently. As per the international research data storage requirements, a USB flash drive and any hardcopy data were only stored by the investigators and kept for a minimum of three years from the completion of the study. No one other than investigators were allowed to view the study data.

2.3. Inclusion and Exclusion Criteria

The study inclusion criteria were patients aged 18 to 60, suffering from any infection, admitted to the ICUs during the study period, and treated with at least one antibiotic. Patients admitted to other wards/departments of the hospitals were excluded from the study. All of the patients who were admitted to ICUs during the study period were strictly assessed to meet the eligibility criteria. All patients meeting the inclusion criteria were included in the study. The study sample (N) of our study was 313, with $n = 82$ in hospital A, $n = 91$ in hospital B, $n = 76$ in hospital C, and $n = 64$ in hospital D.

2.4. Study Setting and Data Collection

All the selected hospitals are categorized as public hospitals in Pakistan. All these hospitals have the capacity of, on average, 800–1000 beds. The average number of beds in the ICUs for infectious diseases is around 30–40 beds in these hospitals. The data were collected from the patient files/records assigned to each patient in the hospitals. The records were further verified by staff nurses. The records of antibiotic treatment of the patients were followed up until their discharge from the ICUs. The number of patients discharged on special request, shifted to the general ward, and shifted to specialized wards were also recorded and included among the outcomes of the antibiotic therapy provided. The demographic details (age and gender), reason for admission, and length of stay were also recorded. The severity of illnesses and physiological and clinical characteristics of ICU-admitted patients were determined using the revised Acute Physiology and Chronic Health Evaluation II (APACHE II) score and Glasgow Coma Scale. Antibiotics were classified using the Anatomical Therapeutic Chemical (ATC) Classification System and their utilization was presented in the form of a daily-defined dose (DDD) per 100 bed days as presented in another study [42]. Further evaluation was made using the type of antibiotic therapy (empirical, definitive, prophylactic), number of antibiotics given, and route of administration. The sensitivity and resistance data were collected from each patient's file/record (which the hospital obtained from the microbiology tests performed and recorded in individual files). Antibiotics were classified using the WHO AWaRe classification system.

2.5. Statistical Analyses

The data were entered in Microsoft Excel version 2023 and analyzed using Statistical Package for the Social Sciences (SPSS) ver. 25. The obtained data were analyzed using Kolmogorov–Smirnov test to confirm the normal distribution of numeric variables. Univariate analyses comprising Chi-square test and Fisher's exact test were used to determine the association between demographic variables and antibiotic usage. Comparisons of categorical variables were also made where appropriate using Chi-square test and Fisher's exact test. A multivariate analyses comprising multinomial logistic regression was also performed to adjust the effects of potential demographic and clinical factors (predictors) that were significant in univariate analyses ($p < 0.05$).

3. Results

Table 1 describes the demographic and clinical characteristics of patients across four selected hospitals. The main demographic and clinical characteristics include age distribution, gender, reasons for admission, length of hospital stay, and therapy outcomes. Total patients included in the study were 313, including $n = 82$ from hospital A, $n = 91$ from hospital B, $n = 76$ from hospital C, and $n = 64$ from hospital D. The number and percentage of males were 28 (34.1%), 38 (41.4%), 29 (38.2%), and 21 (32.8%), while the females were 54 (65.9%), 53 (64.6%), 47 (61.8), and 43 (67.2%) in hospitals A, B, C, and D, respectively. The highest number of patients ($n = 92$, 29.39% of the total) suffered from respiratory tract infection followed by renal infection ($n = 82$, 26.19%). The length of stay in ICUs ranged from 1 to >7 days. The majority of the patients (>50%) stayed for 2–3 days. Our results also showed that 33 (40.2%) patients were shifted to the general ward in hospital A, 36 (39.6%) in hospital B, 31 (40.8%) in hospital C, and 24 (37.5%) in hospital D. Moreover, for hospitals A, B, C, and D, the total number of patients discharged on request were 28 (34.2%), 33 (36.3%), 24 (31.6%), and 22 (34.4%), respectively. The APACHE (II) score of more than 50% of the patients was 11–20. Statistically significant differences were observed for length of stay (days) ($p < 0.001$) and therapy outcomes ($p = 0.036$).

Table 1. Demographic and clinical characteristics of patients ($n = 313$).

Characteristics	Categories	Hospitals								p-Value
		Hospital A ($n = 82$)		Hospital B ($n = 91$)		Hospital C ($n = 76$)		Hospital D ($n = 64$)		
		n	%	n	%	n	%	n	%	
Age	<18	17	20.7	18	19.7	21	27.6	11	17.2	0.301 [a]
	18–35	31	37.8	43	47.3	18	23.7	24	37.5	
	36–55	27	32.9	26	28.6	31	40.8	16	25	
	>55	7	8.6	4	4.4	6	7.9	13	20.3	
Gender	Male	28	34.1	38	41.4	29	38.2	21	32.8	0.122 [a]
	Female	54	65.9	53	64.6	47	61.8	43	67.2	
Reason for admission	Respiratory tract infection	26	31.7	27	29.7	21	27.6	18	28.1	0.097 [a]
	Renal infection	20	24.4	24	26.4	21	27.6	17	26.6	
	CNS infection	16	19.5	17	18.7	14	18.4	12	18.8	
	GIT infection	9	11.0	11	12.1	9	11.8	8	12.5	
	Urinary tract infection	8	11.7	8	8.8	9	11.8	6	9.4	
	Miscellaneous	3	3.7	4	4.4	2	2.6	3	4.7	

Table 1. *Cont.*

Characteristics	Categories	Hospital A (n = 82)		Hospital B (n = 91)		Hospital C (n = 76)		Hospital D (n = 64)		p-Value
		n	%	n	%	n	%	n	%	
Length of stay (days)	1	20	24.4	21	23.1	16	21.1	12	18.8	<0.001 [b]
	2–3	42	51.2	45	49.5	38	49.9	34	53.1	
	4–5	12	14.6	15	16.5	13	17.1	9	14	
	6–7	3	3.7	4	4.4	4	5.3	5	7.8	
	>7	5	6.1	6	6.5	5	6.6	4	6.3	
Therapy outcomes	Death	5	6.1	4	4.3	4	5.2	3	4.7	0.036 [b]
	Discharged on request	28	34.2	33	36.3	24	31.6	22	34.4	
	Shifted to general ward	33	40.2	36	39.6	31	40.8	24	37.5	
	Shifted to specialized ward	16	19.5	18	19.8	17	22.4	15	23.4	
APACHE(II) score	0–10	19	23.3	22	24.5	17	22.6	14	22.1	0.059 [a]
	11–20	48	59.3	51	56.3	44	57.8	38	59.4	
	21–30	12	14.2	13	13.4	12	15.8	9	13.8	
	31–40	3	3.2	5	5.8	3	3.8	3	4.7	
GCS Score	3–5	4	4.9	5	5.5	6	7.9	6	9.4	0.053 [a]
	6–8	15	18.3	19	20.9	15	19.7	10	15.6	
	9–12	42	51.2	43	47.3	36	47.4	27	42.2	
	13–15	21	25.6	24	26.4	19	25.0	21	32.8	

[a] Chi-square test; [b] Fisher's exact test: n = total number of patients included in the study from each hospital. APACHE: Acute Physiology and Chronic Health Evaluation; GCS: Glasgow Coma Scale. Hospital C had a longer patient stay ($p < 0.001$); Hospital A had a higher number of deaths ($p = 0.036$).

According to the obtained results, a statistically significant difference in length of stay ($p < 0.001$) was observed among all four hospitals, with hospital C having a longer patient stay. Additionally, a statistically significant association ($p = 0.036$) was also found in the therapy outcome variable, with hospital A reporting a higher number of deaths.

Total antibiotic consumption based on the DDD(g) and DDD per 100 bed days during the study period was 54.2. Antibiotic types, their consumption based on the DDD/100-bed days, ATC codes, and the number of prescriptions is shown in Table 2.

Table 2. Antibiotic types and their utilization in ICUs of the studied hospitals in DDD(g).

	Types	ATC Code	No. of Prescriptions	%	DDD (g)	ACI (DDD/Bed Days × 100)
Access	Amoxicillin/clavulanic acid	J01CR02	75	9.8	7.6	4.5
	Metronidazole	J01XD01	66	8.6	2.1	4.2
	Ampicillin	J01CA01	59	7.7	1.9	3.1
	Amikacin	J01GB06	44	5.6	9.9	7.5
Watch	Cefoperazone	J01DB09	21	2.7	2	2.8
	Ceftazidime	J01DB05	20	2.6	2	2.6
	Ciprofloxacin	J01MA02	38	4.9	1	1.3
	Cefotaxime	J01DD01	60	7.8	4	2.3
	Azithromycin	J01FA10	37	4.8	0.3	1.1
	Lincomycin	J01FF02	29	3.8	1.8	4.1

Table 2. *Cont.*

	Types	ATC Code	No. of Prescriptions	%	DDD (g)	ACI (DDD/Bed Days × 100)
Watch	Meropenem	J01DH02	29	3.8	2	2.3
	Cefuroxime	J01DC02	48	6.3	0.5	1.8
	Vancomycin	J01XA01	25	3.3	1.9	2.2
	Imipenem/cilastatin	J01DH51	48	6.3	2	1.5
	Ceftriaxone	J01DD04	57	7.4	2	1.6
	Piperacillin/tazobactam	J01CR05	45	5.9	14	8.3
Reserve	Linezolid	J01XX08	38	4.9	1.2	2.3
	Colistin	J01XB01	29	3.8	9 (MU)	0.7
Total antibiotic consumption			768	100		54.2

Furthermore, it was also observed that hospital D followed more appropriate antibiotic prescribing patterns, with prescribers generally adhering to WHO AWaRe classification, i.e., prescribing fewer antibiotics from the Reserve group. However, the percentage of antibiotic usage from the Watch group was similar among all four of the studied hospitals. Antibiotic types, their consumption in each hospital, and the number (percentage) of prescriptions are shown in Table 3.

Table 3. Antibiotic type and their utilization in ICUs of the studied hospitals.

AWaRe Classification 2021	Types	Hospital A	No. of Prescriptions (%)	Hospital B	No. of Prescriptions (%)	Hospital C	No. of Prescriptions (%)	Hospital D	No. of Prescriptions (%)	p-Value
Access	Amoxicillin/clavulanic acid	17	49 (28)	14	49 (21.7)	20	68 (37.8)	24	78 (41.7)	<0.001 [b]
	Metronidazole	13		13		19		21		
	Ampicillin	11		12		17		19		
	Amikacin	8		10		12		14		
Watch	Cefoperazone	4	106 (60.6)	9	150 (66.4)	5	99 (55)	3	102 (54.5)	
	Ceftazidime	4		9		4		3		
	Ciprofloxacin	9		17		7		5		
	Cefotaxime	13		26		10		11		
	Azithromycin	8		10		9		10		
	Lincomycin	7		9		8		5		
	Meropenem	6		4		9		10		
	Cefuroxime	10		12		12		14		
	Vancomycin	5		9		6		5		
	Imipenem/cilastatin	14		15		9		10		
	Ceftriaxone	12		20		11		14		
	Piperacillin/tazobactam	14		10		9		12		
Reserve	Linezolid	11	20 (11.4)	18	27 (11.9)	6	13 (7.2)	3	7 (3.8)	
	Colistin	9		9		7		4		
	Total antibiotic consumption	768	175 (100)		226 (100)		180 (100)		187 (100)	

[b] Fisher's exact test: Hospital B and Hospital C consumed more "Watch" antibiotics.

Our study findings showed a statistically significant difference ($p < 0.001$) in the utilization of Watch category antibiotics, indicating variation in prescription patterns across hospitals. The highest consumption of Watch antibiotics was reported in hospital B and hospital C, suggesting differences in ICU antibiotic stewardship policies. Additionally, the use of Reserve antibiotics was relatively low in all hospitals, reflecting restricted usage for last-resort antibiotics.

Among antibiotic therapy types, the majority of patients were on definitive therapy in all four hospitals, with 34 (41.5%), 37 (40.6%), 34 (44.7%), and 27 (42.2%) patients on definitive therapy in hospitals A, B, C, and D, respectively. The total number of patients on empirical therapy were 29 (35.4%), 33 (36.3%), 24 (31.6%), and 24 (37.5%) and as prophylaxis were 19 (23.1%), 21 (23.1%), 18 (23.7%) and 13 (20.3%) in hospitals A, B, C, and D, respectively. More than 40% of the total studied patients were treated with two antibiotics and the route of administration in the majority of the cases (>50%) was intravenous. These results are presented in Table 4.

Table 4. Antibiotic administration.

Characteristics	Categories	Hospitals								*p*-Value
		Hospital A (*n* = 82)		Hospital B (*n* = 91)		Hospital C (*n* = 76)		Hospital D (*n* = 64)		
		n	%	*n*	%	*n*	%	*n*	%	
Antibiotic therapy type	Empirical	29	35.4	33	36.3	24	31.6	24	37.5	0.039 [b]
	Definitive (after C&S test)	34	41.5	37	40.6	34	44.7	27	42.2	
	Prophylaxis	19	23.1	21	23.1	18	23.7	13	20.3	
Number of antibiotics given per day	1	17	20.7	19	20.9	14	18.4	14	21.9	<0.001 [b]
	2	35	42.7	38	41.8	35	46.1	26	40.6	
	3	16	19.5	15	16.5	16	21.1	14	21.9	
	≥4	14	17.1	19	20.9	11	14.5	10	15.6	
Route of administration	Parenteral (intravenous)	67	81.7	74	81.3	57	75	53	82.8	0.021 [b]
	Oral	15	18.3	17	18.7	19	25	11	17.2	

[b] Fisher's exact test: *n* = total number of patients included in the study from each hospital.

A statistically significant association (<0.001) in the number of antibiotics used per day was observed among the studied hospitals. In hospital B, the highest number of antibiotics used was two (41.8% of patients), while in hospital D, the highest number was also two (40.6% of patients).

According to the results of the C&S test of hospital D, isolates of gram-positive bacteria showed highest sensitivity to meropenem (100%), followed by imipenem/cilastatin (75%), ceftazidime (75%), piperacillin/tazobactam (66.7%), amikacin (66.7%), and lincomycin (60%). Gram-negative bacteria in hospital D showed the highest sensitivity to imipenem/cilastatin (75%), meropenem (66.6%), amikacin (60%), and azithromycin (56.3%) among the total prescriptions sent for C&S analysis. These results are presented in Tables 5 and 6.

Table 5. Antibiotic sensitivity and resistance against gram-positive bacteria.

AWaRe Classification 2021	Types			Gram-Positive (Sensitivity)					Gram-Positive (Resistance)			
		n	N_1	Hospital A	Hospital B	Hospital C	Hospital D	N_2	Hospital A	Hospital B	Hospital C	Hospital D
				n (%)	*n* (%)	*n* (%)	*n* (%)		*n* (%)	*n* (%)	*n* (%)	*n* (%)
Access	Amoxicillin/clavulanic acid	17	13	4 (30.7)	3 (23.1)	3 (23.1)	3 (23.1)	4	1 (25)	1 (25)	1 (25)	1 (25)
	Metronidazole	5	4	1 (25)	3 (75)	0 (0)	0 (0)	1	0 (0)	1 (100)	0 (0)	0 (0)
	Ampicillin	11	9	1 (11.1)	5 (55.6)	2 (22.2)	1 (11.1)	2	1 (50)	1 (50)	0 (0)	0 (0)
	Amikacin	4	3	1 (33.3)	0 (0)	0 (0)	2 (66.7)	1	0 (0)	0 (0)	1 (100)	0 (0)
Watch	Cefoperazone	9	8	2 (25)	1 (12.5)	2 (25)	3 (37.5)	1	1 (100)	0 (0)	0 (0)	0 (0)
	Ceftazidime	7	4	0 (0)	0 (0)	1 (25)	3 (75)	3	1 (33.3)	0 (0)	1 (33.4)	1 (33.3)
	Ciprofloxacin	5	1	0 (0)	1 (100)	0 (0)	0 (0)	4	1 (25)	3 (75)	0 (0)	0 (0)
	Cefotaxime	3	2	0 (0)	0 (0)	1 (50)	1 (50)	1	1 (100)	0 (0)	0 (0)	0 (0)
	Azithromycin	9	7	1 (14.3)	1 (14.3)	1 (14.3)	4 (57.1)	2	0 (0)	0 (0)	1 (50)	1 (50)
	Lincomycin	5	5	0 (0)	1 (20)	1 (20)	3 (60)	0	0 (0)	0 (0)	0 (0)	0 (0)

Table 5. *Cont.*

AWaRe Classification 2021	Types			Gram-Positive (Sensitivity)					Gram-Positive (Resistance)			
		n	N_1	Hospital A	Hospital B	Hospital C	Hospital D	N_2	Hospital A	Hospital B	Hospital C	Hospital D
Watch	Meropenem	4	4	0 (0)	0 (0)	0 (0)	4 (100)	0	0 (0)	0 (0)	0 (0)	0 (0)
	Cefuroxime	12	9	2 (22.2)	4 (44.5)	1 (11.1)	2 (22.2)	3	1 (33.3)	1 (33.3)	0 (0)	1 (33.4)
	Vancomycin	7	6	1 (16.7)	1 (16.7)	1 (16.6)	3 (50)	1	0 (0)	0 (0)	0 (0)	1 (100)
	Imipenem/cilastatin	8	8	1 (12.5)	0 (0)	1 (12.5)	6 (75)	0	0 (0)	0 (0)	0 (0)	0 (0)
	Ceftriaxone	22	14	3 (21.4)	4 (28.6)	3 (21.4)	4 (28.6)	8	1 (12.5)	2 (25)	2 (25)	3 (37.5)
	Piperacillin/tazobactam	4	3	0 (0)	0 (0)	1 (33.3)	2 (66.7)	1	0 (0)	0 (0)	0 (0)	1 (100)
Reserve	Linezolid	11	9	3 (33.3)	0 (0)	3 (33.3)	3 (33.4)	2	0 (0)	0 (0)	1 (50)	1 (50)
	Colistin	4	2	0 (0)	0 (0)	1 (50)	1 (50)	2	1 (50)	0 (0)	0 (0)	1 (50)

N_1 = prescriptions where gram-positive (sensitivity) was checked; N_2 = prescriptions where gram-positive (resistance) was checked. *n* = total prescriptions where gram-positive (sensitivity) and gram-positive (resistance) were checked; NP = not performed.

Table 6. Antibiotic sensitivity and resistance against gram-negative bacteria.

AWaRe Classification 2021	Types			Gram-Negative (Sensitivity)					Gram-Negative (Resistance)			
		n	N_1	Hospital A	Hospital B	Hospital C	Hospital D	N_2	Hospital A	Hospital B	Hospital C	Hospital D
				n (%)	*n* (%)	*n* (%)	*n* (%)		*n* (%)	*n* (%)	*n* (%)	*n* (%)
Access	Amoxicillin/clavulanic acid	32	14	3 (21.4)	4 (28.6)	3 (21.4)	4 (28.6)	18	4 (22.2)	5 (27.8)	5 (27.8)	4 (22.2)
	Metronidazole	6	2	0 (0)	2 (100)	0 (0)	0 (0)	4	0 (0)	2 (50)	0 (0)	2 (50)
	Ampicillin	9	6	1 (16.7)	3 (50)	1 (16.7)	1 (16.6)	3	1 (33.4)	1 (33.3)	1 (33.3)	0 (0)
	Amikacin	14	10	2 (20)	0 (0)	2 (20)	6 (60)	4	0 (0)	0 (0)	2 (50)	2 (50)
Watch	Cefoperazone	10	9	2 (22.2)	3 (33.4)	2 (22.2)	2 (22.2)	1	1 (100)	0 (0)	0 (0)	0 (0)
	Ceftazidime	8	6	1 (16.7)	1 (16.7)	1 (16.6)	3 (50)	2	0 (0)	0 (0)	1 (50)	1 (50)
	Ciprofloxacin	11	8	1 (12.5)	5 (62.5)	1 (12.5)	1 (12.5)	3	1 (33.3)	2 (66.7)	0 (0)	0 (0)
	Cefotaxime	10	8	2 (25)	2 (25)	2 (25)	2 (25)	2	0 (0)	0 (0)	1 (50)	1 (50)
	Azithromycin	17	16	2 (12.5)	2 (12.5)	3 (18.7)	9 (56.3)	1	0 (0)	0 (0)	1 (100)	0 (0)
	Lincomycin	11	4	0 (0)	0 (0)	2 (50)	2 (50)	7	1 (14.3)	1 (14.3)	2 (28.6)	3 (42.8)
	Meropenem	7	6	1 (16.7)	0 (0)	1 (16.7)	4 (66.6)	1	0 (0)	0 (0)	0 (0)	1 (100)
	Cefuroxime	9	6	1 (16.7)	2 (33.3)	2 (33.3)	1 (16.7)	3	1 (33.4)	1 (33.3)	1 (33.3)	0 (0)
	Vancomycin	6	4	1 (25)	0 (0)	1 (25)	2 (50)	2	0 (0)	0 (0)	0 (0)	2 (100)
	Imipenem/cilastatin	8	8	0 (0)	1 (12.5)	1 (12.5)	6 (75)	0	0 (0)	0 (0)	0 (0)	0 (0)
	Ceftriaxone	13	8	3 (37.5)	2 (25)	2 (25)	1 (12.5)	5	1 (20)	2 (40)	1 (20)	1 (20)
	Piperacillin/tazobactam	11	8	1 (12.5)	1 (12.5)	2 (25)	4 (50)	3	0 (0)	0 (0)	1 (33.3)	2 (66.7)
Reserve	Linezolid	0	NP	NP	NP	NP	NP	NP	NP	NP	NP	NP
	Colistin	4	4	2 (50)	0 (0)	1 (25)	1 (25)	0	0 (0)	0 (0)	0 (0)	0 (0)

N_1 = prescriptions where gram-negative (sensitivity) was checked; N_2 = prescriptions where gram-negative (resistance) was checked. *n* = total prescriptions where gram-negative (sensitivity) and gram-negative (resistance) were checked; NP = not performed.

In univariate analyses, among the studied demographic and clinical characteristics variables, only gender, length of stay (days), number of antibiotics given per day, and route of administration were found to be statistically significant ($p < 0.05$) and showed statistically significant differences in AWaRe classification-based usage of antibiotics. These statistically significant variables (predictors) were further analyzed in multivariate analyses using multinomial logistic regression to find pure predictors of antibiotic usage according to the WHO AWaRe categorization among the patients studied. Table 7 presents the multinomial logistic regression analyses results which revealed that for any change in length of stay (days), i.e., >1 day, the scores were 0.197, 0.276, 0.569, and 0.914, for 2–3 days, 4–5 days, 6–7 days, and >7 days, respectively, in relation to the Reserve category antibiotics usage ($p < 0.05$), when adjusted for other variables. Similarly, a change in the number of antibiotics given per day, i.e., one or more antibiotics, was associated with an increase of 0.219, 0.787, and 1.293 for two antibiotics, three antibiotics, and four or more antibiotics, respectively, in the Reserve category ($p < 0.05$), when other demographic and clinical variables kept constant. The variables of gender and route of administration were not statistically significant ($p > 0.05$).

Table 7. Multinomial logistic regression analyses of factors associated with AWaRe classification and the usage pattern of antibiotics.

Total = 768 (100%)		Access 244 (31.8%)			Watch 457 (59.5%)			Reserve 67 (8.7%)	
Characteristics	**β**	**AOR (95% CI)**	***p*-Value**	**β**	**AOR (95% CI)**	***p*-Value**	**β**	**AOR (95% CI)**	***p*-Value**
Gender									
Male		Referent			Referent			Referent	
Female	0.34	0.267 (0.078–1.298)	0.448	−0.13	0.185 (0.041–0.977)	0.058	0.16	0.356 (0.298–1.718)	0.103
Length of stay (days)									
1		Referent			Referent			Referent	
2–3	0.21	0.218 (0.074–0.778)	0.116	−0.24	0.193 (0.048–0.387)	0.063	0.17	0.197 (0.067–0.989)	0.035
4–5	0.32	0.378 (0.055–1.927)	0.238	0.23	0.378 (0.055–1.927)	0.082	0.28	0.276 (0.359–2.174)	0.029
6–7	−0.12	0.514 (0.298–1.718)	0.137	−0.23	0.876 (0.359–2.174)	0.096	0.19	0.569 (0.144–0.891)	0.047
>7	−0.18	0.389 (0.117–1.498)	0.143	−0.36	0.444 (0.363–0.875)	0.059	0.15	0.914 (0.298–1.718)	0.041
Number of antibiotics given per day									
1		Referent			Referent			Referent	
2	0.12	0.391 (0.192–0.767)	0.319	0.11	1.091 (0.581–2.561)	0.278	0.05	0.219 (0.192–0.767)	0.014
3	−0.14	0.485 (0.185–1.317)	0.174	−0.09	0.485 (0.185–1.317)	0.094	0.08	0.787 (0.178–0.956)	0.032
≥4	−0.16	0.289 (0.078–0.456)	0.152	−0.12	0.671 (0.612–1.781)	0.198	0.07	1.293 (0.185–0.478)	0.048
Route of administration									
Parenteral (intravenous)		Referent			Referent			Referent	
Oral	0.25	0.478 (0.362–0.991)	0.231	0.26	1.091 (0.581–2.561)	0.173	0.22	0.719 (0.451–1.981)	0.155

AOR = Adjusted Odds ratio.

4. Discussion

4.1. Demographics and Clinical Characteristics

The global consumption of antibiotics has reached 65% in the last decade and the major cause behind this is the irrational use of antibiotics, especially in developing countries including Pakistan. The reason behind this could be that antibiotics are usually considered a relatively fast remedy to treat infections by numerous prescribers, especially fresh graduates from developing countries [42]. The current study aimed to determine the type, utilization pattern, sensitivity, and resistance pattern of antibiotics used in ICUs of four different hospitals after the third wave of COVID-19 in Pakistan.

In the current study, out of 313 patients, more than 35% were 18 to 35 years old and more than 60% were females. The majority of the patients in ICUs suffered from respiratory tract infections, i.e., they were 31.7%, 29.7%, 27.6%, and 28.1% in hospitals A, B, C, and D, respectively. The presence of renal infections was 24.4%, 26.4%, 27.6%, and 26.6% in hospitals A, B, C, and D, respectively. The other infections include CNS infections, renal, UTIs, and miscellaneous. Length of stay for the maximum number of patients was 2–3 days, i.e., 51.2%, 49.5%, 49.9%, and 53.1% for hospitals A, B, C, and D, respectively. According to the results of this study, there was no statistically significant association observed between some of the studied patients' demographics and the hospital types, i.e., hospital A, B, C, and hospital D. For instance, in age, gender, and reason for admission variables, there were statistically non-significant associations observed ($p = 0.301$, $p = 0.122$, and $p = 0.097$, respectively). In all four studied hospitals, to control all possible confounders and ensure the similarity between them, all of the demographic characteristics of the patients were matched to obtain the actual usage pattern of the antibiotics among patients admitted to the ICUs.

In the literature, it is reported that most of the prescribers consider the use of broad-spectrum antibiotics as empirical therapy which is similar to our study findings. In the current study, it was found that 54.3% of patients were provided with at least one DDD of antibiotics each day. This was higher than the DDD found in the study conducted by Marasine et al. (2021) in ICUs in Nepal [42]. It was found that the DDD/100 bed days for the four most frequently prescribed antibiotics were 7.6 (amoxicillin/clavulanic acid), 4 (cefotaxime), 1.9 (ampicillin), and 2 (ceftriaxone). In another study [43] by Saleem et al. (2021), it was observed that co-amoxiclav, ciprofloxacin, azithromycin, and levofloxacin were the four most commonly dispensed antibiotics in community pharmacies in Pakistan with DDD percentages of 24.3%, 11.6%, 6%, and 8.2%, respectively. The increased DDDs can be attributed to the fact that in Pakistan most physicians prescribe antibiotics based on the assumption of increased AMR among the public due to their irrational overuse.

There were statistically significant differences observed between some of the clinical characteristics of the patients and the hospital types, i.e., hospital A, B, C, and hospital D. For example, regarding the length of stay (days), the association was statistically significant ($p < 0.001$), which showed that hospital D employed better antibiotic prescription practices (prescribing antibiotics appropriately) as per the WHO AWaRe classification. It is worth mentioning that there was also a statistically significant ($p < 0.001$) relationship observed between the type of the hospital and length of stay (days) among the patients of the studied hospitals. We found that in hospital D, where more appropriate use of antibiotics was observed, the length of stay for patients in ICUs was less than in the rest of the hospitals. A statistically significant association ($p = 0.036$) was observed between the therapy outcomes and the studied hospitals, with hospital D showing better therapy outcomes compared to hospitals A, B, and C. These included deaths, discharge on request, and shifting to the wards from ICUs. These study results corroborate the findings of other studies where a higher rate of antibiotic consumption and prolonged hospital stays were observed [42–44]. There could be many reasons/factors that caused non-adherence to practice guidelines (WHO or local) among the prescribers in hospitals A, B, and C. These factors include limited resources, where healthcare systems may not be able to implement prescribing guidelines effectively, lack of awareness where providers may be unaware of or unfamiliar with WHO guidelines, and inadequate training where providers may not receive adequate training, i.e., Continuing Medical Education (CME) about AMR, and AMS [45,46]. In hospital D, according to the hospital practice manual for physicians, all of the prescribers were highly encouraged by the top management to attend at least two CMEs annually, which could be another reason for their better adherence to WHO practice guidelines.

It was observed that in hospital D, the conditions of the patients improved rapidly and were shifted to general wards more frequently compared to the rest of the hospitals. From our study findings, it was also observed that in hospital D, patients' length of stay in ICUs was shorter, and shifting to the general wards from the ICUs (indicating improved recovery) was more frequent compared to the rest of the hospitals. Comparatively, a better prescription pattern was observed among prescribers in hospital D, which may be attributed to their strong adherence to the WHO practice guidelines. However, in our results, some prescribers tend to prioritize their own experience over the guidelines. This justification is further supported by a recent study (2024) conducted by Dobrowolski et al., which suggested that certain prescribers rely on their own perceptions of patients, diseases, and treatment plans over the recommended WHO guidelines when evaluated for reasons of non-adherence to practice guidelines [47]. Other potential reasons may include clinical factors like complicated cases, patients with multiple comorbidities, local resistance patterns where prescribers may adjust prescriptions based on local antibiotic resistance patterns, and patient-specific factors where physicians may consider allergies or organ dysfunction while prescribing antibiotics to their patients [48,49].

4.2. Antibiotic Types and Utilization

The most prescribed antibiotics were amoxicillin/clavulanic acid (n = 75) followed by metronidazole (n = 66), cefotaxime (n = 60), ampicillin (n = 59), ceftriaxone (n = 57), cefuroxime (n = 48), and imipenem (n = 48). The higher rate of antibiotic prescription could be due to a lack of precise and relevant knowledge about antibiotics among physicians and non-compliance among patients. A study in Punjab, Pakistan, regarding antibiotic usage concluded that 60.2% of participants did not have appropriate knowledge about antibiotics utilization, and 59.6% of participants were in favor of using antibiotics for self-medications [46]. AMR is a leading healthcare concern that often results in decreased efficacy and increased treatment expenditures [48–50]. In another study conducted in Nepal by Marasine et al. (2021), it was found that piperacillin was the most frequently used antibiotic because of an increased prevalence of respiratory infections in ICUs, which is also parallel to the results found in the current study [42]. In a study conducted by Sozen et al. (2013) in Turkey [51], cephalosporins were found to constitute about 57% of all antibiotics used in the hospitals followed by fluoroquinolones (14.7%) and penicillin (10%), which is also in line with the findings of our study.

Lack of diagnostic resources, non-compliance with the WHO AWaRe classification usage, and less information about antibiotic sensitivity patterns are among the major problems of AMR that Pakistan currently facing in general [14,15]. This makes it harder to prescribe antibiotics according to the WHO AWaRe recommendation, which could lead to a further increase in AMR [18,19,40]. According to our study results, hospital B was found to be less adherent to WHO AWaRe recommendations, as there was more frequent usage of Watch category antibiotics when compared to the rest of the hospitals. The reason could be that practicing physicians considered it more convenient and timesaving to prescribe antibiotics, irrespective of AMR issues in the country [47–52]. These results corroborate the findings of other studies where the highest rate of antibiotic consumption was observed [41–43]. These results are deeply concerning in light of worries about Pakistan's rising AMR threshold, an increasing rate of irrational antibiotic prescription trends without C&S testing, and the lack of national antibiotic prescribing guidelines at present [22–24].

It was noted that the majority of patients were treated with definitive antibiotic therapies and were prescribed more than two or more antibiotics. Dohou et al. (2022) reported that 57% of patients in ICUs were prescribed two to five antibiotics [53]. Their study findings are parallel to the findings of the current study. It has also been reported that antibiotics are often used as prophylaxis for various diseases in many countries [53–55]. The results of this study can be compared with those from other countries, though some differences may exist due to geographical variations. In Western Europe, 71% of patients in ICUs were observed to have received various antibiotics as prophylaxis for various illnesses, which is similar to the findings of this study [54,55]. Recently, a study conducted in Belgium found that 42% of the studied patients were prescribed prophylactic antibiotic therapy [54]. Patient-related factors like patient expectations, where prescribers may prescribe antibiotics due to patient expectations or pressure, and lack of patient education, where patients may not understand the risks and benefits of antibiotics, can also lead to overprescription [53–59]. Some cultural factors, such as patient beliefs and values, can also influence prescribers' antibiotic prescribing practices [57–60]. Our study results are also in line with another study conducted in Japan where it was noted that 34% of patients in ICUs were prescribed antibiotics for prophylaxis [56]. Regarding empirical and prophylactic usage of antibiotics among patients admitted in ICUs, the utilization of antibiotics was greater in hospital A compared to hospital D. In Pakistan, empirical and definitive antibiotics therapies are more commonly prescribed, similar to what is reported in our study [57,61]. These findings were similar to other findings, where their perception of the rational use of antibiotics was also poor [59–61].

Undeniably, AMR is a major concern regarding high morbidity, mortality, and increased treatment costs worldwide. However, it is particularly important to address AMR in developing nations like the Asia-Pacific region. Antibiotic-resistant microorganisms are thought to be abundant in third-world countries like Pakistan. AMR is predicted to rise in the Asia-Pacific region by 70%, posing a global and local threat [57–59]. Globally, South Asian developing nations like Pakistan pose a serious healthcare concern due to increasing AMR. Numerous initiatives from the WHO like AWaRe classification and the importance of AMS are ongoing, but, unfortunately, the actual implementation of AMS in developing countries like Pakistan has not been initiated or completed so far.

There were statistically significant differences observed among the studied hospitals and their usage of antibiotics in terms of AWaRe classification. According to the obtained results, Access category antibiotics usage in ICUs was almost double (41.7%) in hospital D than in hospitals A (28%) and B (21.7%). The difference was also statistically significant ($p < 0.001$). In the Watch category, all of the ICUs in the studied hospitals used almost similar numbers of antibiotics, i.e., hospitals A (60.6%), B (66.4%), C (55%), and D (54%). In terms of the Reserve category, hospitals A and B used antibiotics almost 2–3 times more i.e., 11.4% and 11.9%, respectively, than hospital D (3.8%). The difference was also statistically significant ($p < 0.001$). It can be said that hospital D was more cautious in using antibiotics from the Reserve category in the ICU. Various miscellaneous factors like time constraints, where prescribers may not have time to thoroughly evaluate patients and follow guidelines, defensive prescribing where prescribers may prescribe antibiotics to avoid potential lawsuits or criticism, and the lack of accountability where prescribers may not be held accountable for their prescribing habits can significantly contribute towards irrational antibiotic prescribing practices.

Similarly, it can also be said that patients' self-preferences were not entertained in hospital D as compared to the hospital B and prescribers were strict about prescribing the antibiotics. For instance, in therapy outcomes, discharge on the request was less in hospital D as compared to the other hospitals like hospitals A and B. Hospital D was also found to be better than the rest of the hospitals, as the length of the stay in ICUs among the admitted patients was less ($p < 0.001$) than the hospital B, C and A. According to the obtained results, there was a statistically significant association observed ($p = 0.039$) between antibiotic therapy-type usage and the studied hospitals. Likewise, in the number of antibiotics given per day, the association was statistically significant ($p < 0.001$) between the studied hospitals, which also showed that hospital D was somehow adherent to WHO AWaRe classification compared to the rest of the hospitals. In terms of route of administration of antibiotics, a statistically significant association ($p = 0.021$) was observed whereby hospital A used more parenteral administrations than the other hospitals.

According to the WHO 30th General Program of Work 2021, a country-level target of a maximum of 60% of total antibiotics consumption should be from the Access category. This means that Access antibiotics should be used more widely than the other 2 categories as per the WHO recommendations, but not more than 60%. The Access category lists the recommended antibiotics for the top 25 infections [4,62]. These antibiotics have to be always accessible, reasonably priced, and of guaranteed quality. The Watch category comprises the majority of the "highest-priority and critically important antibiotics" that should be used to control/treat particular infections that the Access category fails to control. Watch antibiotics should only be used in certain, and restricted situations. Another reason could be that the results of the Watch group antibiotics are better in efficacy than Access group, but they are generally expensive, broad-spectrum, and are more prone to be resistant. Therefore, the WHO recommends their usage to be reduced and only for particular cases, to avoid potential resistance. The Reserve category contains the antibiotics that the WHO recommends only be used as a last resort. These antibiotics ought to be reserved for extreme situations in which all other options have been exhausted. Watch and Reserve categories are nine to 32 times more expensive, respectively, than the Access category antibiotics [4,62].

4.3. Antibiotic Sensitivity and Resistance

This study showed that gram-positive bacteria were more sensitive to amikacin, azithromycin, meropenem, and imipenem/cilastatin. Furthermore, it was also inferred that gram-positive bacteria were resistant to vancomycin, ceftazidime, ciprofloxacin, and cefuroxime. Regarding gram-negative bacteria, this study showed that gram-negative bacteria were more sensitive to azithromycin, colistin, lincomycin, and cefotaxime. Furthermore, it was also inferred that gram-negative bacteria were resistant to amoxicillin/clavulanic acid, ampicillin, ciprofloxacin, and cefuroxime. It was also observed that carbapenems were among the most sensitive antibiotics against all bacterial isolates.

Not only physicians but also the general public play an important role in the increase of AMR [63,64]. In line with our study results, similar findings were reported in a study done in Nepal, where gram-negative bacteria were found to be highly resistant to amoxicillin/clavulanic acid, ampicillin, ciprofloxacin, and cefuroxime [65]. Similarly, they also found that gram-negative bacteria were most sensitive to azithromycin, colistin, lincomycin, and cefotaxime, which is also observed in our study [66]. Similar to our study's findings, two other studies also reported that carbapenems were among the most sensitive antibiotics against all bacterial isolates [47,66].

In Pakistan, another paramount factor that profoundly contributes to decreased sensitivity and increased AMR is the easy access of the general public to antibiotics at drug stores and pharmacies. Sadly, it is a common practice that various types of antibiotics can be accessed and purchased without a prescription from a registered medical practitioner [65–67]. Moreover, customer service in the majority of medicine stores and pharmacies in Pakistan is also untrained and non-professional, leading to an increased practice of inappropriate sales of antibiotics which ultimately results in increased AMR [63–67]. According to a recent study (2020), more than 97% of pharmacies and medicine stores in Pakistan contribute enormously to AMR by giving/providing antibiotics without a valid medical prescription. This malpractice plays a significant role in furthering the irrational use and overuse of antibiotics and promoting antibiotic self-medication [57]. A study reported that more than 70% of antibiotic prescriptions were for minor ailments and some were even for viral infections [61]. Several other studies also reported that in Pakistan, more than 70% of the antibiotics were dispensed without valid prescriptions [57,61,68].

In Pakistan, resistance to some antibiotics like ceftriaxone and quinolone, which are often used to treat non-typhoidal Salmonellae, is also rising [64–67]. Another study reported that around 70% of AMR was present against cefaclor, novobiocin, amoxicillin, and ampicillin [69]. In addition, multidrug resistance (MDR) is also on the rise in Pakistan [69–71]. According to another study, nearly 78% of the screened isolates were resistant to at least three antibiotics [70]. A study conducted in Pakistan also reported an overall increase in AMR in different areas of Pakistan, including the appearance of MDR [71]. This increased AMR strongly supports the impression that the Pakistani nation is experiencing a sharp rise in AMR or is perhaps at the advent of MDR [69–71]. Another study also reported that >80% of various Escherichia coli isolates were resistant to beta-lactam antibiotics in Lahore, Pakistan [70]. Many of these isolates were also resistant to trimethoprim-sulfamethoxazole and fluoroquinolones [69–71]. Overall, our study findings underscore the urgent need for the implementation of AMS programs in all healthcare facilities. Our findings also emphasize strictly adhering to WHO AWaRe classifications of antibiotics usage to ensure appropriate and optimal use of antibiotics in all healthcare facilities across Pakistan, especially in ICUs, to combat AMR.

The daunting problem of AMR in Pakistan can be significantly reduced with the support of strict government policies at the federal, provincial, and local levels, by implementing a code of conduct for the prescribers regarding the prescription of antibiotics according to WHO AWaRe classification, and by arranging CMEs and allied refresher courses like AMS programs. Priority must be given right away to strategies and initiatives that emphasize the responsible use of antimicrobials and restrict their unwanted and irrational use in all healthcare settings. It is anticipated that these actions will significantly lower current infection rates, alter resistance patterns, lower treatment costs, and enhance therapeutic outcomes. In addition to these regulations, the AMR threat can also be mitigated by enhancing public awareness about infectious diseases, providing pure (hygienic) drinking water, and establishing infection control units/centers at the grassroots level in Pakistan.

4.4. Factors Influencing AWaRe Classification-Based Usage of Antibiotics

In our study, pure predictors of AWaRe classification-based use of antibiotics were identified by adjusting or controlling confounders using a multinomial logistic regression model. In multinomial logistic regression analyses, it was inferred that in the Reserve category, the 'length of stay (days)' variable for 2–3 days (AOR 0.197; $p = 0.035$), 4–5 days (AOR 0.276; $p = 0.029$), 6–7 days (AOR 0.569; $p = 0.047$), and >7 days (AOR 0.914; $p = 0.041$) was statistically significant when 1 day was considered as 'referent'. Likewise, in the Reserve category, the 'number of antibiotics given per day' variable for two antibiotics (AOR 0.219; $p = 0.014$), three antibiotics (AOR 0.787; $p = 0.032$), and four or more antibiotics (AOR 1.293; $p = 0.048$) was statistically significant when one antibiotic use was considered as 'referent'. These findings affirmed that in the Reserve category, length of stay (days) and number of antibiotics given per day were the pure predictors of AWaRe classification-based usage of antibiotics among the studied patients when adjusted for the other demographic and clinical characteristics variables/confounders. Both of the predictors showed a statistically significant positive association in the Reserve category with AWaRe classification-based usage of antibiotics among the studied patients in ICUs.

In our study, for any change in length of stay (days), i.e., 2–3 days, 4–5 days, 6–7 days, and >7 days, the odds of usage of antibiotics in the Reserve category were increased to 0.197, 0.276, 0.569, and 0.914, respectively. Our results are in accordance with another study, conducted in Nepal, where it was reported that usage of antibiotics was significantly increased with the increase in the length of the hospital stay (days) [42]. Another study conducted in Sweden also presented similar findings regarding length of the hospital stays [72]. Our results in terms of hospital stay (days) also corroborate with the findings of another study that reported prolonged usage of antibiotics with prolonged hospital stays [73]. Regarding the number of antibiotics given per day, our study findings are in line with studies conducted by Marasine et al. [42] and Walther et al. [72], where it was observed that whenever the Reserve category was more frequently used in ICUs, the total number of antibiotics administrated significantly increased. Similar findings to our study results were also reported by another study in terms of the total number of antibiotics administered per day [73]. Our study results indicated that the odds of Reserve category antibiotics usage in ICUs significantly increased for longer hospital stays and simultaneous administration (overuse) of more than two antibiotics. Multivariate analyses indicated that in the study sample, the usage of Reserve category antibiotics increased with the increase in length of stay (days) and increase in number of antibiotics per day.

The inappropriate utilization of antibiotics in ICUs in Pakistan further endangers human lives since uncontrolled increasing bacterial infections have a considerably high negative impact on human health [29,72,73]. Implementing the AWaRe classification system in hospitals in Pakistan, especially in ICUs, can have numerous benefits. It can enable prescribers to make informed decisions about antibiotic prescription, reducing the misuse of broad-spectrum antibiotics. Additionally, by promoting the Access category (narrow-spectrum, first-line options), hospitals can minimize the risk of AMR and reduce the risk of adverse reactions, like Clostridioides difficile infections, allergic reactions, and antibiotic-associated diarrhea. This, in turn, will enhance patient safety, improve health outcomes, and slow the development of AMR. Moreover, by reserving broad-spectrum antibiotics (Watch and Reserve categories) for specific situations, hospitals can also help preserve antibiotics' effectiveness, reducing the risk of antibiotic failure and improving patient outcomes. Implementing the AWaRe classification system can also lead to reduced costs and shorter hospital stays, as patients are more likely to receive effective, targeted antibiotic therapy, reducing the need for prolonged hospitalization. The AWaRe classification system can further help hospitals manage MDR organisms more effectively, reducing the risk of transmission and improving the overall health-related quality of life of patients.

Therefore, there is a greater need for the development of strict policies as well as their implementation regarding the appropriate and precise utilization of antibiotics in Pakistan. In Pakistan, prescribers predominantly face challenges when prescribing antibiotics due to a lack of AMS programs, developing healthcare systems, and a dearth of diagnostic facilities [29,69–73]. The results of the study could be used not only to evaluate the current healthcare situation in ICUs in some hospitals of Pakistan but would also help to design, implement, and standardize policies and practices regarding safe use of antibiotics, especially according to the WHO AWaRe classification. This necessitates the need to adapt AMS programs similar to those of developed nations. Our study recommends the Ministry of Health, Pakistan, to instruct and enforce all the healthcare facilities to design and implement continuous AMS programs and instruct all prescribers to attend. Authorities can also declare that such programs will be part of their CMEs and will be compulsory to attend for their practice license renewals. This will ultimately promote and encourage prescribers to strictly adhere to the rational use of antibiotics according to WHO AWaRe classification.

4.5. Strengths and Limitations of the Study

Strengths of the study include that it can help understand the prevalence of antibiotics utilization patterns, sensitivity, and resistance in ICUs of four different hospitals after the third wave of COVID-19 in Pakistan. This study's results would also aid in identifying and defining suitable AMS programs for proper antibiotic utilization to combat AMR in hospitals, especially in ICUs in Pakistan. The study results would also help in developing awareness among people about antibiotic irrational use and its consequences in the form of increased AMR.

The current study has a few limitations. Firstly, data was collected from the patients' records/files, which may not be very accurate, and results may be affected due to imprecise accuracy of the records (incomplete data or missing data) and prone to selection bias as compared to prospective studies. Second, this type of study could be prone to misclassification bias. Third, retrospective studies could also be subject to unavoidable variables, i.e., some other related factors may also be present that were ignored or not evaluated. Fourth, increasing the sample size or study sample can further improve the outcome of the study, though we tried to increase it by making a comparative study of four different hospitals. Fifth, the study results cannot be perfectly generalized for overall antibiotic consumption in all provinces of Pakistan since only four hospitals were included in this study. Sixth, our results do not exactly reflect the availability and the cost of the antibiotics used in different hospitals, as cheaper antibiotics are more frequently available and used than expensive antibiotics in third-world countries like Pakistan. In this study, some of the patients were already on antibiotics when they were admitted to a hospital, and the hospital was required to complete that particular antibiotic course, which could mislead the results, making it unfair to accuse a particular hospital. In the future, drug utilization studies (DUS) should be conducted to determine the exact level of adherence of prescribers to the local, regional, or WHO antibiotics' prescribing guidelines.

5. Conclusions

This study clearly shows that in managing various types of infections (even if they are of an analog origin), physicians or medical practitioners, regardless of their experience and education, often choose different antibiotics, which further results in increased hospitalizations and complications among patients suffering from various infections. This strongly necessitates the adoption of national, regional, or WHO protocols for antibiotic utilization in an apt way. There is also a need to strengthen awareness and education programs on proper antibiotic use among healthcare providers, patients, and the general public. More studies are needed in Pakistan to strengthen the apt usage of antibiotics, especially according to the WHO guidelines, particularly the AWaRe classification. In response to the growing AMR crisis, the implementation of AMS has become increasingly imperative as AMS strongly advocates for the sensible use of antibiotics, optimizing treatment outcomes, and minimizing the development of AMR. Additionally, implementing AMS programs in ICUs can also help optimize antibiotic use, monitor prescribing practices, and promote adherence to the WHO guidelines and protocols.

The majority of the studied hospitals in Pakistan are not fully following the WHO Committee of 2019 recommendations or the WHO 30th General Program of Work 2021 regarding apt antibiotic usage, which should be followed and practiced. Prescribers should adopt WHO guidelines, especially the AWaRe classification, to ensure the rational use of antibiotics in Pakistan and to be in line with the WHO initiatives for implementing AMS programs for antibiotics worldwide. In fact, some hospitals in Pakistan have already taken initiatives to make it compulsory for prescribers to strictly adhere to the WHO AWaRe classification and to use antibiotics accordingly to avoid increasing trends of AMR in Pakistan.

Author Contributions: Conceptualization, M.S.I., S.-U.-D.K. and M.Z.I.; methodology, M.S.I., M.F.K., S.F., S.Q. and S.V.; formal analysis, M.S.I., S.V., S.R., S.Q. and M.Z.I.; investigation, M.S.I., M.F.K., S.-U.-D.K., S.Q. and S.R.; resources, S.F., S.V., S.R. and M.Z.I.; data curation, M.S.I., S.V. and M.Z.I.; writing—original draft preparation, M.S.I., M.F.K., S.F., S.R. and M.Z.I.; writing—review and editing, S.-U.-D.K. and S.V.; supervision, S.R., S.V., S.Q. and S.-U.-D.K.; project administration, M.S.I., M.F.K., S.F., S.Q. and M.Z.I.; funding acquisition, M.F.K., S.F., S.V., S.Q. and S.R. All authors have read and agreed to the published version of the manuscript.

Funding: The authors extend their appreciation to Prince Sattam bin Abdulaziz University for funding this research work through the project number (PSAU/2024/03/31658).

Institutional Review Board Statement: The study was conducted according to the guidelines of the Declaration of Helsinki, and approved by the Research Ethics Committee, Lahore Pharmacy College, Lahore Medical & Dental College (ref: ETH/LPC/06/01/21, approval date: 6 January 2021).

Informed Consent Statement: Not applicable.

Data Availability Statement: Data are available upon a reasonable request.

Conflicts of Interest: The authors declare no conflicts of interest.

References

1. Abdelsalam Elshenawy, R.; Umaru, N.; Aslanpour, Z. WHO AWaRe classification for antibiotic stewardship: Tackling antimicrobial resistance—A descriptive study from an English NHS Foundation Trust prior to and during the COVID-19 pandemic. *Front. Microbiol.* **2023**, *14*, 1298858. [CrossRef] [PubMed]
2. Adedeji, W.A. The Treasure Called Antibiotics. *Ann. Ibadan Postgrad. Med.* **2016**, *14*, 56–57.
3. Darkwah, T.O.; Afriyie, D.K.; Sneddon, J.; Cockburn, A.; Opare-Addo, M.N.A.; Tagoe, B.; Amponsah, S.K. Assessment of Prescribing Patterns of Antibiotics Using National Treatment Guidelines and World Health Organization Prescribing Indicators at the Ghana Police Hospital: A Pilot Study. *Pan Afr. Med. J.* **2021**, *39*, 222. [CrossRef] [PubMed]
4. Sharland, M.; Zanichelli, V.; Ombajo, L.A.; Bazira, J.; Cappello, B.; Chitatanga, R.; Chuki, P.; Gandra, S.; Getahun, H.; Harbarth, S.; et al. The WHO Essential Medicines List AWaRe Book: From a List to a Quality Improvement System. *Clin. Microbiol. Infect.* **2022**, *28*, 1533–1535. [CrossRef]
5. World Health Organization (WHO). The WHO AWaRe (Access, Watch, Reserve) Antibiotic Book—Infographics. Available online: https://www.who.int/publications/i/item/WHO-MHP-HPS-EML-2022.02 (accessed on 12 December 2024).
6. Sharland, M.; Pulcini, C.; Harbarth, S.; Zeng, M.; Gandra, S.; Mathur, S.; Magrini, N. Classifying Antibiotics in the WHO Essential Medicines List for Optimal Use—Be AWaRe. *Lancet Infect. Dis.* **2018**, *18*, 18–20. [CrossRef]
7. World Health Organization. 2021 AWaRe Classification. Available online: https://www.who.int/publications/i/item/2021-aware-classification (accessed on 12 December 2024).
8. Hsia, Y.; Lee, B.R.; Versporten, A.; Yang, Y.; Bielicki, J.; Jackson, C.; Newland, J.; Goossens, H.; Magrini, N.; Sharland, M. Use of the WHO Access, Watch, and Reserve Classification to Define Patterns of Hospital Antibiotic Use (AWaRe): An Analysis of Paediatric Survey Data from 56 Countries. *Lancet Glob. Health* **2019**, *7*, e861–e871. [CrossRef]
9. Budd, E.; Cramp, E.; Sharland, M.; Hand, K.; Howard, P.; Wilson, P.; Wilcox, M.; Muller-Pebody, B.; Hopkins, S. Adaptation of the WHO Essential Medicines List for National Antibiotic Stewardship Policy in England: Being AWaRe. *J. Antimicrob. Chemother.* **2019**, *74*, 3384–3389. [CrossRef]
10. Martens, E.; Demain, A.L. The Antibiotic Resistance Crisis, with a Focus on the United States. *J. Antibiot.* **2017**, *70*, 520–526. [CrossRef]
11. Pacios, E. Antibiotic Stewardship in the Real World. *Lancet Infect. Dis.* **2022**, *22*, 448–449. [CrossRef]
12. Godman, B.; Egwuenu, A.; Haque, M.; Malande, O.O.; Schellack, N.; Kumar, S.; Saleem, Z.; Sneddon, J.; Hoxha, I.; Islam, S.; et al. Strategies to Improve Antimicrobial Utilization with a Special Focus on Developing Countries. *Life* **2021**, *11*, 528. [CrossRef]
13. Hardefeldt, L.Y.; Weese, J.S.; Page, S.W. General Concepts in Antimicrobial Stewardship. *Antimicrob. Ther. Vet. Med.* **2024**, *30*, 401–423.
14. Liu, S.; Yu, C.; Tu, Q.; Zhang, Q.; Fu, Z.; Huang, Y.; He, C.; Yao, L. Bacterial co-infection in COVID-19: A call to stay vigilant. *PeerJ* **2024**, *12*, e18041. [CrossRef] [PubMed]
15. Rahman, M.M.; Alam Tumpa, M.A.; Zehravi, M.; Sarker, M.T.; Yamin, M.D.; Islam, M.R.; Harun-Or-Rashid, M.; Ahmed, M.; Ramproshad, S.; Mondal, B.; et al. An overview of antimicrobial stewardship optimization: The use of antibiotics in humans and animals to prevent resistance. *Antibiotics* **2022**, *11*, 667. [CrossRef] [PubMed]
16. Aslam, B.; Asghar, R.; Muzammil, S.; Shafique, M.; Siddique, A.B.; Khurshid, M.; Ijaz, M.; Rasool, M.H.; Chaudhry, T.H.; Aamir, A.; et al. AMR and Sustainable Development Goals: At a crossroads. *Glob. Health* **2024**, *20*, 73. [CrossRef]
17. Abrar, S.; Hussain, S.; Khan, R.A.; Ul Ain, N.; Haider, H.; Riaz, S. Prevalence of extended-spectrum-β-lactamase-producing Enterobacteriaceae: First systematic meta-analysis report from Pakistan. *Antimicrob. Resist. Infect. Control.* **2018**, *7*, 1–11. [CrossRef]
18. Yasmin, F.; Akhtar, N.; Hameed, A. In vitro synergistic effect of ciprofloxacin with aminoglycosides against multidrug resistant-Pseudomonas aeruginosa. *Pak. J. Pharm. Sci.* **2013**, *26*, 1041–1045.
19. Qamar, F.N.; Yousafzai, M.T.; Khalid, M.; Kazi, A.M.; Lohana, H.; Karim, S.; Khan, A.; Hotwani, A.; Qureshi, S.; Kabir, F.; et al. Outbreak investigation of ceftriaxone-resistant Salmonella enterica serotype Typhi and its risk factors among the general population in Hyderabad, Pakistan: A matched case-control study. *Lancet Infect. Dis.* **2018**, *18*, 1368–1376. [CrossRef]
20. Latif, S.; Anwar, M.S.; Ahmad, I. Bacterial pathogens responsible for blood stream infection (BSI) and pattern of drug resistance in a tertiary care hospital of Lahore. *Biomedica* **2009**, *25*, 101–105.
21. Faizullah, M.; Umar, M.I.; Anwar, M.; Sarfraz, M.K. A cross-sectional study on knowledge, attitude and practices of medical doctors towards antibiotic prescribing patterns and resistance in Khyber Pakhtun Khawah, Pakistan. *J. Appl. Pharm. Sci.* **2017**, *7*, 38–46.

22. Mirha, H.T.; Ali, S.H.; Aamar, H.; Sadiq, M.; Tharwani, Z.H.; Habib, Z.; Malikzai, A. The impact of antibiotic resistance on the rampant spread of infectious diseases in Pakistan: Insights from a narrative review. *Health Sci. Rep.* **2024**, *7*, e2050. [CrossRef]
23. Akhtar, H.; Akhtar, S.; Rahman, F.U.; Afridi, M.; Khalid, S.; Ali, S.; Akhtar, N.; Khader, Y.S.; Ahmad, H.; Khan, M.M. An overview of the treatment options used for the management of COVID-19 in Pakistan: Retrospective observational study. *JMIR Public Health Surveill* **2021**, *7*, e28594. [CrossRef] [PubMed]
24. Hayat, K.; Mustafa, Z.U.; Ikram, M.N.; Ijaz-Ul-Haq, M.; Noor, I.; Rasool, M.F.; Ishaq, H.M.; Rehman, A.U.; Hasan, S.S.; Fang, Y. Perception, attitude, and confidence of physicians about antimicrobial resistance and antimicrobial prescribing among COVID-19 patients: A cross-sectional study from Punjab, Pakistan. *Front. Pharmacol.* **2022**, *12*, 794453. [CrossRef] [PubMed]
25. Saleem, Z.; Hassali, M.A.; Versporten, A.; Godman, B.; Hashmi, F.K.; Goossens, H.; Saleem, F. A multicenter point prevalence survey of antibiotic use in Punjab, Pakistan: Findings and implications. *Expert Rev. Anti-Infect Ther.* **2019**, *17*, 285–293. [CrossRef] [PubMed]
26. Khilnani, G.C.; Zirpe, K.; Hadda, V.; Mehta, Y.; Madan, K.; Kulkarni, A.; Mohan, A.; Dixit, S.; Guleria, R.; Bhattacharya, P. Guidelines for Antibiotic Prescription in Intensive Care Unit. *Indian J. Crit. Care Med.* **2019**, *23* (Suppl. S1), S1–S63.
27. Silva, A.R.O.; Salgado, D.R.; Lopes, L.P.N.; Castanheira, D.; Emmerick, I.C.M.; Lima, E.C. Increased Use of Antibiotics in the Intensive Care Unit During Coronavirus Disease (COVID-19) Pandemic in a Brazilian Hospital. *Front. Pharmacol.* **2021**, *12*, 778386. [CrossRef]
28. Ul Mustafa, Z.; Salman, M.; Aldeyab, M.; Kow, C.S.; Hasan, S.S. Antimicrobial consumption among hospitalized patients with COVID-19 in Pakistan. *SN Compr. Clin. Med.* **2021**, *3*, 1691–1695. [CrossRef]
29. Saleem, Z.; Saeed, H.; Hassali, M.A.; Godman, B.; Asif, U.; Yousaf, M.; Ahmed, Z.; Riaz, H.; Raza, S.A. Pattern of Inappropriate Antibiotic Use among Hospitalized Patients in Pakistan: A Longitudinal Surveillance and Implications. *Antimicrob. Resist. Infect. Control* **2019**, *8*, 188. [CrossRef]
30. Saleem, Z.; Godman, B.; Azhar, F.; Kalungia, A.C.; Fadare, J.; Opanga, S.; Markovic-Pekovic, V.; Hoxha, I.; Saeed, A.; Al-Gethamy, M.; et al. Progress on the national action plan of Pakistan on antimicrobial resistance (AMR): A narrative review and the implications. *Expert Rev. Anti-Infect. Ther.* **2022**, *20*, 71–93. [CrossRef]
31. Grau, S.; Hernandez, S.; Echeverria-Esnal, D.; Almendral, A.; Ferrer, R.; Limon, E.; Horcajada, J.P.; Catalan Infection Control Antimicrobial Stewardship Program (VINCat-PROA). Antimicrobial Consumption Among 66 Acute Care Hospitals in Catalonia: Impact of the COVID-19 Pandemic. *Antibiotics* **2021**, *10*, 943. [CrossRef]
32. Young, D.; McKenzie, C.A.; Gupta, S.; Sparkes, D.; Beecham, R.; Browning, D.; Dushianthan, A.; Saeed, K. Exploring Antibacterial Usage and Pathogen Surveillance over Five Years in a Tertiary Referral Teaching Hospital Adult General Intensive Care Unit (ICU). *Pathogens* **2024**, *13*, 961. [CrossRef]
33. Pandolfo, A.M.; Horne, R.; Jani, Y.; Reader, T.W.; Bidad, N.; Brealey, D.; Enne, V.I.; Livermore, D.M.; Gant, V.; Brett, S.J. Understanding decisions about antibiotic prescribing in ICU: An application of the necessity concerns framework. *BMJ Qual. Saf.* **2022**, *31*, 199–210. [CrossRef] [PubMed]
34. Volz, E.; Mishra, S.; Chand, M.; Barrett, J.C.; Johnson, R.; Geidelberg, L.; Hinsley, W.R.; Laydon, D.J.; Dabrera, G.; O'Toole, Á.; et al. Transmission of SARS-CoV-2 Lineage B. 1.1. 7 in England: Insights from linking epidemiological and genetic data. *medRxiv* **2021**, *2021*, 20249034.
35. Umair, M.; Ikram, A.; Salman, M.; Alam, M.M.; Badar, N.; Rehman, Z.; Tamim, S.; Khurshid, A.; Ahad, A.; Ahmad, H.; et al. Importation of SARS-CoV-2 variant B. 11 7 in Pakistan. *J. Med. Virol.* **2021**, *93*, 2623–2625. [CrossRef] [PubMed]
36. Nori, P.; Cowman, K.; Chen, V.; Bartash, R.; Szymczak, W.; Madaline, T.; Katiyar, C.P.; Jain, R.; Aldrich, M.; Weston, G.; et al. Bacterial and fungal coinfections in COVID-19 patients hospitalized during the New York City pandemic surge. *Infect. Control Hosp. Epidemiol.* **2021**, *42*, 84–88. [CrossRef]
37. Rawson, T.M.; Wilson, R.C.; Holmes, A. Understanding the role of bacterial and fungal infection in COVID-19. *Clin. Microbiol. Infect.* **2021**, *27*, 9–11. [CrossRef]
38. Langford, B.J.; So, M.; Raybardhan, S.; Leung, V.; Soucy, J.P.R.; Westwood, D.; Daneman, N.; MacFadden, D.R. Antibiotic prescribing in patients with COVID-19: Rapid review and meta-analysis. *Clin. Microbiol. Infect.* **2021**, *27*, 520–531. [CrossRef]
39. O' Neill, J. The Review on Antimicrobial Resistance: Tackling Drug-Resistant Infections Globally: Final Report and Recommendations. Available online: https://apo.org.au/node/63983 (accessed on 15 February 2025).
40. Świder, K.; Babicki, M.; Biesiada, A.; Suszko, M.; Mastalerz-Migas, A.; Kłoda, K. Factors Influencing Antibiotic Prescribing and Antibiotic Resistance Awareness Among Primary Care Physicians in Poland. *Antibiotics* **2025**, *14*, 212. [CrossRef]
41. El-Shabasy, R.M.; Nayel, M.A.; Taher, M.M.; Abdelmonem, R.; Shoueir, K.R. Three waves changes, new variant strains, and vaccination effect against COVID-19 pandemic. *Int. J. Biol. Macromol.* **2022**, *204*, 161–168. [CrossRef]
42. Marasine, N.R.; Shrestha, S.; Sankhi, S.; Paudel, N.; Gautam, A.; Poudel, A. Antibiotic utilization, sensitivity, and cost in the medical intensive care unit of a tertiary care teaching hospital in Nepal. *SAGE Open Med.* **2021**, *9*, 20503121211043710. [CrossRef]

43. Saleem, Z.; Faller, E.M.; Godman, B.; Malik, M.S.A.; Iftikhar, A.; Iqbal, S.; Hassali, M.A. Antibiotic consumption at community pharmacies: A multicenter repeated prevalence surveillance using WHO methodology. *Med. Access@ Point Care* **2021**, *5*, 23992026211064714. [CrossRef]
44. Christensen, I.; Haug, J.B.; Berild, D.; Bjørnholt, J.V.; Skodvin, B.; Jelsness-Jørgensen, L.-P. Factors Affecting Antibiotic Prescription among Hospital Physicians in a Low-Antimicrobial-Resistance Country: A Qualitative Study. *Antibiotics* **2022**, *11*, 98. [CrossRef] [PubMed]
45. Kasse, G.E.; Humphries, J.; Cosh, S.M.; Islam, M.S. Factors contributing to the variation in antibiotic prescribing among primary health care physicians: A systematic review. *BMC Prim. Care* **2024**, *25*, 8. [CrossRef] [PubMed]
46. Xin, S.; Chen, W.; Yu, Q.; Gao, L.; Lu, G. Effect of the number of coronavirus disease 2019 (COVID-19) vaccination shots on the occurrence of pneumonia, severe pneumonia, and death in SARS-CoV-2-infected patients. *Front. Public Health* **2024**, *11*, 1330106. [CrossRef]
47. Dobrowolski, P.; Prejbisz, A.; Szyndler, A.; Olszanecka, A.; Kapłon-Cieślicka, A.; Wełnicki, M.; Jankowski, P.; Narkiewicz, K.; Wolf, J. Physician–patient partnership—Can it help increase adherence to the therapeutic recommendations in cardiovascular disease? *Arter. Hypertens.* **2024**, *28*, 50–70. [CrossRef]
48. Schwartz, K.L.; Brown, K.A.; Etches, J.; Langford, B.J.; Daneman, N.; Tu, K.; Johnstone, J.; Achonu, C.; Garber, G. Predictors and variability of antibiotic prescribing amongst family physicians. *J. Antimicrob. Chemother.* **2019**, *74*, 2098–2105. [CrossRef]
49. Sharaf, N.; Al-Jayyousi, G.F.; Radwan, E.; Shams Eldin, S.M.E.; Hamdani, D.; Al-Katheeri, H.; Elawad, K.; Habib, S.A. Barriers of appropriate antibiotic prescription at PHCC in Qatar: Perspective of physicians and pharmacists. *Antibiotics* **2021**, *10*, 317. [CrossRef]
50. Khurram, M.; Umar, M.; Akhter, T.S.; Faheem, M. Frequently isolated bacteria and their culture and sensitivity pattern in a medical ICU. *J. Coll. Physicians Surg. Pak.* **2013**, *23*, 681–683.
51. Sözen, H.; Gönen, I.; Sözen, A.; Kutlucan, A.; Kalemci, S.; Sahan, M. Application of ATC/DDD methodology to evaluate of antibiotic use in a general hospital in Turkey. *Ann. Clin. Microbiol. Antimicrob.* **2013**, *12*, 1–6. [CrossRef]
52. Saleem, Z.; Haseeb, A.; Abuhussain, S.S.A.; Moore, C.E.; Kamran, S.H.; Qamar, M.U.; Azmat, A.; Pichierri, G.; Raees, F.; Asghar, S.; et al. Antibiotic Susceptibility Surveillance in the Punjab Province of Pakistan: Findings and Implications. *Medicina* **2023**, *59*, 1215. [CrossRef]
53. Dohou, A.M.; Buda, V.O.; Yemoa, L.A.; Anagonou, S.; Van Bambeke, F.; Van Hees, T.; Dalleur, O. Antibiotic Usage in Patients Having Undergone Caesarean Section: A Three-Level Study in Benin. *Antibiotics* **2022**, *11*, 617. [CrossRef]
54. Vincent, J.L.; Rello, J.; Marshall, J.; Silva, E.; Anzueto, A.; Martin, C.D.; Epic II Group of Investigators. International study of the prevalence and outcomes of infection in intensive care units. *JAMA* **2009**, *302*, 2323–2329. [CrossRef] [PubMed]
55. De Bus, L.; Gadeyne, B.; Steen, J.; Boelens, J.; Claeys, G.; Benoit, D.; Depuydt, P. A complete and multifaceted overview of antibiotic use and infection diagnosis in the intensive care unit: Results from a prospective four-year registration. *Crit. Care* **2018**, *22*, 1–10. [CrossRef] [PubMed]
56. Ohnuma, T.; Hayashi, Y.; Yamashita, K.; Marquess, J.; Lefor, A.K.; Sanui, M.; Andoh, K.; Egi, M.; Fujita, M.; Fujitani, S.; et al. A nationwide survey of intravenous antimicrobial use in intensive care units in Japan. *Int. J. Antimicrob. Agents* **2018**, *51*, 636–641. [CrossRef] [PubMed]
57. Iqbal, S.; Bhatti, S.M.; Amir, M.; Zaman, Q.U.; Raza, A. Scenario of Antibiotic Resistance in Pakistan: A Systematic Review. *Pak. J. Med. Health Sci.* **2022**, *16*, 643–649. [CrossRef]
58. Sulis, G.; Sayood, S.; Gandra, S. Antimicrobial Resistance in Low- and Middle-Income Countries: Current Status and Future Directions. *Expert Rev. Anti Infect. Ther.* **2022**, *20*, 147–160. [CrossRef]
59. Impact of COVID-19 on People's Livelihoods, Their Health and Our Food Systems. Available online: https://www.eurofoodbank.org/what-s-new-2020-10-19-impact-of-covid-19-on-people-s-livelihoods-their-health-and-our-food-systems/ (accessed on 15 February 2025).
60. Mancuso, G.; Midiri, A.; Gerace, E.; Biondo, C. Bacterial antibiotic resistance: The most critical pathogens. *Pathogens* **2021**, *10*, 1310. [CrossRef]
61. Nausheen, S.; Hammad, R.; Khan, A. Rational use of antibiotics--a quality improvement initiative in hospital setting. *J. Pak. Med. Assoc.* **2013**, *63*, 60.
62. World Health Organization. *The WHO AWaRe (Access, Watch, Reserve) Antibiotic Book*; World Health Organization: Geneva, Switzerland, 2022. Available online: https://www.who.int/publications/i/item/9789240062382 (accessed on 12 December 2024).
63. Kamran, K.; Ali, A. Challenges and Strategies for Pakistan in the Third Wave of COVID-19: A Mini Review. *Front. Public Health* **2021**, *9*, 690820. [CrossRef]
64. Anand, N.; Nayak, I.N.; Advaitha, M.V.; Thaikattil, N.J.; Kantanavar, K.A.; Anand, S. Antimicrobial agents' utilization and cost pattern in an Intensive Care Unit of a Teaching Hospital in South India. *Indian J. Crit. Care Med.* **2016**, *20*, 274–279. [CrossRef]
65. Shankar, P.R.; Partha, P.; Dubey, A.K.; Mishra, P.; Deshpande, V.Y. Intensive care unit drug utilization in a teaching hospital in Nepal. *Kathmandu Univ. Med. J. (KUMJ)* **2005**, *3*, 130–137.

66. Hawkings, N.J.; Butler, C.C.; Wood, F. Antibiotics in the community: A typology of user behaviours. *Patient Educ. Couns.* **2008**, *73*, 146–152. [CrossRef] [PubMed]
67. Parajuli, N.P.; Acharya, S.P.; Mishra, S.K.; Parajuli, K.; Rijal, B.P.; Pokhrel, B.M. High burden of antimicrobial resistance among gram negative bacteria causing healthcare associated infections in a critical care unit of Nepal. *Antimicrob. Resist. Infect. Control* **2017**, *6*, 67. [CrossRef] [PubMed]
68. Ali, I.; Ahmad, J.; Khan, A.U.; Khan, T.M.; Khan, J.; Ul-Haq, Z. Self-medication and non-adherence with antibiotics: The current situation in Pakistan. *J. Pharm. Pract. Res.* **2016**, *46*, 34–37. [CrossRef]
69. Arshad, H.; Gillani, A.H.; Akbar, J.; Abbas, H.; Bashir Ahmed, A.; Gillani, S.N.H.; Anum, R.; Ji, W.; Fang, Y. Knowledge on Multi-Drug Resistant Pathogens, Antibiotic Use and Self-Reported Adherence to Antibiotic Intake: A Population-Based Cross Sectional Survey From Pakistan. *Front. Pharmacol.* **2022**, *13*, 903503. [CrossRef]
70. Kaleem, F.; Usman, J.; Hassan, A.; Khan, A. Frequency and susceptibility pattern of metallo-beta-lactamase producers in a hospital in Pakistan. *J. Infect. Dev. Ctries.* **2010**, *4*, 810–813. [CrossRef]
71. Afzal, A.; Sarwar, Y.; Ali, A.; Maqbool, A.; Salman, M.; Habeeb, M.A.; Haque, A. Molecular evaluation of drug resistance in clinical isolates of Salmonella enterica serovar Typhi from Pakistan. *J. Infect. Dev. Ctries.* **2013**, *7*, 929–940. [CrossRef]
72. Walther, S.M.; Erlandsson, M.; Burman, L.G.; Cars, O.; Gill, H.; Hoffman, M.; Isaksson, B.; Kahlmeter, G.; Lindgren, S.; Nilsson, L.; et al. Antibiotic prescription practices, consumption and bacterial resistance in a cross section of Swedish intensive care units. *Acta Anaesthesiol. Scand.* **2002**, *46*, 1075–1081. [CrossRef]
73. Weber, R.J.; Kane, S.L.; Oriolo, V.A.; Saul, M.; Skledar, S.J.; Dasta, J.F. Impact of intensive care unit (ICU) drug use on hospital costs: A descriptive analysis, with recommendations for optimizing ICU pharmacotherapy. *Crit. Care Med.* **2003**, *31* (Suppl. S1), S17–S24. [CrossRef]

medicina

MDPI

Article

Etiological Aspects of Infectious Endocarditis in a Tertiary Hospital in Northeastern Romania

Isabela Ioana Loghin [1,2,*], Amelia Elena Surdu [3,*], Şerban Alin Rusu [2], Ion Cecan [2], Victor Daniel Dorobăţ [4], Amelia Andreea Mihăescu [2] and Carmen Mihaela Dorobăţ [2]

1 Department of Infectious Diseases, "Grigore T. Popa" University of Medicine and Pharmacy, 700115 Iasi, Romania
2 Department of Infectious Diseases, "St. Parascheva" Clinical Hospital of Infectious Diseases, 700116 Iasi, Romania; rususerbanalin@yahoo.com (Ş.A.R.); ion11cecan@gmail.com (I.C.); ameliamihaescu@gmail.com (A.A.M.); carmendorobat@yahoo.com (C.M.D.)
3 Department of Implantology, Removable Prostheses and Technology, Faculty of Dental Medicine, "Grigore T. Popa" University of Medicine and Pharmacy, 700115 Iasi, Romania
4 Department of Intensive Care, University Hospital of Emergency, 050098 Bucharest, Romania; victordorobat@yahoo.com
* Correspondence: isabelabegezsan@yahoo.com (I.I.L.); amelia.surdu@dentesse.ro (A.E.S.)

Abstract: *Background and Objectives*: Infective endocarditis (IE) is a severe, life-threatening infection of the endocardial surface. Its incidence has shifted towards older, immunocompromised patients and those with cardiac devices. *Materials and Methods*: This study was conducted at the "Sf. Parascheva" Clinical Hospital of Infectious Diseases in Iasi, Romania, and retrospectively analyzed cases of IE from 1 January 2019, to 30 September 2024. It received ethical approval (Approval No. 7/17 June 2024). *Results*: The study included 130 patients with infectious endocarditis, predominantly men (75.38%), with a median age of 55 years. The most affected age groups were 50–59 and over 60 years, each representing 30.76% of cases. The most frequently implicated etiological agent was *Staphylococcus aureus* in 33% of cases. The most common antibiotic regimen combined glycopeptides and fluoroquinolones/polymyxins (27% cases). *Conclusions*: A multidisciplinary approach involving infectious disease specialists, cardiologists, and cardiovascular surgeons is essential for effective treatment. Immediate combined antibiotic therapy is vital for presumed IE cases. Despite advances in diagnosis and treatment, the high mortality rates highlight the importance of timely intervention. Future research should focus on improving preventive and therapeutic strategies for IE.

Keywords: infective endocarditis; etiological agents; antibiotics; duke criteria; echocardiography

1. Introduction

Infective endocarditis (IE) is defined as a microbial infection of the endocardial surface. It represents "infection of the endocardium with the presence of microorganisms at the level of the lesion", specifying that it may be in the valvular endocardium, parietal or septal defects, or a persistent arterial channel. This descriptive formulation emphasizes the initial endocardial changes, which are more common in approaches to the condition from a cardiological perspective [1,2].

In the last 50 years, there have been major changes in IE. Thus, a significant decrease in mortality was observed, the etiological spectrum changed, new antibiotics and new laboratory techniques appeared, echocardiography was developed, and the susceptible population changed, increasing the proportion of immunocompromised people and those with valve prostheses or pacemakers at the expense of those with rheumatic valvular diseases [3,4].

Over the last decades, shifts in etiology and epidemiology have been observed. The accurate incidence of IE is difficult to establish due to the variability in diagnostic criteria and reporting methodologies. IE continues to be a rare condition in Western countries, with its incidence influenced by geographic factors, predisposing risk factors, and the presence of underlying health conditions. Early diagnosis and appropriate initial management of IE remain particularly challenging, especially in the emergency department setting. Although the overall annual incidence of IE remained relatively stable, from 9 to 15 cases per 100,000 per year, this condition has progressively become more prevalent among older adults, with a significant increase in incidence observed in patients over the age of 60 and those with multiple comorbidities. It is important to note that the incidence of IE is higher in men than in women, with male-to-female ratios ranging. The incidence rate is greater in older individuals and shows an upward trend over time. In the younger population, congenital heart disease continues to be the predominant risk factor for IE, whereas intravenous drug use has emerged as a growing concern [5,6].

Community-acquired native valve IE is attributable to staphylococci, streptococci, or enterococci in approximately 90% of cases. These microorganisms are commensal species, commonly residing in the skin, oropharynx, and urogenital and gastrointestinal tracts [7,8].

IE involves a variety of etiological agents, which can vary depending on specific clinical scenarios. Acute IE is most commonly caused by *Staphylococcus aureus* (meticillin-sensitive *Staphylococcus aureus*—MSSA—or meticillin-resistant *Staphylococcus aureus*—MRSA), *Streptococcus pneumoniae,* and *Haemophilus influenzae*. Subacute IE, on the other hand, is typically associated with *Streptococcus viridans*, *Enterococcus* spp., and *Staphylococcus aureus*. Among intravenous drug users, the most frequently implicated pathogens include *Staphylococcus aureus*, *Pseudomonas aeruginosa*, *Candida* spp., and *Enterococcus* spp. In the case of the prosthetic valve, the primary causative agents of IE are *Staphylococcus epidermidis*, *Staphylococcus aureus*, and group B streptococci [9,10].

The main risk factors associated with IE are poor dental hygiene, diabetes mellitus, immunosuppression, systemic sepsis, and recent surgical or non-surgical invasive procedures [11,12]. The clinical diagnosis involves a combination of major criteria (positive blood cultures, evidence of valvular damage in the echocardiographic examination) and minor criteria (fever, manifestations of glomerulonephritis, Osler nodules, predisposing cardiac factors, suggestive but not conclusive echocardiographic images to be considered a major criterion, splenomegaly, elevated erythrocyte sedimentation rate (ESR), elevated C-Reactive Protein (CRP), presence of venous catheters, microscopic hematuria).

Bacteriological diagnosis consists of highlighting the etiological agent in blood cultures (three samples are recommended), and dynamic transthoracic and/or transesophageal echocardiography allows the definite confirmation of valvular changes [13,14].

Given that IE continues to be a significant concern and the associated risk factors are becoming increasingly prevalent, it is essential to adopt a comprehensive approach that emphasizes commonly encountered aspects. This will facilitate enhanced understanding and enable prompt intervention [15,16].

The goal of this study is to illustrate the traits and development of IE patients. Also, we aim to highlight the etiology of infective endocarditis in the northeastern region of Romania, along with the evaluation skills needed to evaluate possible cases, the available treatment and management options for IE in our country, and the interprofessional team strategies for enhancing communication and care coordination to enable better outcomes and more efficient care for IE patients.

2. Materials and Methods

2.1. Database Description

To highlight the characteristics and related comorbidities of IE cases, we conducted a retrospective clinical study on patients who were hospitalized at the "Sf. Parascheva" Clinical Hospital of Infectious Diseases from Iasi in the northeastern region of Romania. The time frame under investigation was 1 January 2019, to 30 September 2024.

2.2. Ethical Approval

The "St. Parascheva" Clinical Hospital of Infectious Diseases in Iasi, Romania, gave the study its clearance (17 June 2024; Approval No. 7/2024). Written informed consent was obtained from the patients when they were admitted to our hospital, according to the hospital's policy.

2.3. Study Design

Data on demographics specific to age and gender, individual pathological histories, clinical characteristics, blood tests, assessments of possible bacteriological infections, patient comorbidities, the initiation of antibiotic therapy, and the course and prognosis of infectious endocarditis patients were all collected. Modified Duke criteria were used for the diagnosis of IE. Further, the presence of 2 major criteria, 1 major and 3 minor criteria, or 5 minor criteria suggests definite IE, while the presence of 1 major and 1 minor or 3 minor criteria suggests possible IE.

2.4. Study Setting

The "St. Parascheva" Clinical Hospital of Infectious Disease Iasi is a primary referral medical facility in the northeastern region of Romania, with a capacity of 300 beds. It is divided into six pavilions. The enrolled patients were evaluated by echocardiographic imaging (transthoracic echocardiography and transesophageal echocardiography). Contact was maintained with the cardiologist and cardiovascular surgeon regarding the evolution of the cases.

The "St. Parascheva" Clinical Hospital of Infectious Disease Iasi laboratory benefits from accreditation by the Romanian Accreditation Association with ISO 15189/2013 standards, an obligation that is unique in Europe [17].

All blood tests were performed by the hospital's central laboratory. Blood cultures were collected and antibiograms were made after the etiologic agent was found.

2.5. Statistical Analysis

The Pearson test in the XLSTAT version 2019 program was used to determine the correlation between demographic characteristics, clinical data, and the results. Kendall's Tau correlation coefficients were established. Statistical Software for Excel (XLSTAT 2019.4) version 2019 was used to conduct the statistical analysis. The descriptive data are displayed as means, percentages, and absolute values. The $\chi 2$ and unpaired Student *t*-tests were used to determine whether the differences between the groups were statistically significant.

3. Results

In our clinical hospital in the northeastern part of Romania, 130 patients diagnosed with IE were recorded from 1 January 2019, to 30 September 2024.

Men most frequently presented with infectious endocarditis (98 cases, 76%) compared with women (32 cases, 24%). Most of the instances involved adults aged between 50 and 59—40 patients (31%)—and over 60—40 cases (31%). Next were the age groups

40–49 years—30 patients (23%); 30–39 years—15 patients (11%); and 20–29 years—5 patients (4%). The study group's median age was 55 years old (Table 1).

Table 1. Distribution of the study cases according to age and gender.

Age (Years)	Male (*n*, %)	Female (*n*, %)	Total Number of Cases (*n*, %)
20–29	3 (2%)	2 (2%)	5 (4%)
30–39	10 (7%)	5 (4%)	15 (11%)
40–49	20 (16%)	10 (7%)	30 (23%)
50–59	30 (24%)	10 (7%)	40 (31%)
Over 60	35 (27%)	5 (4%)	40 (31%)
Total	98 (76%)	32 (24%)	130 (100%)

Due to the SARS-CoV2 pandemic, we registered low admissions between 2020 and 2021, with 7 cases (5%) and 10 cases (8%), respectively. The year with the most admissions, in the study period, was 2019 with 45 cases (35%) (Table 2).

Table 2. Distribution of the cases according to the year of hospitalization and gender.

Hospitalization Year	Number of Cases (*n*, %)	Male (*n*, %)	Female (*n*, %)
2019	45 (35%)	35 (28%)	10 (7%)
2020	7 (5%)	5 (4%)	2 (1%)
2021	10 (8%)	7 (5%)	4 (3%)
2022	21 (16%)	18 (14%)	3 (2%)
2023	25 (19%)	17 (13%)	7 (6%)
2024	22 (17%)	16 (12%)	6 (5%)

The portal of entry (POE) for the present IE cases was identified in 93 patients (71%). Among the identified POEs, 42% were cutaneous, 27% were oral or dental, and 23% were gastrointestinal (Figure 1).

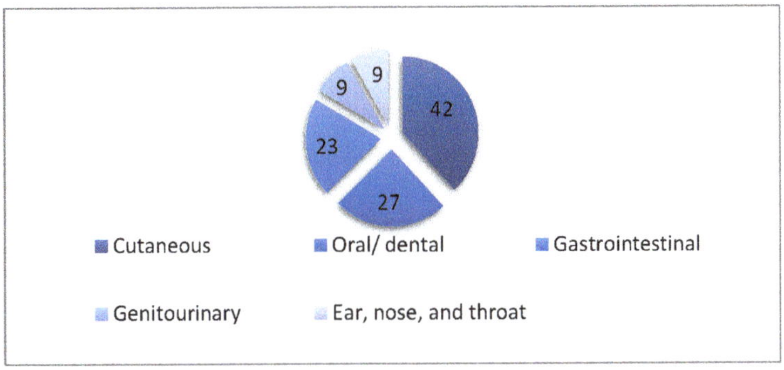

Figure 1. Portal of entry for the present IE cases.

At admission, the most frequent symptoms were cardiac murmurs, noted in 117 patients (90%), followed by fever and chills in 110 patients (85%), and physical and mental fatigue in 104 patients (80%). Dyspnea on minimal exertion was reported in 90 patients (69%), while precordial pain was present in 52 patients (40%). Neurological symptoms, such as obnubilation, paresis, and paresthesias, were rare, affecting only five patients (4%). These data highlight cardiac murmurs and fever as key clinical indicators for diagnosis (Table 3).

Table 3. Distribution of the cases according to the symptoms at admission.

Clinical Symptoms and Signs	Number of Cases (%)
cardiac murmurs	117 (90%)
physical and mental asthenia	104 (80%)
fever, chills	110 (85%)
dyspnea on light exertion	90 (69%)
chest pain	52 (40%)
cough	39 (30%)
headache	45 (35%)
numbness, paresis, paresthesias	5 (4%)

Modified Duke criteria were used to diagnose or presumptively diagnose IE. Further, the presence of two major criteria, one major and three minor criteria, or five minor criteria suggests definite IE, while the presence of one major and one minor or three minor criteria suggests possible IE (Table 4).

Table 4. Applied Duke criteria for the study cases.

Modified Duke Criteria	Number of Cases (*n*, %)
Definite IE	
- 2 major criteria	80 cases, 61%
- 1 major criterion + 3 minor criteria	20 cases, 15%
- 5 minor criteria	3 cases, 4%
Possible IE	
- 1 major criterion + 1 minor criterion	12 cases, 9%
- 3 minor criteria	15 cases, 11%

The localization of vegetation detected through transthoracic or transesophageal echocardiography showed a higher frequency on the mitral valve, observed in 51% of cases, followed by the aortic and tricuspid valves, each with an incidence of 15% and 12%. Vegetations located on the pulmonary valve were less frequent (11%). There were 15 cases (12%) that had presented normal echocardiographic findings, but according to the modified Duke criteria were registered as possible IE (Table 5). Ten patients (8%) had prosthetic mitral valve implantation before the IE episode.

Table 5. Echocardiographic distribution of the valve vegetation of the study patients.

Echocardiographic Locations of Vegetation	Number of Cases (%)
Tricuspid valve	15 (12%)
Aortic valve	20 (15%)
Mitral valve	66 (51%)
Pulmonary valve	14 (11%)

Cardiac IE-predisposing factors were found in 23% of patients (30 cases), 5% (6 cases) presented mitral valve prolapse, 10% (13 cases) had hypertrophic cardiomyopathy, and 8% (11 cases) had an anterior episode of endocarditis. The percentage of patients with primary IE was 77% (100 cases).

The characterizations of vegetation revealed that most were mobile, observed in 88% of cases. Regarding size, 81% of vegetation was smaller than 10 mm, while only 12% was classified as large (>10 mm). Ten cases presented multiple vegetations in various locations (7%) (Table 6).

Table 6. The characteristics of the vegetation are related to the number of cases.

Vegetation Character	Number of Cases (%)
Mobile vegetation	114 (88%)
Vegetation < 10 mm	105 (81%)
Large vegetation (>10 mm)	15 (12%)
Multiple vegetations	10 (7%)

Blood cultures were collected and an etiologic agent was found in 103 cases (84%). The most frequently implicated etiological agent was *Staphylococcus aureus* with 33% of total strains and identified in 43 of patients, followed by *Enterococcus faecalis* with 20% of total strains and identified in 26 patients; *Viridans Group Streptococci* were found in 15% of total strains and identified in 20 patients; and coagulase-negative *Staphylococcus epidermidis* was found in 10 patients (13%). It should be noted that the Gram-negative bacterium involved was *Klebsiella pneumoniae* in four cases (3.07%), (Table 7).

Table 7. Etiology spectrum in study patients with infectious endocarditis.

Etiologic Agent	Number of Cases (*n*, %)
Staphylococcus aureus	43 cases, 33%
Enterococcus faecalis	26 cases, 20%
Viridans Group Streptococci	20 cases, 15%
Staphylococcus epidermidis	10 cases, 13%
Klebsiella pneumoniae	4 cases, 3%

Broad-spectrum antibiotic therapy for which the antibiogram showed sensitivity to beta-lactams, cephalosporins, glycopeptides, trimethoprim-sulfamethoxazole, rifampicin, quinolones, lincosamides, oxazolidinones, and thus specific treatment was initiated according to the antibiogram.

The therapeutic regimens were with glycopeptide + fluoroquinolone/polymyxin (27%), aminopenicillins and quinolones administered (19%), third-generation cephalosporins + quinolones/aminopenicillins (15%), oxazolidinone + quinolones (8%), carbapenem + quinolones (6%), and lincosamide + quinolone (4%) (Table 8).

Table 8. Comparative analysis of therapeutic regimens.

Therapeutic Regimen	Number of Cases (*n*, %)
Glycopeptide + fluoroquinolone/polymyxin	35 (27%)
Aminopenicillin/aminoglycoside + fluoroquinolone	25 (19%)
Third-generation cephalosporins + fluoroquinolone/aminoglycoside	20 (15%)
Oxazolidinone + quinolone	10 (8%)
Carbapenem + quinolone	8 (6%)
Lincosamide + quinolone	5 (4%)

For the cases with negative blood cultures, treatment was initiated with aminopenicillins/aminoglycosides + fluoroquinolons (14 cases, 11%) and glycopeptides + fluoroquinolone/polymyxin (13 cases, 10%), with positive clinical and biological response.

The treatment instituted led to negative blood cultures in the first 4–7 days, but an extension of antibiotic therapy was necessary to sterilize the vegetation present on echocardiography.

Between the years of the SARS-CoV2 pandemic (2020 and 2021), there were 17 cases (13%) recorded, from which 7 cases (6%) presented SARS-CoV2 coinfection (4 cases (3%) were male and 3 (2%) were female). Regardless of the small number of SARS-CoV2 coinfection cases during this period, the identified spectrum was the same, with positive hemocultures for *Staphylococcus aureus* (three cases, 2%), *Viridans Group Streptococci* (two cases, 1%) and *Enterococcus faecalis* (two cases, 1%). Broad-spectrum antibiotic therapy for which the antibiogram showed sensitivity to glycopeptide + fluoroquinolone/polymyxin (three cases, 2%) and aminopenicillin/aminoglycoside + fluoroquinolone (four cases, 3%) was administered. Also, the imaging criteria were met—echocardiography was performed for these cases and four cases (3%) presented normal cardiac valves, while in the other three cases (2%), mobile and < 10 mm vegetations were recorded.

Pathogenic and antithrombotic treatment was used (low-molecular-weight heparin, calculated per kg) in collaboration and recommended by the cardiologist, with favorable outcomes.

In the studied cases, a favorable evolution was most frequently observed in 58 cases (45%). A reserved prognosis was noted in 13% of the investigated patients, with the registration of death in 5% (seven cases). The share of patients with endocarditis transferred for cardiological consultation was 28 (22%). Patients were evaluated by the cardiovascular surgeon, and 20 (15%) of the subjects were transferred to cardiovascular surgery services for intervention (following the cardiovascular surgeon's recommendation) (Table 9).

Table 9. Prognosis of the study cases.

Evolution	Number of Cases (*n*, %)
Favorable	58 (45%)
Reserved	17 (13%)
Deceased	7 (5%)
Transfer of cardiovascular surgery services	20 (15%)
Cardiology transfer	28 (22%)

Major complications included heart failure (seven cases, 5%), pericarditis (three cases, 2%), and thromboembolic events (three cases, 2%). Although their incidence was low, these complications significantly contributed to increased mortality and morbidity (Table 10).

Table 10. Complications during the evolution of the patients.

Major Complications	Number of Cases (n, %)
Heart failure	7 (5%)
Pericarditis	3 (2%)
Thromboembolic events	3 (2%)

4. Discussion

Rajani R. et al. stated that despite advancements in microbiological and diagnostic methods, infectious endocarditis is linked to a high rate of morbidity and mortality. Prompt surgical intervention when necessary and early diagnoses with the early inclusion of a specialized IE team are proven strategies that enhance patient outcomes. To provide fair IE care across various clinical networks, further patient pathway development is needed [18].

Holland T.L. et al. concluded that imaging technology will continue to advance, and further research is needed to define which patients with suspected IE should undergo transoesophageal echocardiography and which patients may benefit from newer imaging modalities. Novel Gram-positive antibiotics are promising but as yet untested in IE. If proven to be effective, they might enable simpler and more patient-friendly treatment regimens. The debate around IE prophylaxis will likely continue until prophylaxis strategies are compared prospectively. Vaccine development has not yet yielded an effective and commercially available product, but numerous candidates are in the pipeline [19].

Since infectious endocarditis is a complicated condition, experts from a variety of disciplines must contribute. In both IE research and disease management, it is imperative to prioritize a multidisciplinary approach. Even though IE has been diagnosed and treated more effectively in recent decades, there are still many unsolved issues, and randomized clinical studies are desperately needed to learn more about this difficult illness. There is potential for better patient outcomes thanks to advancements in AI-powered machine learning and imaging technologies [20].

Endocarditis is becoming more common as the population ages, invasive medical device use rises, and the opioid crisis persists. The illness is still deadly and challenging to identify. Thankfully, we are still learning more about the illness. New imaging and immunoassay methods are available to help with diagnosis. The recently updated modified Duke criteria are still applicable. The guidelines for antibiotic treatment are always changing, and newer drugs—particularly dalbavancin—have the potential to enhance treatment. All healthcare professionals should be aware of the continuous modifications to our strategy for treating infective endocarditis [21].

Lindberg H. et al. observed that in 4050 episodes of bacteremia, the modified Duke criteria assigned 307 episodes (7.6%) as confirmed IE, 1190 (29%) as possible IE, and 2553 (63%) as rejected IE. Using the Duke-ISCVID criteria, 13 episodes (0.3%) were reclassified from possible to definite IE, and 475 episodes (12%) were reclassified from rejected to possible IE. With the modified Duke criteria, 79 episodes that were treated as IE were classified as possible IE, and 11 of these episodes were reclassified to definite IE with Duke-ISCVID. Applying the decision to treat IE as a reference standard, the sensitivity of the Duke criteria was 80% [22].

One limitation of our study is that we did not record rare etiologic agents, particularly members of the HACEK group. This is probably due to the limited possibilities of the bacteriological laboratory of the hospital, which uses hemocultures tests.

5. Conclusions

The co-occurrence of bacteremia and a murmur in a feverish patient strongly suggests the possible presence of IE from the standpoint of solely clinical signs. To properly evaluate the type of valvular lesion, identify vegetation, and determine the severity of any problems related to IE, an echocardiography must be performed as soon as feasible. It is wise to start with transthoracic echocardiography (TTE) because of its non-invasiveness, simplicity, and superior myocardial function information (such as ejection fraction), even though transesophageal echocardiography (TEE) has a higher sensitivity for detecting valvular vegetation and paravalvular problems. Given the high likelihood that the patient may have IE, a TEE should be performed if a TTE is determined to be negative or inconclusive [23].

The most frequently implicated etiological agents found in blood cultures were *Staphylococcus aureus*, followed by *Enterococcus, Viridans Group Streptococci*, and *Staphylococcus epidermidis*. The Gram-negative bacteria involved *Klebsiella pneumoniae*. We did not record rare etiologic agents, particularly members of the HACEK group. This is probably due to the limited possibilities of the bacteriological laboratory of the hospital, which uses hemoculture tests.

According to the antibiogram, a particular treatment was started for broad-spectrum antibiotic therapy with beta-lactams, cephalosporins, glycopeptides, trimethoprim-sulfamethoxazole, rifampicin, quinolones, lincosamides, and oxazolidinones.

To deliver care, a multidisciplinary team would be assembled, comprising experts in infectious disease, cardiology, and cardiovascular surgery. To treat presumed IE, combined antibiotic therapy must be administered as soon as possible.

Despite advancements in microbiological and diagnostic methods, IE is linked to a high rate of morbidity and mortality in our country. Prompt surgical intervention when necessary and early diagnosis with the early inclusion of a specialized IE team are proven strategies that enhance patient outcomes. To provide fair IE care across various clinical networks, further patient pathway development is needed. When treating feverish patients, clinicians should be on the lookout for signs including bacteremia and heart murmurs.

In conclusion, we are emphasizing the necessity of early diagnosis and vigorous treatment to address the ongoing high fatality rates of IE. When treating feverish patients, clinicians should be on the lookout for signs including bacteremia and heart murmurs. Future studies should concentrate on creating preventative measures and treatment plans that are more successful.

Author Contributions: Conceptualization, I.I.L. and C.M.D.; Methodology, Ș.A.R. and A.A.M.; Software, Ș.A.R., I.C., and A.A.M.; Validation, I.I.L., C.M.D., and A.E.S.; Formal analysis, V.D.D.; Investigation, I.I.L., Ș.A.R., and I.C.; Resources, I.I.L. and Ș.A.R.; Data curation, A.A.M.; Writing—original draft preparation, I.I.L. and Ș.A.R.; Writing—review and editing, A.E.S. and V.D.D.; Visualization, I.I.L.; Supervision, C.M.D.; Project administration, A.E.S.; Funding acquisition, C.M.D. All authors have read and agreed to the published version of the manuscript.

Funding: This research received no external funding.

Institutional Review Board Statement: The study was conducted according to the Declaration of Helsinki and approved by the Ethics Committee of the "St. Parascheva" Clinical Hospital of Infectious Diseases, Iasi, Romania (Approval No.7/17 June 2024).

Informed Consent Statement: This was a retrospective study, and written informed consent was obtained from the patients when they were admitted to our hospital, according to the hospital policy.

Data Availability Statement: All data generated or analyzed during this study are included in this published article.

Conflicts of Interest: The authors declare no conflicts of interest.

Abbreviations

The following abbreviations are used in this manuscript:

IE	infective endocarditis
MSSA	meticillin-sensitive *Staphylococcus aureus*
MRSA	meticillin-resistant *Staphylococcus aureus*
ESR	erythrocyte sedimentation rate
CRP	C-Reactive Protein
POE	portal of entry
TTE	transthoracic echocardiography
TEE	transesophageal echocardiography

References

1. Kellerman, R.D.; Rakel, D.P.; Heidelbaugh, J.J. *Conn's Current Therapy 2024*; Elsevier: Amsterdam, The Netherlands, 2024.
2. Fowler, V.G.; Bayer, A.S.; Baddour, L.M. Infective Endocarditis. In *Goldman-Cecil Medicine*, 27th ed.; Elsevier Inc.: Amsterdam, The Netherlands, 2024.
3. Bradley, W.; Frazee, M.E.M. Infective endocarditis and valvular heart disease. In *Rosen's Emergency Medicine: Concepts and Clinical Practice*; Elsevier: Amsterdam, The Netherlands, 2023.
4. Li, M.; Kim, J.B.; Sastry, B.K.S.; Chen, M. Infective endocarditis. *Lancet* **2024**, *404*, 377–392. [CrossRef] [PubMed]
5. Fort, G.G. End ocarditis, Infective. In *Ferri's Clinical Advisor 2025*; Elsevier Inc.: Amsterdam, The Netherlands, 2025.
6. Kirsty Lloyd, E.-W.T. Cardiovascular system. In *Underwood's Pathology*; Elsevier Inc.: Amsterdam, The Netherlands, 2025.
7. Maleki, M.; Alizadehasl, A.; Haghjoo, M. *Practical Cardiology: Principles and Approaches*; Elsevier Inc.: Amsterdam, The Netherlands, 2022.
8. Nappi, F. Native Infective Endocarditis: A State-of-the-Art-Review. *Microorganisms* **2024**, *12*, 1481. [CrossRef] [PubMed]
9. Vogkou, C.T.; Vlachogiannis, N.I.; Palaiodimos, L.; Kousoulis, A.A. The causative agents in infective endocarditis: A systematic review comprising 33,214 cases. *Eur. J. Clin. Microbiol. Infect. Dis.* **2016**, *35*, 1227–1245. [CrossRef] [PubMed]
10. Scheggi, V.; Del Pace, S.; Ceschia, N.; Vanni, F.; Merilli, I.; Sottili, E.; Salcuni, L.; Zoppetti, N.; Alterini, B.; Cerillo, A.; et al. Infective endocarditis in intravenous drug abusers: Clinical challenges emerging from a single-centre experience. *BMC Infect. Dis.* **2021**, *21*, 1010. [CrossRef] [PubMed]
11. Cahill, T.J.; Dayer, M.; Prendergast, B.; Thornhill, M. Do patients at risk of infective endocarditis need antibiotics before dental procedures? *BMJ* **2017**, *223*, 692. [CrossRef] [PubMed]
12. Martico, M.; Kapageridis, H.; Ouanounou, A. Infective Endocarditis: Etiology, Epidemiology and Current Recommendations for the Dental Practitioner. *J. Can. Dent. Assoc.* **2024**, *90*, 64. [PubMed]
13. Pierce, D.; Calkins, B.C.; Thornton, K. Infectious endocarditis: Diagnosis and treatment. *Am. Fam. Physician* **2012**, *85*, 981–986. [PubMed]
14. Liesman, R.M.; Pritt BSMaleszewski, J.J.; Patel, R. Laboratory Diagnosis of Infective Endocarditis. *J. Clin. Microbiol.* **2017**, *55*, 2599–2608. [CrossRef] [PubMed]
15. Roy, A.S.; Hagh-Doust, H.; Abdul Azim, A.; Caceres, J.; Denholm, J.T.; Dong, M.Q.; King, M.; Yen, C.F.; Lee, T.C.; McDonald, E.G. Multidisciplinary Teams for the Management of Infective Endocarditis: A Systematic Review and Meta-analysis. *Open Forum Infect. Dis.* **2023**, *10*, ofad444. [CrossRef] [PubMed]
16. Khan, U.A.; Zaidi, S.H.; Majeed, H.; Lopez, E.; Tofighi, D.; Andre, P.; Schevchuck, A.; Garcia, M.E.; Sheikh, A.B.; Raizada, V.; et al. Clinical Risk Factors for Infective Endocarditis Patients With Staphylococcus Aureus Bacteremia and the Diagnostic Utility of Transesophageal Echocardiogram. *Curr. Probl. Cardiol.* **2022**, *47*, 101331. [CrossRef] [PubMed]
17. Available online: https://european-accreditation.org/wp-content/uploads/2018/10/ea-4-20-g-rev00-may-2015-rev.pdf (accessed on 8 December 2024).
18. Rajani, R.; Klein, J.L. Infective endocarditis: A contemporary update. *Clin. Med.* **2020**, *20*, 31–35. [CrossRef] [PubMed] [PubMed Central]
19. Holland, T.L.; Baddour, L.M.; Bayer, A.S.; Hoen, B.; Miro, J.M.; Fowler, V.G., Jr. Infective endocarditis. *Nat. Rev. Dis. Primers* **2016**, *2*, 16059. [CrossRef] [PubMed]
20. Hubers, S.A.; DeSimone, D.C.; Gersh, B.J.; Anavekar, N.S. Infective Endocarditis: A Contemporary Review. *Mayo Clin. Proc.* **2020**, *95*, 982–997. [CrossRef] [PubMed]
21. Dale, S.; Tayyem, Z.; Maceyko, S. Endocarditis: A Review of Recent Literature. *Curr. Emerg. Hosp. Med. Rep.* **2024**, *12*, 67–73. [CrossRef]

22. Lindberg, H.; Berge, A.; Jovanovic-Stjernqvist, M.; Hagstrand Aldman, M.; Krus, D.; Öberg, J.; Kahn, F.; Bläckberg, A.; Sunnerhagen, T.; Rasmussen, M. Performance of the 2023 Duke-International Society of Cardiovascular Infectious Diseases Diagnostic Criteria for Infective Endocarditis in Relation to the Modified Duke Criteria and to Clinical Management—Reanalysis of Retrospective Bacteremia Cohorts. *Clin. Infect. Dis.* **2024**, *78*, 956–963. [CrossRef] [PubMed]
23. N'cho-Mottoh, M.B.; Erpelding, M.L.; Roubaud, C.; Delahaye, F.; Fraisse, T.; Dijos, M.; Ennezat, P.-V.; Fluttaz, A.; Richard, B.; Beaufort, C.; et al. The impact of transoesophageal echocardiography in elderly patients with infective endocarditis. *Arch. Cardiovasc. Dis.* **2023**, *116*, 258–264. [CrossRef] [PubMed]

medicina

MDPI

Article

Comparative Analysis of the Prevalence of Dysphagia in Patients with Mild COVID-19 and Those with Aspiration Pneumonia Alone: Findings of the Videofluoroscopic Swallowing Study

Junhyung Kim, Byungju Ryu, Yunhee Kim, Yireh Choi and Eunyoung Lee *

Department of Physical Medicine and Rehabilitation, Sahmyook Medical Center, Seoul 02500, Republic of Korea; caumed2832@naver.com (J.K.); btjrbj@gmail.com (B.R.); yhkim76@hanmail.net (Y.K.)
* Correspondence: euneun9204@naver.com; Tel.: +82-2-2210-3133

Abstract: *Background and Objectives:* Patients recovering from mild coronavirus disease (COVID-19) reportedly have dysphagia or difficulty in swallowing. We compared the prevalence of dysphagia between patients diagnosed with mild COVID-19 and those diagnosed with aspiration pneumonia alone. *Materials and Methods:* A retrospective study was conducted from January 2020 to June 2023 in 160 patients referred for a videofluoroscopic swallowing study (VFSS) to assess for dysphagia. The cohort included 24 patients with mild COVID-19 and aspiration pneumonia, 30 with mild COVID-19 without aspiration pneumonia, and 106 with aspiration pneumonia alone. We reviewed the demographic data, comorbidities, and VFSS results using the penetration–aspiration scale (PAS) and functional dysphagia scale (FDS). *Results:* In a study comparing patients with mild COVID-19 (Group A) and those with aspiration pneumonia alone (Group B), no significant differences were observed in the baseline characteristics, including the prevalence of dysphagia-related comorbidities between the groups. Group A showed milder dysphagia, as evidenced by lower PAS and FDS scores, shorter oral and pharyngeal transit times ($p = 0.001$ and $p = 0.003$, respectively), and fewer residues in the vallecula and pyriform sinuses ($p < 0.001$ and $p < 0.03$, respectively). When Group A was subdivided into those with COVID-19 with (Group A1) and without aspiration pneumonia (Group A2), both subgroups outperformed Group B in terms of specific VFSS metrics, such as oral transit time ($p = 0.01$), pharyngeal transit time ($p = 0.04$ and $p = 0.02$, respectively), and residue in the vallecula ($p = 0.04$ and $p = 0.02$, respectively). However, Group B showed improved triggering of the pharyngeal swallowing reflex compared with Group A2 ($p = 0.02$). *Conclusion:* Mild COVID-19 patients showed less severe dysphagia than those with aspiration pneumonia alone. This finding was consistent across VFSS parameters, even when the COVID-19 group was subdivided based on the status of aspiration pneumonia.

Keywords: COVID-19; swallowing disorders; dysphagia; aspiration pneumonia; videofluoroscopic swallowing study

1. Introduction

Since December 2019, coronavirus disease (COVID-19) has caused various medical problems worldwide. The atypical symptoms of COVID-19 include fever, cough, dyspnea, muscle pain, fatigue, occasional diarrhea, and vomiting [1]. The World Health Organization (WHO) classifies the severity of COVID-19 into four levels, mild, moderate, severe, and critical, based on the severity degree of clinical and respiratory symptoms, including increased oxygen demand [2]. In some patients with acute respiratory distress syndrome (ARDS), low oxygen saturation levels and inadequate oxygen delivery to organs may necessitate the need for invasive interventions, such as intubation or tracheotomy [3,4], and these interventions may increase the incidence of dysphagia [5,6]. Dysphagia is a medical condition characterized by difficulty in swallowing and poses significant challenges to patients' nutritional intake and overall wellbeing [7]. Dysphagia can occur due to several factors, including neuromuscular conditions, structural abnormalities, esophageal motility anomaly, oropharyngeal dysfunction, and postoperative changes [8]. In particular, studies investigating COVID-19-related dysphagia have mainly focused on severely ill patients [9,10]. Approximately 60% of patients who are mechanically ventilated experience dysphagia even after extubation [11,12], and the risk of developing dysphagia increases as the duration of intubation and age increase [13]. In addition, patients with severe COVID-19 exhibit a higher degree of dysphagia than those with aspiration pneumonia [14].

However, the proportion of severe and critical cases of COVID-19 is considerably lower than that of mild-to-moderate cases [15]. Research on the incidence of dysphagia in patients with mild COVID-19 is scant. A study conducted by Can et al. [16] suggested that the risk of dysphagia in patients with mild COVID-19 should be considered. Shadi et al. [17] reported a high prevalence of self-reported swallowing difficulties among COVID-19 patients who were not intubated. Furthermore, studies comparing the characteristics of dysphagia in COVID-19 patients with mild-to-moderate symptoms and those with aspiration pneumonia are limited. Therefore, this study aimed to compare the swallowing function between patients with mild-to-moderate COVID-19, who comprise the majority of COVID-19 patients, and those with aspiration pneumonia. We formulated the hypothesis that patients with mild COVID-19 are likely to exhibit mild dysphagia.

2. Materials and Methods

2.1. Participants

We retrospectively collected the data of patients with dysphagia who were admitted to Sahmyook Medical Center from January 2020 to June 2023. A total of 358 patients were referred for a videofluoroscopic swallowing study (VFSS) to evaluate dysphagia. Patients who were (i) eating by mouth prior to hospitalization and (ii) referred for swallowing disorders that occurred after aspiration pneumonia or COVID-19 were included in the study. Patients who (i) were previously diagnosed with oropharyngeal cancer and had undergone tumor removal; (ii) were unable to complete the required examination due to poor cooperation or cognition; (iii) were on Levin tube feeding or had undergone percutaneous endoscopic gastrostomy due to a previous stroke; (iv) with severe to critical COVID-19; (v) with a history of admissions to the intensive care unit; and (vi) were admitted in the hospital within >180 days prior to their confirmed COVID-19 date were excluded. Only 160 patients were included in the final analysis. The patients were initially divided into two distinct groups: 54 patients with mild COVID-19 irrespective of pneumonia status (Group A) and 106 patients with aspiration pneumonia in the absence of COVID-19 (Group B). Additionally, patients with mild COVID-19 (Group A) were further subdivided into two groups based on the status of aspiration pneumonia to evaluate the variations in swallowing function across all subsets. Among these, 24 were diagnosed with mild COVID-19 aspiration pneumonia with dysphagia (Group A1), 30 were diagnosed with mild COVID-19 without aspiration pneumonia (Group A2), and 106 were diagnosed with aspiration pneumonia alone. COVID-19 was confirmed through a positive result in the reverse transcriptase polymerase chain reaction test, and pneumonia was diagnosed by conducting various imaging tests, such as chest radiography or computed tomography, along with the assessment of clinical signs of oxygen saturation in room air. This study was approved by the Institutional Review Board of the Sahmyook Medical Center (116286-202307-HR-01; 6 July 2023). Patient consent was waived due to the retrospective nature of the study. A flowchart of the study participants is shown in Figure 1.

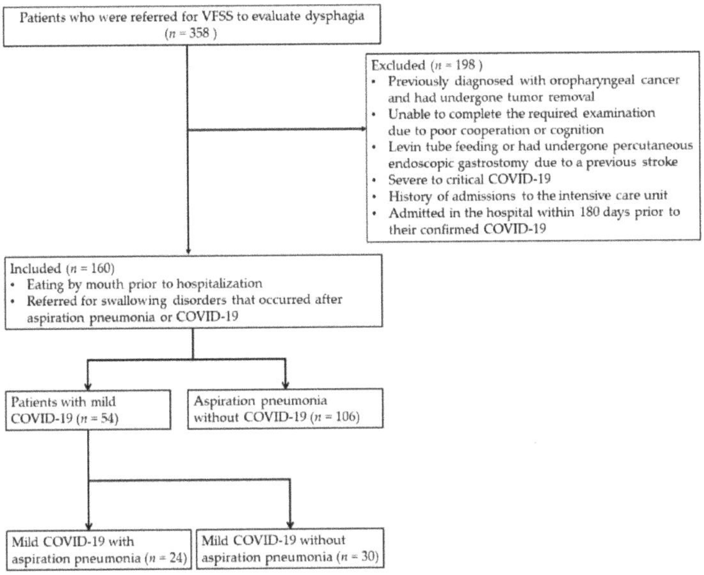

Figure 1. Flowchart of study participants.

2.2. VFSS

The normal process of swallowing proceeds through the oral preparatory and propulsive stages and then advances to the pharyngeal and esophageal stages [7]. VFSS is a radiographic procedure that provides a dynamic view of swallowing. It evaluates oropharyngeal swallowing in various anatomical regions using 11 distinct factors: lip closure, bolus formation, transition time, post-swallowing residue, and aspiration [18]. Rehabilitation medicine specialists and residents participated in this study. After positioning the patient on a chair, lateral fluoroscopic imaging was performed using a fluoroscopy device (Brivo OEC 850, Milwaukee, WI, USA). First, the patients were instructed to initially swallow 2 mL of barium contrast solution. Subsequently, they were asked to swallow 5 mL of barium contrast solution. If no aspiration occurred, the patients were asked to swallow each of following thin porridge, thick porridge, and boiled rice, all of which were combined with a barium contrast solution. For patients with no swallowing dysfunction, the swallowing procedure was performed once, and then they proceeded to the next step. In cases with penetration, the procedure was repeated twice for confirmation. If aspiration occurred at any point, the study was terminated. All the processes were recorded at a rate of 30 frames per second, and the recorded videos were analyzed frame-by-frame to assess the swallowing function after completing the examination.

2.3. Penetration–Aspiration Scale Measurement

The penetration–aspiration scale (PAS) is an 8-point interval scale designed to assess the severity of penetration and aspiration [19]. The PAS scores are categorized as follows: normal swallowing (PAS 1), penetration above the vocal folds (PAS 2–3), contact with the vocal folds (PAS 4–5), aspiration below the vocal folds (PAS 6–7), and silent aspiration (PAS 8), with increasing scores indicating higher severity and risk of complications. In our study, each patient's PAS score was determined by identifying the highest stage observed during VFSS. A higher PAS score indicated decreased swallowing function.

2.4. Functional Dysphagia Scale Measurement

The functional dysphagia scale (FDS) is a tool based on the VFSS developed to evaluate the swallowing function in patients (Table 1).

Table 1. FDS parameters based on VFSS.

Factor	Assigned Value		Score
Lip closure	Intact Inadequate None	0 5 10	10
Bolus formation	Intact Inadequate None	0 3 6	6
Residue in oral cavity	None ≤10% 10–50% ≥50%	0 2 4 6	6
Oral transit time	≤1.5 s >1.5 s	0 6	6
Triggering of pharyngeal swallow	Normal Delayed	0 10	10
Laryngeal elevation and epiglottic closure	Normal Reduced	0 12	12
Nasal penetration	None ≤10% 10–50% ≥50%	0 4 8 12	12
Residue in vallecula	None ≤10% 10–50% ≥50%	0 4 8 12	12
Residue in pyriform sinuses	None ≤10% 10–50% ≥50%	0 4 8 12	12
Coating of pharyngeal wall after swallow	No Yes	0 10	10
Pharyngeal transit time	≤1.0 s >1.0 s	0 4	4
Total			100

FDS, functional dysphagia scale; VFSS, videofluoroscopic swallowing study.

It is a sensitive and specific method for diagnosing and assessing the severity of dysphagia [20]. Eleven distinct factors were used to evaluate the swallowing function in individual anatomical regions. The total score is 100 points, with a higher score indicating deterioration in swallowing function.

2.5. Statistical Analysis

Descriptive statistics, Fisher's exact test, or Pearson's chi-square test were used to compare the categorical data, while the Kruskal–Wallis test and Mann–Whitney U test were used for comparisons of continuous variables. Subsequent post hoc analyses were conducted to distinguish the differences among the three groups. A p value of <0.05 was considered significant, and all statistical analyses were performed using commercial software (IBM SPSS Statistics. Version 27.0. Armonk, NY, USA: IBM Corp.).

3. Results

3.1. Baseline Characteristics

The demographic and clinical characteristics of the study participants are presented in Tables 2 and 3. In a comparison between patients with mild COVID-19 (Group A1 and A2) and those with aspiration pneumonia alone (Group B), no significant differences were observed in the prevalence of dysphagia-related comorbidities, such as stroke, Parkinson's disease, dementia, asthma, and chronic obstructive pulmonary disease.

Table 2. Demographic characteristics of patients.

	Group A1 (n = 24)	Group A2 (n = 30)	Group B (n = 106)
Age (years)	82.62 ± 1.41	84.43 ± 1.73	81.58 ± 0.72
Sex			
Male	12 (50%)	11 (36.7%)	71 (67.0%)
Female	12 (50%)	19 (63.3%)	35 (33.0%)
Vaccination			
Yes	17 (70.8%)	19 (63.3%)	45 (42.4%)
No	7 (29.2%)	11 (36.7%)	61 (57.6%)
Antiviral treatment			
Yes	19 (79.2%)	13 (43.3%)	
No	5 (20.8%)	17 (56.7%)	

Continuous variables are presented as mean ± standard deviation (SD) and categorical variables as number and percentage.

Table 3. Comorbidities of patients with COVID-19 or aspiration pneumonia.

	Group A1 (n = 24)	Group A2 (n = 30)	Group B (n = 106)	p-Value
Stroke				0.84
No	15 (62.5%)	21 (70%)	70 (66.0%)	
Yes	9 (37.5%)	9 (30%)	36 (34.0%)	
Parkinson				0.74
No	21 (87.5%)	28 (93.3%)	97 (91.5%)	
Yes	3 (12.5%)	2 (6.7%)	9 (8.5%)	
Dementia				0.31
No	14 (58.3%)	19 (63.3%)	77 (72.6%)	
Yes	10 (41.7%)	11 (36.7%)	29 (27.4%)	
Asthma				0.37
No	23 (95.8%)	26 (86.7%)	99 (93.4%)	
Yes	1 (4.2%)	4 (13.3%)	7 (6.6%)	
COPD				0.26
No	22 (91.7%)	30 (100%)	97 (91.5%)	
Yes	2 (8.3%)	0 (0%)	9 (8.5%)	

Categorical variables are presented as number and percentage. Variables were compared using Fisher's exact test or Pearson's chi-square test as appropriate. COPD, chronic obstructive pulmonary disease; COVID-19, coronavirus disease.

3.2. Comparison of VFSS Parameter by Group

Table 4 and Figure 2 depict the differences in the VFSS parameters between Groups A and B. Group A tended to have lower PAS and FDS scores than Group B, indicating milder dysphagia. Among the FDS sub-scores, oral transit time (p = 0.001) and pharyngeal transit time (p = 0.003) were significantly shorter in Group A. Additionally, the prevalence rates of bolus formation (p = 0.04), nasal penetration (p = 0.02), residue in the vallecula (p < 0.001), and residue in the pyriform sinus (p = 0.03) were lower in Group A (Table 4 and Figure 2).

Table 4. Comparison of PAS and FDS scores based on VFSS between Groups A and B.

	Group A (n = 54)	Group B (n = 106)	p-Value
PAS	4.31 (2.73)	4.88 (2.83)	0.21
Lip closure	1.02 (2.975)	0.57 (1.87)	0.64
Bolus formation	2.5 (2.84)	3.45 (2.58)	**0.04**
Residue in oral cavity	1.74 (1.456)	2.15 (1.87)	0.23
Oral transit time	2.11 (2.892)	3.74 (2.92)	**0.001**
Triggering of pharyngeal swallow	4.44 (5.016)	2.92 (4.57)	0.06
Laryngeal elevation and epiglottic closure	6.44 (6.04)	4.87 (5.92)	0.12
Nasal penetration	0.07 (0.544)	0.53 (1.36)	**0.02**
Residue in vallecula	4.52 (3.391)	6.83 (3.94)	**<0.001**
Residue in pyriform sinuses	4 (3.645)	5.51 (4)	**0.03**
Coating of pharyngeal wall after swallow	4.81 (5.043)	5.38 (5.01)	0.50
Pharyngeal transit time	0 (0)	0.6 (1.44)	**0.003**
Total	31.67(21.466)	36.55(21.39)	0.20

Continuous variables are presented as mean ± standard deviation (SD). Bold numbers depict significant difference (p-value < 0.05). FDS, functional dysphagia scale; PAS, penetration–aspiration scale; VFSS, videofluoroscopic swallowing study.

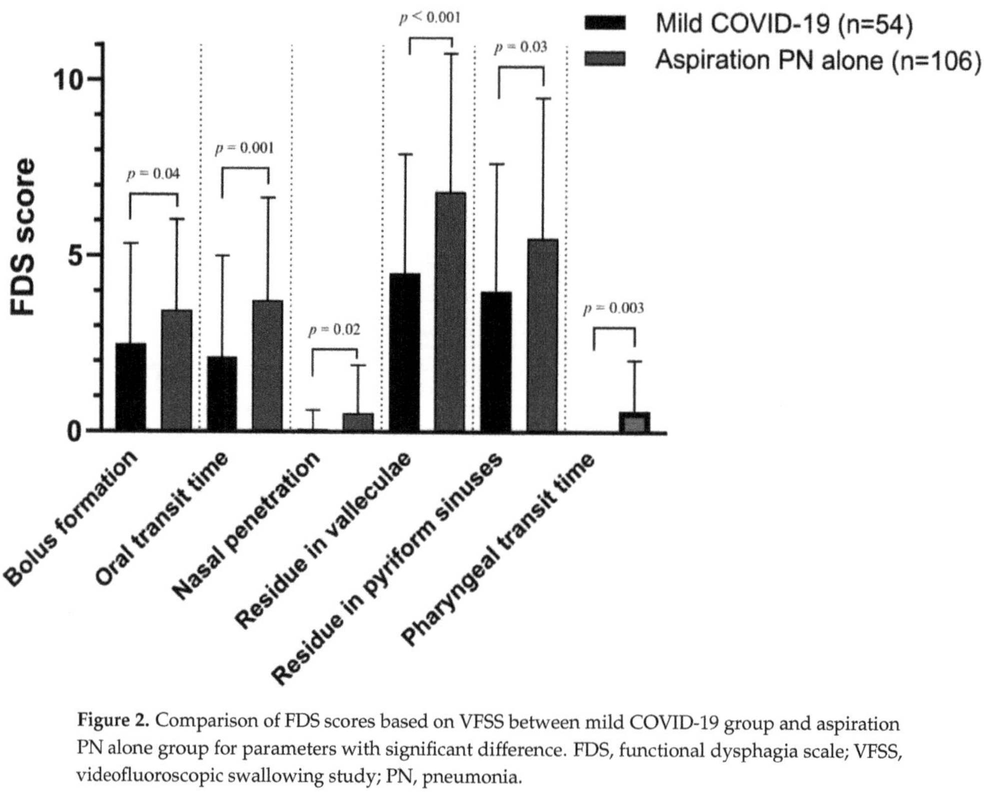

Figure 2. Comparison of FDS scores based on VFSS between mild COVID-19 group and aspiration PN alone group for parameters with significant difference. FDS, functional dysphagia scale; VFSS, videofluoroscopic swallowing study; PN, pneumonia.

3.3. Comparison of VFSS Parameters by Subgroup

The patients were subdivided into COVID-19 with aspiration pneumonia (Group A1), COVID-19 without aspiration pneumonia (Group A2), and aspiration pneumonia alone (Group B) (Table 5 and Figure 3). The bolus formation was better in Group A1 than in Group B (p = 0.009). The oral transit times in Groups A1 and A2 were shorter than that in Group B (p = 0.01). The amount of vallecular residues was lower in Groups A1 and A2 than in Group B (p = 0.005 and p = 0.008, respectively). Similarly, the pharyngeal transit time was shorter in Groups A1 and A2 than in Group B (p = 0.02 and p = 0.04, respectively). Nasal penetration also differed between Groups A1 and B ($p = 0.04$). Group B showed improvement in the triggering of pharyngeal swallowing compared with Group A2 ($p = 0.02$).

Table 5. Comparison of PAS and FDS scores based on VFSS among Groups A1, A2, and B.

	Group A1 (*n* = 24)	Group A2 (*n* = 30)	Group B (*n* = 106)	*p*-Value	Group 1–2	Group 2–3	Group 1–3
PAS	3.90 (2.64)	4.83 (2.79)	4.88 (2.83)	0.23	0.22	0.86	0.09
Lip closure	1.04 (2.94)	1 (3.05)	0.57 (1.87)	0.87	0.81	0.60	0.83
Bolus formation	3.13 (3)	2 (2.65)	3.45 (2.58)	**0.04**	0.17	0.66	**0.009**
Residue in oral cavity	1.67 (1.4)	1.8 (1.52)	2.15 (1.87)	0.47	0.81	0.3	0.4
Oral transit time	2 (2.89)	2.2 (2.94)	3.74 (2.92)	**0.005**	0.80	**0.01**	**0.01**
Triggering of pharyngeal swallow	5.42 (5.09)	3.67 (4.9)	2.92 (4.57)	0.07	0.20	**0.02**	0.439
Laryngeal elevation and epiglottic closure	6 (6.13)	6.8 (6.05)	4.87 (5.92)	0.26	0.63	0.4	0.118
Nasal penetration	0.17 (0.82)	0 (0)	0.53 (1.36)	0.06	0.26	0.212	**0.04**
Residue in vallecula	4.5 (3.19)	4.53 (3.6)	6.83 (3.94)	**0.002**	0.99	**0.008**	**0.005**
Residue in pyriform sinuses	4 (3.54)	4 (3.79)	5.51 (4)	0.09	0.94	0.10	0.07
Coating of pharyngeal wall after swallow	5 (5.11)	4.67 (5.07)	5.38 (5.01)	0.78	0.81	0.74	0.49
Pharyngeal transit time	0 (0)	0 (0)	0.6 (1.44)	**0.01**	1	**0.04**	**0.02**
Total	32.92(22)	30.67(21.35)	36.55(21.39)	0.42	0.72	0.46	0.23

Kruskal–Wallis test was used to compare the three groups, while Mann–Whitney U test was used to compare two groups. Continuous variables are presented as mean ± standard deviation (SD). Bold numbers depict significant difference (p-value < 0.05). FDS, functional dysphagia scale; PAS, penetration–aspiration scale; VFSS, videofluoroscopic swallowing study.

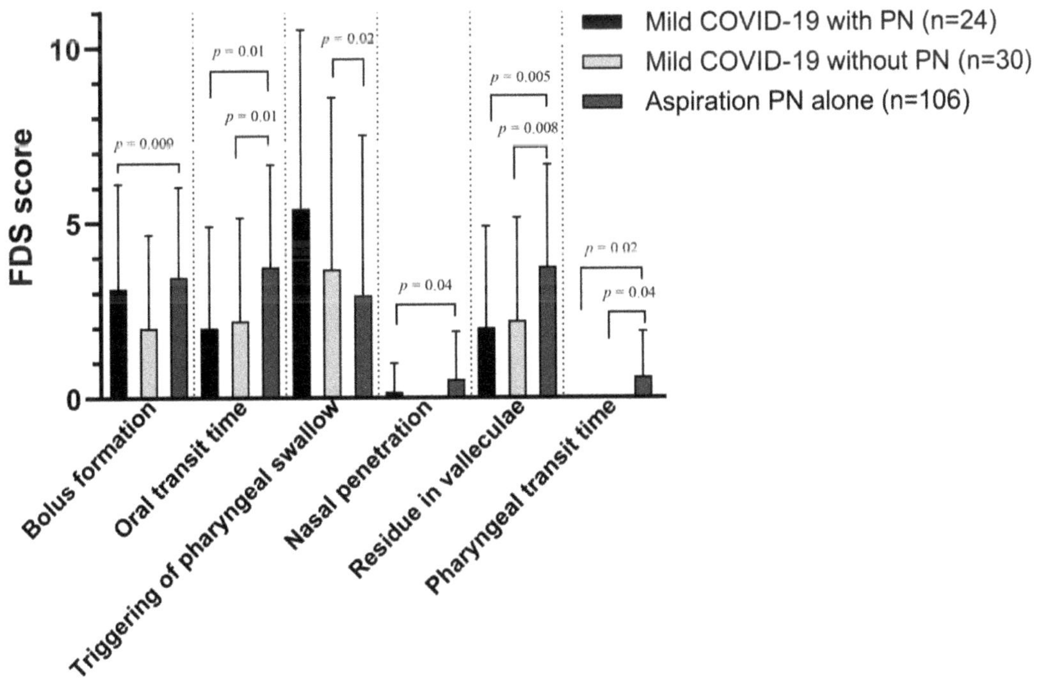

Figure 3. Comparison of FDS scores based on VFSS among mild COVID-19 with PN group, mild COVID-19 without PN, and aspiration pneumonia alone group for parameters with significant difference. FDS, functional dysphagia scale; VFSS, videofluoroscopic swallowing study; PN, pneumonia.

4. Discussion

This study primarily aimed to identify the differences in swallowing dysfunction between patients with mild COVID-19 and those with aspiration pneumonia using VFSS. The mild COVID-19 group exhibited lower PAS and FDS scores, showing less severe dysphagia, compared with the scores in the aspiration pneumonia-only group. This trend was evident in several VFSS parameters, such as transit time and post-swallowing residue. When the mild COVID-19 group was subdivided into COVID-19 with aspiration pneumonia (Group A1) and without aspiration pneumonia (Group A2), both subgroups A1 and A2 showed better VFSS parameters than Group B, with specific differences in oral and pharyngeal transit times, vallecular residues, and nasal penetration. These findings indicate that patients with mild COVID-19 experience mild degrees of dysphagia, irrespective of the status of aspiration pneumonia, compared with those with aspiration pneumonia alone.

According to the WHO classification, mild COVID-19 has less severe symptoms compared with severe COVID-19 [2]. Shadi et al. [17] reported that complications of COVID-19 are associated with the degree of severity. Jeon et al. [14] reported that patients with severe COVID-19 exhibited more pronounced dysphagia compared to those with aspiration pneumonia. Based on these previous studies, our research finding that mild COVID-19 is associated with milder dysphagia compared to aspiration pneumonia confirms our hypothesis.

Severe acute respiratory syndrome coronavirus 2 (SARS-CoV-2), the causative pathogen for COVID-19, demonstrates a predilection for binding to angiotensin-converting enzyme 2 (ACE2) [21], a receptor found across multiple organ systems, including neural tissues [22]. Previous studies have reported cases of cranial nerve infections following COVID-19, as well as cognitive impairment due to diffuse white matter damage [23,24]. Symptoms such as loss of smell and Bell's palsy also result from olfactory and facial nerve involvement [25,26].

Among the cranial nerves involved in swallowing, damage to the trigeminal nerve can affect mastication because it innervates the masticatory muscles [7]. The facial nerve plays a role in preventing food leakage during swallowing by controlling lip movement [27]. Damage to the glossopharyngeal and vagus nerves can adversely affect pharyngeal swallowing [27,28]. Similarly, hypoglossal nerve damage may affect tongue movement, which can influence bolus formation [29]. This could mean that the virus directly affects the nerves responsible for swallowing, thus contributing to the emergence of dysphagia in patients with COVID-19 [30,31]. The possibility of nerve damage could also explain the delays in the triggering of pharyngeal swallowing in Group A2 compared with that in Group B.

When the SARS-CoV-2 virus binds to the ACE2 receptors in the respiratory epithelium, it triggers an inflammatory response via a cytokine storm. This response can range from asymptomatic to severe, which may progress to ARDS [3], potentially necessitating mechanical ventilation (MV) [31]. Invasive respiratory support, such as endotracheal intubation or MV, has been associated with the increased prevalence and severity of swallowing difficulty [11–14]. Frajkova et al. [5] reported that dysphagia during intubation can be attributed to various factors, such as the duration of MV, which is linked to the incidence of dysphagia; worsening of nutritional status due to reduced food intake while on MV; and the possibility of injury to oral structures during the intubation process. Considering that MV has been linked to a higher risk of dysphagia [5,6], the fact that the mild COVID-19 group did not require invasive treatments and had a lower risk of nerve damage than the severe-to-critical group implies that their dysphagia was probably less severe.

Age was a significant factor in the occurrence of dysphagia [13,32,33]. Presbyphagia is a swallowing disorder that can occur due to aging, even in otherwise healthy individuals [34]. This is due to the weakening of swallowing-related muscles caused by sarcopenia [35]. Martín et al. [36] reported that as the average age increased, frailty became more severe, and the swallowing function declined. However, the existing literature comparing the incidence of presbyphagia and dysphagia resulting from COVID-19 is limited. Considering that the average age of Groups A1 (82.62 ± 1.41) and A2 (84.43 ± 1.73) was higher than that of Group B (81.58 ± 0.72), Groups A1 and A2 were expected to have a poorer swallowing function when considering the effects of presbyphagia. However, our observation that Groups A1 and A2 demonstrated better swallowing function might imply that the effect of mild COVID-19 on swallowing disorders is less severe than that of presbyphagia.

Sarcopenia is defined by a reduction in both the quantity and strength of skeletal muscles [37], leading to impaired respiratory and swallowing muscle functions, malnutrition, and a weakened immune system [38]. The impaired functions can increase susceptibility to COVID-19. Of note, isolation in a hospital or at home for several days following COVID-19 diagnosis, along with a decrease in activity levels due to deconditioning, promotes muscle loss and contributes to the onset of sarcopenia [39]. Sarcopenia experienced by the elderly can lead to muscle loss and subsequently trigger dysphagia, creating a vicious cycle [40]. To break this detrimental cycle, appropriate post-infection dysphagia rehabilitation is essential to facilitate functional recovery. Dysphagia emerging after COVID-19 shows rapid improvement with short-term therapy [41], and speech therapists can provide swallowing rehabilitation with several speech–language therapies and oral motor facilitation techniques [42]. However, the rehabilitation procedures were considered aerosol-generating procedures. Therefore, when evaluating and treating swallowing disorders in patients with COVID-19, healthcare professionals and patients are at risk of infection, emphasizing the importance of the thorough use of personal protective equipment [43].

While the WHO continues to classify the pandemic as ongoing, certain nations are shifting their public health strategies to treat COVID-19 as an endemic disease. Safety restrictions that have been impeding dysphagia treatment will gradually be loosened, allowing for more proactive treatment. Our research findings may be useful in developing treatment strategies for dysphagia accompanying mild COVID-19.

Our study has several limitations. First, owing to the retrospective nature of our study, we were unable to control the time interval between the onset of symptoms and the timing of the tests, leading to potential bias and limitations in data collection. Also, we were unable to verify the spontaneous resolution of COVID-19-induced dysphagia via follow-up evaluations. Considering the relatively early recovery of swallowing function in patients who developed dysphagia after COVID-19 [16,44], using a prospective study design could help overcome these limitations and yield more objective and precise findings. Second, the limited sample size hindered in-depth subgroup evaluations; participants were exclusively recruited from a secondary medical institute, and patients with suspected aspiration pneumonia or COVID-19, who were more likely to experience dysphagia, were exclusively included in the study. Patients without respiratory symptoms were not part of the research, which further limits the generalizability of our study findings. Third, the study failed to account for additional medical conditions which could potentially influence dysphagia. In our study, no significant differences were found between the groups in terms of the incidence of stroke or Parkinson's disease, both of which are known to influence swallowing difficulty. However, a more detailed comparison of the dysphagia-related factors, including sex, age, and presence of diseases, such as multiple sclerosis, myopathy, and Guillain–Barré syndrome, would have been possible if neurological assessments had been included.

5. Conclusions

Patients with mild COVID-19 had lower PAS and FDS scores, suggesting milder dysphagia than for those with aspiration pneumonia. This pattern persisted in multiple VFSS parameters. When the patients were further divided into subgroups of COVID-19 with and without aspiration pneumonia, both subgroups outperformed the aspiration pneumonia group in specific VFSS parameters, including oral and pharyngeal transit times and vallecular residue. During the COVID-19 pandemic, there have been limitations on treatment. However, if COVID-19 changes to an endemic disease with fewer treatment limitations, proactive dysphagia rehabilitation for mild COVID-19 patients could be enabled, potentially aiding in the rapid recovery of swallowing disorders.

Author Contributions: Conceptualization, J.K., B.R., Y.K., Y.C. and E.L.; data curation, J.K. and Y.C.; formal analysis, J.K. and E.L.; investigation, J.K. and Y.C.; methodology, B.R. and Y.K.; project administration, E.L.; supervision, B.R. and Y.K.; validation, B.R., Y.K. and E.L.; writing—original draft, J.K.; writing—review and editing, E.L. All authors have read and agreed to the published version of the manuscript.

Funding: This research received no external funding.

Institutional Review Board Statement: The study was conducted in accordance with the Declaration of Helsinki and approved by the Institutional Review Board of the Sahmyook Medical Center (ethical approval reference No. 116286-202307-HR-01 from 6 July 2023).

Informed Consent Statement: Patient consent was waived due to the retrospective nature of the study.

Data Availability Statement: The data used and/or analyzed during the current study are available from the corresponding author upon reasonable request.

Conflicts of Interest: The authors declare no conflict of interest.

References

1. Zhang, J.J.; Dong, X.; Cao, Y.Y.; Yuan, Y.D.; Yang, Y.B.; Yan, Y.Q.; Akdis, C.A.; Gao, Y.D. Clinical characteristics of 140 patients infected with SARS-CoV-2 in Wuhan, China. *Allergy* **2020**, *75*, 1730–1741. [CrossRef] [PubMed]
2. World Health Organization. COVID-19 Clinical Management: Living Guidance, 18 August 2023. Available online: https://www.who.int/publications/i/item/WHO-2019-nCoV-clinical-2023.2 (accessed on 30 August 2023).
3. Aleksova, A.; Gagno, G.; Sinagra, G.; Beltrami, A.P.; Janjusevic, M.; Ippolito, G.; Zumla, A.; Fluca, A.L.; Ferro, F. Effects of SARS-CoV-2 on cardiovascular system: The dual role of angiotensin-converting enzyme 2 (ACE2) as the virus receptor and homeostasis regulator-review. *Int. J. Mol. Sci.* **2021**, *22*, 4526. [CrossRef] [PubMed]
4. Ochani, R.; Asad, A.; Yasmin, F.; Shaikh, S.; Khalid, H.; Batra, S.; Sohail, M.R.; Mahmood, S.F.; Ochani, R.; Hussham Arshad, M.; et al. COVID-19 pandemic: From origins to outcomes. A comprehensive review of viral pathogenesis, clinical manifestations, diagnostic evaluation, and management. *Infez. Med.* **2021**, *29*, 20–36. [PubMed]
5. Frajkova, Z.; Tedla, M.; Tedlova, E.; Suchankova, M.; Geneid, A. Postintubation dysphagia during COVID-19 outbreak-contemporary review. *Dysphagia* **2020**, *35*, 549–557. [CrossRef] [PubMed]
6. Grilli, G.M.; Giancaspro, R.; Del Colle, A.; Quarato, C.M.I.; Lacedonia, D.; Foschino Barbaro, M.P.; Cassano, M. Dysphagia in non-intubated patients affected by COVID-19 infection. *Eur. Arch. Otorhinolaryngol.* **2022**, *279*, 507–513. [CrossRef] [PubMed]
7. Matsuo, K.; Palmer, J.B. Anatomy and physiology of feeding and swallowing: Normal and abnormal. *Phys. Med. Rehabil. Clin. N. Am.* **2008**, *19*, 691–707. [CrossRef]
8. Carucci, L.R.; Turner, M.A. Dysphagia revisited: Common and unusual causes. *RadioGraphics* **2015**, *35*, 105–122. [CrossRef]
9. Dziewas, R.; Hufelschulte, L.M.; Lepper, J.; Sackarnd, J.; Minnerup, J.; Teismann, I.; Ahring, S.; Claus, I.; Labeit, B.; Muhle, P.; et al. Dysphagia in patients with severe coronavirus disease 2019-potential neurologic etiologies. *Crit. Care Explor.* **2021**, *3*, e0332. [CrossRef]
10. Osbeck Sandblom, H.; Dotevall, H.; Svennerholm, K.; Tuomi, L.; Finizia, C. Characterization of dysphagia and laryngeal findings in COVID-19 patients treated in the ICU-An observational clinical study. *PLoS ONE* **2021**, *16*, e0252347. [CrossRef]
11. Brodsky, M.B.; Huang, M.; Shanholtz, C.; Mendez-Tellez, P.A.; Palmer, J.B.; Colantuoni, E.; Needham, D.M. Recovery from dysphagia symptoms after oral endotracheal intubation in acute respiratory distress syndrome survivors. A 5-year longitudinal study. *Ann. Am. Thorac. Soc.* **2017**, *14*, 376–383. [CrossRef]
12. Ceruti, S.; Glotta, A.; Galli, A.; Biggiogero, M.; Bona, G.; Mauri, R.; Saporito, A.; Capdevila, X. Dysphagic disorder in a cohort of COVID-19 patients: Evaluation and evolution. *Ann. Med. Surg.* **2021**, *69*, 102837. [CrossRef] [PubMed]
13. Skoretz, S.A.; Yau, T.M.; Ivanov, J.; Granton, J.T.; Martino, R. Dysphagia and associated risk factors following extubation in cardiovascular surgical patients. *Dysphagia* **2014**, *29*, 647–654. [CrossRef] [PubMed]
14. Jeon, H.-E.; Ku, Y.-S.; Lee, Y.-G.; Jung, H.-Y.; Lee, J.-H.; Joa, K.-L. The comparison of dysphagia between COVID-19 pneumonia and aspiration pneumonia. *J. Korean Dysphagia Soc.* **2023**, *13*, 24–33. [CrossRef]
15. Herrera-Esposito, D.; de Los Campos, G. Age-specific rate of severe and critical SARS-CoV-2 infections estimated with multi-country seroprevalence studies. *BMC Infect. Dis.* **2022**, *22*, 311. [CrossRef]
16. Can, B.; İsmagulova, N.; Enver, N.; Tufan, A.; Cinel, İ. Sarcopenic dysphagia following COVID-19 infection: A new danger. *Nutr. Clin. Pract.* **2021**, *36*, 828–832. [CrossRef]
17. Shadi, M.S.; Farahat, M. Self-perceived dysphagia in non-invasively ventilated COVID-19 patients. *Eur. Arch. Otorhinolaryngol.* **2022**, *279*, 5929–5937. [CrossRef] [PubMed]
18. Stokely, S.L.; Molfenter, S.M.; Steele, C.M. Effects of barium concentration on oropharyngeal swallow timing measures. *Dysphagia* **2014**, *29*, 78–82. [CrossRef] [PubMed]

19. Rosenbek, J.C.; Robbins, J.A.; Roecker, E.B.; Coyle, J.L.; Wood, J.L. A penetration-aspiration scale. *Dysphagia* **1996**, *11*, 93–98. [CrossRef] [PubMed]
20. Han, T.R.; Paik, N.J.; Park, J.W. Quantifying swallowing function after stroke: A functional dysphagia scale based on videofluoroscopic studies. *Arch. Phys. Med. Rehabil.* **2001**, *82*, 677–682. [CrossRef]
21. Kirtipal, N.; Kumar, S.; Dubey, S.K.; Dwivedi, V.D.; Gireesh Babu, K.; Malý, P.; Bharadwaj, S. Understanding on the possible routes for SARS CoV-2 invasion via ACE2 in the host linked with multiple organs damage. *Infect. Genet. Evol.* **2022**, *99*, 105254. [CrossRef]
22. Liu, L.; Ni, S.Y.; Yan, W.; Lu, Q.D.; Zhao, Y.M.; Xu, Y.Y.; Mei, H.; Shi, L.; Yuan, K.; Han, Y.; et al. Mental and neurological disorders and risk of COVID-19 susceptibility, illness severity and mortality: A systematic review, meta-analysis and call for action. *EClinicalmedicine* **2021**, *40*, 101111. [CrossRef] [PubMed]
23. Gelpi, E.; Klotz, S.; Beyerle, M.; Wischnewski, S.; Harter, V.; Kirschner, H.; Stolz, K.; Reisinger, C.; Lindeck-Pozza, E.; Zoufaly, A.; et al. Multifactorial white matter damage in the acute phase and pre-existing conditions may drive cognitive dysfunction after SARS-CoV-2 infection: Neuropathology-based evidence. *Viruses* **2023**, *15*, 908. [CrossRef] [PubMed]
24. Huang, S.; Zhou, X.; Zhao, W.; Du, Y.; Yang, D.; Huang, Y.; Chen, Y.; Zhang, H.; Yang, G.; Liu, J.; et al. Dynamic white matter changes in recovered COVID-19 patients: A two-year follow-up study. *Theranostics* **2023**, *13*, 724–735. [CrossRef] [PubMed]
25. Tonkal, A.; Alamri, A.A.; AlMaghrabi, S.J.; Mozahim, N.F.; Mozahim, S.F.; Alsubaie, S.A.; Alsehly, A.A.; Alshuaibi, R.O.; Alotaibi, L.A.; Qashgari, F.S. Cranial nerve impairment associated with COVID-19 infections: A systematic review. *Cureus* **2022**, *14*, e31997. [CrossRef]
26. Doblan, A.; Kaplama, M.E.; Ak, S.; Basmacı, N.; Tarini, E.Z.; Göktaş, Ş.E.; Güler, S.; Müderris, T. Cranial nerve involvement in COVID-19. *Am. J. Otolaryngol.* **2021**, *42*, 102999. [CrossRef]
27. Florie, M.G.M.H.; Pilz, W.; Dijkman, R.H.; Kremer, B.; Wiersma, A.; Winkens, B.; Baijens, L.W.J. The effect of cranial nerve stimulation on swallowing: A systematic review. *Dysphagia* **2021**, *36*, 216–230. [CrossRef]
28. Erman, A.B.; Kejner, A.E.; Hogikyan, N.D.; Feldman, E.L. Disorders of cranial nerves IX and X. *Semin. Neurol.* **2009**, *29*, 85–92. [CrossRef]
29. Lee, J.H.; Kim, H.S.; Yun, D.H.; Chon, J.; Han, Y.J.; Yoo, S.D.; Kim, D.H.; Lee, S.A.; Joo, H.I.; Park, J.S.; et al. The relationship between tongue pressure and oral dysphagia in stroke patients. *Ann. Rehabil. Med.* **2016**, *40*, 620–628. [CrossRef]
30. Kim, D.Y. The pathologic mechanisms and epidemiology of dysphagia associated with COVID-19. *J. Korean Dysphagia Soc.* **2021**, *11*, 87–92. [CrossRef]
31. Bourgonje, A.R.; Abdulle, A.E.; Timens, W.; Hillebrands, J.L.; Navis, G.J.; Gordijn, S.J.; Bolling, M.C.; Dijkstra, G.; Voors, A.A.; Osterhaus, A.D.; et al. Angiotensin-converting enzyme 2 (ACE2), SARS-CoV-2 and the pathophysiology of coronavirus disease 2019 (COVID-19). *J. Pathol.* **2020**, *251*, 228–248. [CrossRef]
32. Lindh, M.G.; Mattsson, G.; Koyi, H.; Johansson, M.B.; Razmi, R.; Palm, A. Swallowing function in COVID-19 patients after invasive mechanical ventilation. *Arch. Rehabil. Res. Clin. Transl.* **2022**, *4*, 100177. [CrossRef]
33. Sura, L.; Madhavan, A.; Carnaby, G.; Crary, M.A. Dysphagia in the elderly: Management and nutritional considerations. *Clin. Interv. Aging* **2012**, *7*, 287–298. [CrossRef] [PubMed]
34. Robbins, J.; Hamilton, J.W.; Lof, G.L.; Kempster, G.B. Oropharyngeal swallowing in normal adults of different ages. *Gastroenterology* **1992**, *103*, 823–829. [CrossRef]
35. Mehraban-Far, S.; Alrassi, J.; Patel, R.; Ahmad, V.; Browne, N.; Lam, W.; Jiang, Y.; Barber, N.; Mortensen, M. Dysphagia in the elderly population: A videofluoroscopic study. *Am. J. Otolaryngol.* **2021**, *42*, 102854. [CrossRef]
36. Martín-Martínez, A.; Viñas, P.; Carrillo, I.; Martos, J.; Clavé, P.; Ortega, O. The impact of frailty, oropharyngeal dysphagia and malnutrition on mortality in older patients hospitalized for COVID-19. *Aging Dis.* **2023**, *14*, 6:1–6:12. [CrossRef] [PubMed]
37. Cruz-Jentoft, A.J.; Baeyens, J.P.; Bauer, J.M.; Boirie, Y.; Cederholm, T.; Landi, F.; Martin, F.C.; Michel, J.-P.; Rolland, Y.; Schneider, S.M.; et al. Sarcopenia: European consensus on definition and diagnosis: Report of the European Working Group on Sarcopenia in Older People. *Age Ageing* **2010**, *39*, 412–423. [CrossRef]
38. Morley, J.E.; Kalantar-Zadeh, K.; Anker, S.D. COVID-19: A major cause of cachexia and sarcopenia? *J. Cachexia Sarcopenia Muscle* **2020**, *11*, 863–865. [CrossRef] [PubMed]
39. Maeda, K.; Akagi, J. Treatment of sarcopenic dysphagia with rehabilitation and nutritional support: A comprehensive approach. *J. Acad. Nutr. Diet* **2016**, *116*, 573–577. [CrossRef]
40. Kim, J.; Han, Y.; Han, S.J.; Shim, H.; Choi, H.J.; Suh, J.H. Rehabilitation in a patient with sarcopenic dysphagia on venovenous extracorporeal membrane oxygenation support following COVID-19 infection: A case report. *J. Korean Dysphagia Soc.* **2023**, *13*, 155–160. [CrossRef]
41. Ko, S.H. Assessment and management of dysphagia during the COVID-19 pandemic. *J. Korean Dysphagia Soc.* **2021**, *11*, 93–98. [CrossRef]
42. Lima, M.S.d.; Sassi, F.C.; Medeiros, G.C.d.; Ritto, A.P.; Andrade, C.R.F.d. Functional development of swallowing in ICU patients with COVID-19. *CoDAS* **2020**, *32*, e20200222. [CrossRef] [PubMed]

43. Schindler, A.; Baijens, L.W.J.; Clave, P.; Degen, B.; Duchac, S.; Dziewas, R.; Farneti, D.; Hamdy, S.; Michou, E.; Pokieser, P.; et al. ESSD commentary on dysphagia management during COVID pandemia. *Dysphagia* **2021**, *36*, 764–767. [CrossRef] [PubMed]
44. Clayton, N.A.; Walker, E.; Freeman-Sanderson, A. Clinical profile and recovery pattern of dysphagia in the COVID-19 patient: A prospective observational cohort within NSW. *Aust. Crit. Care* **2023**, *36*, 262–268. [CrossRef] [PubMed]

medicina

MDPI

Article

Barriers and Motivators toward Childhood COVID-19 Vaccination: A Cross-Sectional Study Conducted among Saudi Population

Hind M. AlOsaimi [1,*], Ali M. Alqahtani [1], Nadia M. Alanazi [2], Nouf N. Alotibi [3], Mohammed S. Alrazog [4], Hanoof A. Aljameel [3], Raghad M. Alshehri [5], Sarah J. Alhusayni [6] and Mohammed K. Alshammari [1,*]

1 Pharmacy Services Administration, King Fahad Medical City, Riyadh Second Health Cluster, Riyadh 12211, Saudi Arabia; amalqahtani1@kfmc.med.sa
2 Department of Pharmacy Rumah General Hospital, Riyadh 12211, Saudi Arabia; naianazi@moh.gov.sa
3 Department of Pharmacy, Qassim University, Qassim Region, Buraidah 56218, Saudi Arabia; noufottibi@gmail.com (N.N.A.); hanoofaljameel@hotmail.com (H.A.A.)
4 Department of Pharmacy, Prince Sultan Military Medical City, Riyadh 12211, Saudi Arabia; malrazog@psmmc.med.sa
5 Department of Pharmacy, King Khalid University, Abha 62217, Saudi Arabia; raghadalshehri.98@gmail.com
6 Department of Pharmacy, Taibah University, Medina 41311, Saudi Arabia; sarah-alhussaini@hotmail.com
* Correspondence: halosaimi@kfmc.med.sa (H.M.A.); mkaalshammari@kfmc.med.sa (M.K.A.)

Abstract: *Background and Objectives:* In 2020, one of the most important steps that were made was to give priority to the development of a COVID-19 vaccine to prevent the rising incidence of COVID-19 from continuing to rise. However, globally, there is a variable acceptance of the level of the COVID-19 vaccine. This study aims to explore Saudi parents' willingness to vaccinate their children against COVID-19. *Materials and Methods*: This was a cross-sectional study; the online questionnaire was used to investigate the views of Saudi parents with children aged under 18 toward the immunization of their children against COVID-19. The data were gathered from 10 May 2022 to 31 October 2022. The data analysis uses SPSS version 20. A p-value of 0.05 or lower was regarded as statistically significant. *Results:* A total of 978 Saudi parents participated in this study. Most of the respondents were from the age group of 36–45 years with the educational qualification of high school and bachelor's degree. Overall, it was observed that the majority, 98.2% of the respondents, disclosed that they needed more information ($p = 0.004$) about COVID-19 vaccine safety among children so that they could decide whether to vaccinate their child. About 91.4% of parents mention that vaccination against COVID-19 is not necessary for children ($p = 0.001$). About 68.3% of respondents agreed that getting vaccinated against COVID-19 could help Saudi Arabia control COVID-19 ($p = 0.007$, RI = 0.76). In terms of negative attitudes toward COVID-19 vaccination, 71.3% think that there will be severe side effects ($p = 0.019$, RI = 0.75); 67.7% think that the vaccine's protection will only last for a short time ($p = 0.055$, RI = 0.72); 80.1% said they were afraid of getting vaccinated because of needle fear ($p = 0.045$, RI = 0.76), and 41.2% said lack of time was the main barrier to not vaccinating their child. *Conclusions:* Parents expressed concerns regarding the safety and efficacy of the COVID-19 vaccine, which might be some of the main factors influencing their decision to vaccinate their children. It is the need of the hour to take action to communicate, educate, and intervene with Saudi parents to enhance COVID-19 vaccination compliance rates across the board.

Keywords: COVID-19; vaccination; children; parents; hesitancy; Saudi Arabia

1. Introduction

The first case of the COVID-19 outbreak was reported on 31 December 2019 in Wuhan, China, and on 13 January 2020, Thailand reported its first case of COVID-19 [1]. Since then, COVID-19 has become a global pandemic [2]. Saudi Arabia is the second most populated country in the Gulf region, with a population of more than 34 million, of whom about 37% are expatriates [3]. The first case of COVID-19 was reported on 2 March 2020; before that, Saudi Arabia was one of the first countries to take preventative measures to stop the propagation of COVID-19 in the Kingdom [4]. Travel restrictions, strict immigration checks, movement control, implementation of sanitization and hygiene practices at workplaces (i.e., use of sanitizer and masks), suspending academic and religious activities, and reducing the number of workers in workplaces were some of the main preventive actions implemented [5]. Perhaps, due to these timely measures, the prevalence of COVID-19 was observed to be lower compared to the neighboring Gulf countries [6].

In 2020, The World Health Organization (WHO) declared COVID-19 a global pandemic, and timely development of a COVID-19 vaccine was prioritized to prevent the rising incidence of COVID-19 [7]. Regardless of these global efforts for vaccine development, however, there was a considerable number of individuals worldwide who refused COVID-19 vaccination [8]. According to the Strategic Advisory Group of Experts on Immunization (SAGE) of the World Health Organization (WHO), vaccine hesitancy (VH) is defined as a "delay in acceptance or refusal of vaccination despite the availability of vaccination services" [9]. WHO emphasized the necessity of the national and international stakeholders to conduct campaigns on the significance of COVID-19 immunizations so that vaccine hesitancy among the public could be reduced and willingness to vaccinate themselves and their children could be increased [10].

High uptake rates are necessary for a successful immunization response [11]. Both the acceptance of vaccines and the demand for them are dependent on the community's perceptions toward vaccination [12]. Recent research has shown that equal access to vaccination across all demographic groups is difficult to achieve because of the complexity of human behavior and the fact that it varies over geography and time. Therefore, the groups willing to get vaccinated should be prioritized for vaccination, and side-by-side efforts should be made to educate and create awareness among those who may have negative perceptions toward vaccination [13]. The COVID-19 vaccine developed by Pfizer and BioNTech (AstraZeneca®) can now be administered in Saudi Arabia specifically to children aged 5 to 11 after receiving approval from the Saudi Food and Drug Authority. However, the willingness of parents toward vaccination is very important; it is observed that overall, in the last few decades, there has been an increase in parents' refusal of immunizations for their children, and this has led to an increase in the number of vaccine-preventable diseases [14]. Belief in conspiracy theories (such as the idea that vaccines might harm or sterilize children or contain contagion) are some of the main factors strengthening vaccine refusal [15,16]. Since the beginning of its development, the COVID-19 vaccination has been linked to many conspiracies as well as rumors concerning its safety and effectiveness [17].

In an attempt to regulate the situation in Saudi Arabia, about 30 million doses of the COVID-19 vaccine (AstraZeneca) have been distributed [18]. It is evident from recent studies that parents have a relatively positive attitude toward vaccinating their children against COVID-19, with an overall vaccine hesitancy ranging between 33% [19] and 21% [20]. To overcome this information gap and ensure that successful vaccine interventions are properly designed and fine-tuned for the community, it is imperative that such attitudes and intentions be understood. This understanding is a pressing necessity [21]. The Health Belief Model may provide the stakeholders with a suitable set of measures for effective interventions to modify parents' behaviors and negative perceptions toward COVID-19 vaccination [22]. If there is a widespread hesitation to get vaccinated against COVID-19, it is critical to identify the factors (i.e., attitudes or reasons) that lie behind the resistance toward vaccination. Public education programs (such as "do it for the herd") can be helpful to some extent; however, identifying factors leading to vaccination hesitancy is essential to improve overall vaccine uptake [23]. The aim of this study is to identify the barriers to COVID-19 vaccination among Saudi parents so that timely interventional measures can be planned to attain "Herd Immunity" in the Saudi Region.

2. Materials and Methods

This cross-sectional study was conducted using an online questionnaire to investigate the Saudi parents' perception of COVID-19 immunization for their children under 18. Online data collection is proven to be an efficient, timely, and rapid method that enables researchers to collect insight on the topic under consideration in a short time with a higher response rate [24,25].

2.1. Tool Development and Validity

A structured questionnaire was developed [26–29], which was subjected to a validation process explained in detail below [30–32]:

- Step one: Preparation of draft and any permission required;
- Step two: Content validity;
- Step three: Finalization of recommendations;
- Step four: Face validity;
- Step five: Final version of the tool.

During the first step, a draft of the study tools was finalized, and permissions of use were taken under the condition that the relevant citations would be given when this paper was published. Wild et al. (2005) stated that, ideally, the authors of the original tool should be invited to participate in the validation of the tool [30]. The entire pattern and the contents of each section were discussed in detail and were well understood by the lead researcher and colleagues. To avoid ambiguities, the draft version of the study tool was submitted to five experts from clinical care and academic settings to finalize the contents of the study tool. Some changes were suggested by these members, which aimed to simplify the language or presentation of the questions and the selection of the option to respond to the study questions. The finalized version was forwarded to the members again, and all agreed with the final version of the tool and recommended this tool be used for an online survey.

The final version was proofread, and some typing errors were then rectified and submitted to face validity of 30 respondents. Internal consistency was measured with coefficient alpha or Cronbach's coefficient alpha (CA) [33,34]. In addition, CA is easy to interpret as its value ranges from 0 to 1, and the CA value for this tool was 0.79. Furthermore, to address any further concerns about the tool's content, its adequacy was measured using Bartlett's test of sphericity. The Kaiser–Meyer–Olkin measure of sampling adequacy is an effective technique for judging content adequacy. If the Kaiser–Meyer–Olkin value is higher than 0.6, it demonstrates that the contents of the instrument are satisfactory to meet the study needs [35,36].

2.2. Construct of Study Tool

An overview of the objectives, methods, confidentiality, and anonymity agreements was provided on the questionnaire's cover page. The questionnaire contained three sections. The first section targets demographic characteristics, including age, gender, marital status, educational level, type of work, history of seasonal influenza vaccination, family history of COVID-19, the informational sources regarding COVID and its vaccine, and child's age. Questions in the second section are intended to gauge parents' perceptions of the decision not to vaccinate their kids against COVID-19. Questions in the third section gauge parents' attitudes toward the COVID-19 vaccination.

2.3. Data Collection Procedure

The online forms were circulated over various social media websites. Online data collection is an effective method to collect data and plan the required interventions, and various international studies conducted on vaccine hesitancy for COVID-19 vaccination have utilized online data collection procedures using different methods [37–40]. In addition, a QR code was printed on a banner explaining participation in this online survey and pasted with permission in the ER departments of the hospitals and nearby pharmacies. QR code is a very convenient method of participation in a study, and it will take the respondent to the questionnaire page with one click. In addition, the link to the online data collection tool was also shared in different social media groups to gather data. Additionally, respondents were requested to share the form with other people in their immediate circle to share their opinions about the questions regarding COVID-19 vaccination among children. The data were gathered over a period of six months, beginning on 10 May 2022 and ending on 31 October 2022.

2.4. Inclusion and Exclusion Criteria

All Saudi residents who were married and had at least one child under 18 were included in this study. All non-Saudi parents are among this study's exclusion criteria. Unmarried individuals and parents without children were excluded from this study.

2.5. Sample Size

Using Rao soft®, the sample size was calculated to be 377 as the minimal effective sample with a 95% confidence interval, 5% margin of error, and a 50% response distribution. An online questionnaire was used to approach potential participants. The distribution of the form was performed via social media platforms or community online social groups.

2.6. Statistical Analysis

This data analysis uses SPSS version 20. Both descriptive (frequency, mean, standard deviation) and inferential statistical techniques (chi-square test) were used to analyze the data. To determine the relationship between the groups and variables, the chi-square test was used. Furthermore, the relative index was also estimated to identify the top priorities of the parents for their willingness to vaccinate their children. A p-value of 0.05 or lower was regarded as statistically significant.

2.7. Ethical Approval

The ethical approval for this study was granted by the institutional review board (IRB) at King Fahad Medical City (IRB Log Number: 23-220, Dated 29 May 2023). A brief introduction to this study was given on the title page of the questionnaire. An online consent was taken before the response was collected from the respondent. It was entirely voluntary to participate. Since no information was gathered that could reveal the respondents' identities, the confidentiality of the responses was guaranteed.

3. Results

A total of N = 978 Saudi parents opted to respond using an online survey form and share their views toward vaccinating their children against COVID-19. The demographic information about the participants is shown in Table 1. The majority (45.6%) of the respondents were from the age group from 36 to 45 years (45.6%), with relatively more men (50.1%) than women. All the respondents who participated in this study were literate, and most disclosed having high school and bachelor's education. In terms of occupation, most had their own businesses (543 [55.5%]). In response to a very specific question regarding flu shots, about 49.3% disclosed noncompliance with the routine seasonal flu vaccination, while 52.6% disclosed that they or someone in their family suffered from COVID-19. Details are described in Table 1. The prime source of information for the majority (73%) of the parents for COVID-19 immunization was social media sites like Facebook, LinkedIn, etc., followed by friend and family groups (70.6%). In addition, 55.7% of parents learned about COVID-19 immunization from television and other electronic media, whereas 59% of parents received messages about COVID-19 vaccination from health authorities. Only 35.8% of parents acquired information from print media, such as newspapers and magazines.

Table 1. Socio-demographics of participants.

Sociodemographic Characteristics of the Parents (n = 978)	N	%
Age group		
<25 years	35	3.6
25–35 years	250	25.6
36–45 years	446	45.6
>46 years	247	25.3
Gender		
Male	490	50.1
Female	488	49.9
Marital status		
Married, having at least one child	937	95.8
Divorced, having children	41	4.2
Educational level		
None	0	0.0
High school or below	361	36.9
Diploma	207	21.2
Bachelor's	340	34.8
Master's	60	6.1
PhD	10	1.0
Type of work		
Private Sector	120	12.3
Public Sector	217	22.2
Non-profit Organization	543	55.5
Retired	97	9.9
History of seasonal influenza vaccination		
No	482	49.3
Yes, within one year	344	35.2
Yes, beyond one year ago	153	15.6
Family history of COVID-19		
Yes	514	52.6
No	464	47.4
Child age		
3 years or under	206	21.1
4–7 years	200	20.4
8–12 years	394	40.3
<18 years	179	18.3
From where you are accruing information about COVID-19 and its vaccination *		
Facebook, social media, LinkedIn, etc.	713	72.9
Newspapers, magazines, print media	350	35.7
Television, electronic media	545	55.7
Friend and family/friend groups	690	70.6
Messages from health authorities	577	59.0

* Multiple options were given to the respondents to disclose their responses.

The next section of this study's questionnaire aimed to explore the parents' willingness to vaccinate their children against COVID-19 (Table 2). In response to the question of whether the COVID-19 vaccine was safe and risk-free for children, 98.2% of parents answered that they needed more information about COVID-19 vaccine safety so that they could decide effectively to vaccinate their children with COVID-19 vaccine ($p = 0.004$). In addition, further information that parents needed to decide on COVID-19 vaccination for their children was proof of the COVID-19 vaccine's advantages (95.1%, $p = 0.015$). Otherwise, most of the parents, 91.4%, had reservations against COVID-19 vaccination, assuming that it was not necessary for children ($p = 0.001$). Details are shown in Table 2.

Table 2. Factors influencing willingness.

What Do You Think About Why Parents May Not Consider Vaccinating Their Child Against COVID-19	Yes	No	*p*-Value
Parents may perceive children are not at risk of COVID-19 and, therefore, do not need vaccination	894	84	<0.001
Parents need more information before I decide about COVID-19 vaccine for my children	940	38	0.005
Parents need more evidence for COVID-19 Vaccine and its benefits for children	930	48	0.015
Parents need more information about the safety and risk of COVID-19 vaccine in children	960	18	0.004

Chi-square. *p*-value < 0.005 was considered statistically significant.

Therefore, the sum of responses for this specific question may not be 100%.

This section was the main part of this study, aiming to explore the potential barriers and motivators to parents' willingness to vaccinate their children against COVID-19. Analysis has revealed that 83.3% of the parents were aware of the fact that the National Health Services Department of Saudi Arabia has ensured the availability of the COVID-19 vaccine in the Kingdom (RI = 0.80; Rank 2; *p*-value < 0.001) and it is convenient for them to vaccinate their child. However, they emphasize that their willingness to vaccinate their children is the main factor in case they want to vaccinate their children against COVID-19 (RI = 0.84; Rank 1; *p*-value < 0.001). Regardless of this fact, the majority, 68.3%, were optimistic that timely vaccination against COVID-19 among children will assist in preventing COVID-19 in Saudi Arabia (RI = 0.76; Rank 3; *p*-value < 0.007). Almost 80.0% of the parents were observed to be reluctant toward vaccination due to the needle fear their children had (RI = 0.76; Rank 3; *p*-value < 0.045), and 71.3% disclosed fear of side effects (RI = 0.75; Rank 4; *p*-value < 0.019) as the main factor hindering COVID-19 vaccination. Other concerns that were limiting willingness toward COVID-19 vaccination were parents' perception that the effect of COVID-19 vaccine might last for a short time in children (RI = 0.72; Rank 6; *p*-value < 0.055) and lack of time to bring children for vaccination (RI = 0.64; Rank 7; *p*-value < 0.029). Nearly 74.8% disclosed that they had sufficient family support in case they wanted to get their child vaccinated. Details regarding the barriers and motivators for vaccination are shown in Table 3.

Table 3. Parents' perception about their children's vaccination.

Statement	Strongly Agree	Agree	Disagree	Strongly Disagree	RI	Ranking	*p*-Value
COVID-19 vaccination is effective in protecting your child from COVID-19	250	200	373	155	0.63	8	0.079
Timely vaccination of COVID-19 among children will assist preventing COVID-19 in Saudi Arabia	455	213	193	117	0.76	3	0.007
There is sufficient supply of COVID-19 vaccine and booster dose in Saudi Arabia	508	273	100	97	0.8	2	<0.001
Fear of side effects hinders my decision to vaccinate my child	413	284	155	126	0.75	4	0.019
The protection of COVID-19 vaccines will last for a short time in children	412	250	113	203	0.72	6	0.055
Due to needle fear, I am reluctant to vaccinate my child against COVID-19	303	480	120	75	0.76	3	0.045
You do not have time to take your child for COVID-19 vaccination	213	190	500	75	0.64	7	0.029
Family members would support you in having your child take up COVID-19 vaccination	342	390	100	146	0.74	5	0.029
Having the child receive COVID-19 vaccination is easy for you if you want them to	597	218	70	93	0.84	1	<0.001

No response was recorded for neutral option; relative index ranking was performed, and level of significance was tested using chi-square. *p*-value < 0.005 was considered statistically significant.

4. Discussion

This is perhaps the first Saudi study that has reported vaccine hesitancy among Saudi parents toward COVID-19 vaccination and their willingness to vaccinate their children. One of the main strengths of this study is the large sample size of 978 parents, which has enabled the researcher to explore the severity of the COVID-19 vaccine in an effective manner. The findings of this study revealed that parents were found relying on social media as a main source of information regarding COVID-19 and its vaccination. Overall, the majority of the parents insisted on the need to provide more information regarding the COVID-19 vaccine and its safety in children; this has resulted in reservations among more than 90% of the parents to vaccinate their children against COVID-19. In addition, needle fear and the lack of benefits of COVID-19 vaccination among children were some of the main barriers revealed by this study.

For the effective outcome of any vaccine program, it is essential that all the members of the community receive the required doses so that the required HERD immunity can be attained. In addition, to achieve this vital task, it is important to assess willingness for vaccination in the community [41]. The current study is a similar effort aiming to explore Saudi parents' willingness to vaccinate their children aged 18 years and younger against COVID-19. Unfortunately, the results of this study have shown a significant level of reluctance/hesitancy among Saudi parents to vaccinate their children aged 18 or younger against COVID-19. Parents who participated in this study were found to emphasize their willingness on whether they wanted to vaccinate their child or not. In addition, the majority reported that if they wanted to go ahead with COVID-19 vaccination for their child, they would have sufficient time and family support for this decision.

The vast majority of parents have reservations about vaccinating their offspring. It could be possible that the skepticism of parents regarding processes of vaccine development and approval highlights the need for ongoing transparency and active public education regarding the development and approval process carried out by the United States Food and Drug Administration, the Advisory Committee on Immunization Practices, and the Centers for Disease Control and Prevention (CDC) [42]. It is crucial to underline the safety profile of vaccines for children, which can be derived from both vaccination trials and post-approval data that will definitely assist in achieving the required vaccination rates for the children [43]. In this situation, there is an urgent need to design interventions that are tailored to Saudi parents to address specific concerns on safety, efficacy, development, and after-vaccination benefits so that national indicators for vaccination can be achieved [44]. Specifically, the level of refusal for COVID-19 vaccination among Saudi parents is somewhat lesser in proportion to the studies that have addressed similar research in France, Germany, Italy, Portugal, the Netherlands, and the United States [45–47] and comparable to reports from Denmark and Australia [48].

One of the main concerns that is observed in this study is perhaps the lack of will to vaccinate the children. About 83.3% of the parents shared that they were aware that the vaccine for COVID-19 was sufficiently available in the Kingdom; however, if they were willing to vaccinate their child, then they would definitely consider visiting the health center for COVID-19 vaccination (RI = 0.84; Rank 1; p-value < 0.001). Parents' willingness to vaccinate their children was observed to be the main barrier to COVID-19 vaccination. The results from this study reported a unique parents' perspective, "If I am willing, I will vaccinate my child". Almost 80.0% of the parents were observed to be reluctant about vaccination due to the needle fear in their children (RI = 0.76; Rank 3; p-value < 0.045), and 71.3% disclosed fear of side effects (RI = 0.75; Rank 4; p-value < 0.019) as the main factor hindering COVID-19 vaccination. The majority of people who refused the COVID-19 vaccine cited concerns over vaccine safety, effectiveness, and the benefits of vaccinating children as their justifications [49]. The parents' concerns regarding the safety and risk of any unproven harm to their children are perhaps the main factors that will hinder their willingness to COVID-19 vaccination. Almost similar initial concerns were reported in other parts of the world; however, upon observing the severity of infection among the geriatric population, European parents feared the worst consequences of COVID-19 for children, and perhaps the seriousness of the disease has elevated their trust in the effect of the vaccine, and they were more receptive to COVID-19 vaccine for children [50]. Large-scale public education efforts have been launched to encourage people to get vaccinated; it is possible that these campaigns have influenced people's faith in vaccines [20,51], and similar approaches can be adopted by Saudi health authorities to increase COVID-19 vaccination among children.

In addition, for a newly developed vaccine for COVID-19, similar results of hesitancy were shown by the parents from the US who requested more reliable information, which will definitely increase their confidence in COVID-19 vaccination [38,52,53]. While some participants thought children were less vulnerable to COVID-19, others pointed out that youngsters were more likely to experience long-term negative effects. Parents said that additional proof is needed to validate the vaccine's safety for young patients. Moreover, the lack of multinational clinical trials and the efficacy of the mRNA vaccine [54] are reported to be the other factors hindering COVID-19 vaccination among children. In addition, the majority of the parents disclosed that they were relying on social media as a source of information for COVID-19 vaccination; in this, the COVID-19 vaccine was massively criticized with false accusations. It is essential to investigate how social media influences the perspectives and worries of parents, as well as what they may believe about a new pandemic or health concern in general, in order to determine the various factors that may affect parents' levels of tolerance to new COVID-19 vaccination [55,56]. The elements that influence the willingness of parents to vaccinate their children.

These findings provide information that can serve as a baseline for future vaccination programs, which can help boost immunization rates. In order for public health officials to establish successful immunization strategies to improve vaccine uptake for the purpose of preventing and controlling COVID-19, it will be helpful for them to investigate both the obstacles to vaccination and the factors that facilitate its use [57]. The fact that the participants are active on many anti-vaccination Facebook sites suggests that the participation of individuals in anti-vaccination is more than just a consequence of Facebook's recommended algorithm [58]. Previous studies in the literature that did not utilize social media to investigate reasons for reluctance were consistent with the reasons for hesitancy, which suggests a consistency in hesitancy reasons regardless of whether they are expressed on social media or not [59]. According to the findings of this study, users of social media in different parts of the world exhibited varying levels of good and negative emotions, and these feelings changed over the course of their interactions with the platform. According to the findings of one study, public opinion is dependent not only on the government but also on the company that makes the vaccine [60].

Limitations of This Study

This study has utilized the online data collection method, which is utilized by most of the international studies exploring vaccine hesitancy toward COVID-19 vaccination for urban population [37–40]. In addition, the prime focus of this research was on the Saudi population residing in the urban areas of Saudi Arabia; therefore, it is possible that the level of hesitancy toward COVID-19 vaccination may be higher or lower in comparison to the perspective of the study population reported in this study. Regardless of this limitation, this study manages to represent the barriers and facilitators toward COVID-19 vaccination in a very effective manner and will assist the public health stakeholders in planning respective interventions effectively.

5. Conclusions

For health policy-makers and healthcare professionals organizing vaccination programs, this study gives current information on parents' opinions about immunizing their children. Concerns expressed by respondents about a prospective COVID-19 vaccine serve as crucial targets for potential international educational campaigns, which are the need of the hour to increase rates of vaccination. Saudi parents' main excuse not to vaccinate their children with the COVID-19 vaccine was their self-perceived willingness, followed by the concerns about the safety and potential adverse effects and the perception that their child was not at risk for COVID-19 were the subjects of the respondents' greatest concerns. The parents were heavily influenced by social media. There is an urgent need to educate patients with evidence-based information so that the effect of unreliable information that is available on various social media platforms can be neutralized. Also, as a scientific community, we must take action to communicate, educate, and intervene to enhance COVID-19 vaccination compliance rates across the board. Overall, most parents reported that if they had time to go for COVID-19 vaccination for their children and if they were willing to go for this decision, there would be sufficient family support.

Recommendations

Tourism (Hajj and Umrah) is one of the main sources of revenue generation for Saudi Arabia. In this case, the possibility of any outbreak will affect not only the Saudi economy but also the health of the residents. Moreover, in Saudi Arabia, more than 85.0% of the population resides in rural areas; thus, there is an immediate need for tailored communication campaigns or approaches to assist in improving health literacy among the residents to enhance acceptance of the COVID-19 vaccination.

In addition, there is an immediate need to train healthcare providers as well so that they can act as effective educators and counselors whenever they identify parents or adults who are hesitant toward COVID-19 vaccination. Moreover, having a trained health task force will also assist in neutralizing the disinformation/negative claims that are shared on various social media sites. Vaccine hesitancy has emerged as a global problem. Since the conditions of every person and society are different, it is essential for Saudi stakeholders to identify and measure vaccine acceptance or reluctance as well as access constraints. In order to combat misinformation, effective community participation and communication tactics are required, with coercive measures being employed as a last choice following less restrictive and trust-building initiatives.

Author Contributions: H.M.A. and A.M.A., conceptualization, methodology, software, data curation, validation, formal analysis, investigation, resources, writing, visualization, and funding acquisition; N.M.A. and N.N.A., investigation, resources, writing, visualization, and funding acquisition; M.S.A., investigation, resources, writing, visualization, and funding acquisition; H.A.A., investigation, resources, writing, visualization, and funding acquisition; R.M.A., investigation, resources, writing, visualization, and funding acquisition; S.J.A., investigation, resources, writing, visualization, and funding acquisition; M.K.A., conceptualization, methodology, software, data curation, validation, formal analysis, resources, writing, visualization, supervision, and project administration; M.K.A., conceptualization, methodology, software, data curation, validation, formal analysis, resources, writing, visualization, supervision, and project administration. All authors have read and agreed to the published version of the manuscript.

Funding: This research received no external funding.

Institutional Review Board Statement: This study protocol was approved by King Fahad Medical City under the ethical approval number H-01-R-12 and Federal Wide Assurance number NIH UAS, FWA00018774, 29 May 2023.

Informed Consent Statement: Written (online) informed consent has been obtained from the patient(s) to publish this paper.

Data Availability Statement: Available on request.

Acknowledgments: The authors would like to thank the Research Center at King Fahd Medical City, Riyadh Second Health Cluster, for their valuable technical support provided for the manuscript.

Conflicts of Interest: The authors declare no conflict of interest.

References

1. Micheal, A.; Mobolaji, O.; Olabisi, O.; Ademola, A. Data Analytics and Visualization of COVID-19 Epidemic in Nigeria based on Recovered and Death Cases. *Int. J. Appl. Inf. Syst.* **2020**, *12*, 32.
2. Hamzah, F.B.; Lau, C.; Nazri, H.; Ligot, D.V.; Lee, G.; Tan, C.L.; Shaib, M.; Zaidon, U.H.B.; Abdullah, A.B.; Chung, M.H. CoronaTracker: Worldwide COVID-19 outbreak data analysis and prediction. *Bull. World Health Organ.* **2020**, *1*, 1–32.
3. Stat, G. General Authority of Statistics. Kingdom of Saudi Arabia. *Riyadh Saudi Arab.* **2019**.
4. Algaissi, A.A.; Alharbi, N.K.; Hassanain, M.; Hashem, A.M. Preparedness and response to COVID-19 in Saudi Arabia: Building on MERS experience. *J. Infect. Public Health* **2020**, *13*, 834–838. [CrossRef]
5. Anaam, M.S.; Alsahali, S. Gender Differences in Knowledge, Attitudes, and Practices toward COVID-19 in Saudi Arabia: A Cross-Sectional Study. *Diseases* **2023**, *11*, 63. [CrossRef]
6. Alahdal, H.; Basingab, F.; Alotaibi, R. An analytical study on the awareness, attitude and practice during the COVID-19 pandemic in Riyadh, Saudi Arabia. *J. Infect. Public Health* **2020**, *13*, 1446–1452. [CrossRef]
7. Pilkington, V.; Keestra, S.M.; Hill, A. Global COVID-19 vaccine inequity: Failures in the first year of distribution and potential solutions for the future. *Front. Public Health* **2022**, *10*, 821117. [CrossRef]
8. Pan American Health Organization (PAHO). *Communicating about Vaccine Safety: Guidelines to Help Health Workers Communicate with Parents, Caregivers, and Patients*; Pan American Health Organization (PAHO): Washington, DC, USA, 2020.
9. Klugar, M.; Riad, A.; Mohanan, L.; Pokorná, A. COVID-19 vaccine booster hesitancy (VBH) of healthcare workers in Czechia: National cross-sectional study. *Vaccines* **2021**, *9*, 1437. [CrossRef]
10. Almoosa, Z.; Alhamoud, H.H.; Alkhalaf, A.B.; Alabdullah, W.A.; Alghafli, J.A.; Albensaad, M.S.; Alghazal, Z.Y. Impact of Coronavirus Disease 2019 (COVID-19) pandemic on routine pediatric vaccination in Eastern Region, Saudi Arabia. *Med. Sci.* **2020**, *24*, 4672–4681.
11. Kim, J.H.; Marks, F.; Clemens, J.D. Looking beyond COVID-19 vaccine phase 3 trials. *Nat. Med.* **2021**, *27*, 205–211. [CrossRef]

12. Xiao, X.; Wong, R.M. Vaccine hesitancy and perceived behavioral control: A meta-analysis. *Vaccine* **2020**, *38*, 5131–5138. [CrossRef] [PubMed]
13. Al-Mohaithef, M.; Padhi, B.K. Determinants of COVID-19 vaccine acceptance in Saudi Arabia: A web-based national survey. *J. Multidiscip. Healthc.* **2020**, *13*, 1657–1663. [CrossRef] [PubMed]
14. Al-Qahtani, A.M.; Mannasaheb, B.A.; Shaikh, M.A.K.; Alajlan, S.A.; Alayed, M.S.Z.; Shaikh, I.A.; Asdaq, S.M.B.; Al-Qahtani, F.S.; Ghazwani, E.Y.; Al-Qahtani, N.S. Parental Willingness for COVID-19 Vaccination among Children Aged 5 to 11 Years in Riyadh City, Saudi Arabia: A Cross-Sectional Study. *Vaccines* **2022**, *10*, 1979. [CrossRef]
15. Soares, P.; Rocha, J.V.; Moniz, M.; Gama, A.; Laires, P.A.; Pedro, A.R.; Dias, S.; Leite, A.; Nunes, C. Factors associated with COVID-19 vaccine hesitancy. *Vaccines* **2021**, *9*, 300. [CrossRef]
16. Temsah, M.H.; Alhuzaimi, A.N.; Aljamaan, F.; Bahkali, F.; Al-Eyadhy, A.; Alrabiaah, A.; Alhaboob, A.; Bashiri, F.A.; Alshaer, A.; Temsah, O.; et al. Parental Attitudes and Hesitancy about COVID-19 vs. Routine Childhood Vaccinations: A National Survey. *Front. Public Health* **2021**, *9*, 752323. [CrossRef]
17. Sallam, M. COVID-19 vaccine hesitancy worldwide: A concise systematic review of vaccine acceptance rates. *Vaccines* **2021**, *9*, 160. [CrossRef] [PubMed]
18. Altulaihi, B.A.; Alaboodi, T.; Alharbi, K.G.; Alajmi, M.S.; Alkanhal, H.; Alshehri, A.; Altulaihi, B.; Alshehri, A.Q. Perception of parents towards COVID-19 vaccine for children in Saudi population. *Cureus* **2021**, *13*, 160. [CrossRef]
19. Alfieri, N.L.; Kusma, J.D.; Heard-Garris, N.; Davis, M.M.; Golbeck, E.; Barrera, L.; Macy, M.L. Parental COVID-19 vaccine hesitancy for children: Vulnerability in an urban hotspot. *BMC Public Health* **2021**, *21*, 1–9. [CrossRef]
20. Ruggiero, K.M.; Wong, J.; Sweeney, C.F.; Avola, A.; Auger, A.; Macaluso, M.; Reidy, P. Parents' Intentions to Vaccinate Their Children against COVID-19. *J. Pediatr. Health Care* **2021**, *35*, 509–517. [CrossRef]
21. Alsulaiman, J.W.; Mazin, M.; Al-Shatanawi, T.N.; Kheirallah, K.A.; Allouh, M.Z. Parental willingness to vaccinate their children against SARS-CoV-2 in Jordan: An explanatory cross-sectional study. *Risk Manag. Healthc. Policy* **2022**, *15*, 955–967. [CrossRef]
22. Hobani, F.; Alhalal, E. Factors related to parents' adherence to childhood immunization. *BMC Public Health* **2022**, *22*, 819. [CrossRef] [PubMed]
23. Taylor, S.; Landry, C.A.; Paluszek, M.M.; Groenewoud, R.; Rachor, G.S.; Asmundson, G.J. A proactive approach for managing COVID-19: The importance of understanding the motivational roots of vaccination hesitancy for SARS-CoV-2. *Front. Psychol.* **2020**, *11*, 575950. [CrossRef] [PubMed]
24. Regmi, P.R.; Waithaka, E.; Paudyal, A.; Simkhada, P.; van Teijlingen, E. Guide to the design and application of online questionnaire surveys. *Nepal. J. Epidemiol.* **2016**, *6*, 640–644. [CrossRef] [PubMed]
25. Reynolds, R.A.; Woods, R.; Baker, J.D. *Handbook of Research on Electronic Surveys and Measurements*; Igi Global: Hershey, PA, USA, 2006.
26. Abed, M.G.; Abdulbaqi, R.F.; Shackelford, T.K. Saudi Arabian Students' Beliefs about and Barriers to Online Education during the COVID-19 Pandemic. *Children* **2022**, *9*, 1170. [CrossRef] [PubMed]
27. Abouzid, M.; El-Sherif, D.M.; Eltewacy, N.K.; Dahman, N.B.H.; Okasha, S.A.; Ghozy, S.; Islam, S.M.S. Influence of COVID-19 on lifestyle behaviors in the Middle East and North Africa Region: A survey of 5896 individuals. *J. Transl. Med.* **2021**, *19*, 129. [CrossRef]
28. Abu Alhommos, A.K.; AlSaad, B.A.; AlRamadan, H.S.; AlAlwan, I.A.; Butayban, L.S.; AlHamad, R.A.; AlSalman, Z.A.; El Hassan, E.L.W. Knowledge of COVID-19 and Its Treatment Among Healthcare Worker in Al-Ahsa Region of Saudi Arabia. *J. Multidiscip. Healthc.* **2022**, *15*, 2481–2492. [CrossRef]
29. Aedh, A.I. Parents'Attitudes, Their Acceptance of the COVID-19 Vaccines for Children and the Contributing Factors in Najran, Saudi Arabia: A Cross-Sectional Survey. *Vaccines* **2022**, *10*, 1264. [CrossRef]
30. Diane, W.; Alyson, G.; Mona, M.; Sonya, E.; Sandra, M.; Aneesa, V.L.; Pennifer, E. Principles of Good Practice for the Translation and Cultural Adaptation Process for Patient-Reported Outcomes (PRO) Measures: Report of the ISPOR Task Force for Translation and Cultural Adaptation. *Value Health* **2005**, *8*, 94–104.
31. Hasson, F.; Keeney, S.; McKenna, H. Research guidelines for the Delphi survey technique. *J. Adv. Nurs.* **2000**, *32*, 1008. [CrossRef]
32. McKenna, H.P. The Delphi technique: A worthwhile research approach for nursing? *J. Adv. Nurs.* **1994**, *19*, 1221–1225. [CrossRef]
33. Cronbach, L.J.; Rajaratnam, N.; Gleser, G.C. Theory of generalizability: A liberalization of reliability theory. *Br. J. Stat. Psychol.* **1963**, *16*, 137–163. [CrossRef]
34. Yang, Y.; Green, S.B. Coefficient Alpha: A Reliability Coefficient for the 21st Century? *J. Psychoeduc. Assess.* **2011**, *29*, 377–392. [CrossRef]
35. Thompson, B. *Exploratory and Confirmatory Factor Analysis: Understanding Concepts and Applications*; American Psychological Association: Washington, DC, USA, 2004.
36. Bowling, A. The Principles of Research. In *Research Methods in Health: Investigating and Health Services*, 2nd ed.; Philadelphia University Press: Philadelphia, PA, USA, 2002.
37. Mundagowa, P.T.; Tozivepi, S.N.; Chiyaka, E.T.; Mukora-Mutseyekwa, F.; Makurumidze, R. Assessment of COVID-19 vaccine hesitancy among Zimbabweans: A rapid national survey. *PLoS ONE* **2022**, *17*, e0266724. [CrossRef] [PubMed]
38. Khan, Z.A.; Allana, R.; Afzal, I.; Ali, A.S.; Mariam, O.; Aslam, R.; Shah, I.A.; Allana, A.; Haider, M.M.; Jandani, R.; et al. Assessment of attitude and hesitancy toward vaccine against COVID-19 in a Pakistani population: A mix methods survey. *Vacunas* **2022**, *23*, S26–S32. [CrossRef]

39. Lazarus, J.V.; Wyka, K.; White, T.M.; Picchio, C.A.; Gostin, L.O.; Larson, H.J.; Rabin, K.; Ratzan, S.C.; Kamarulzaman, A.; El-Mohandes, A. A survey of COVID-19 vaccine acceptance across 23 countries in 2022. *Nat. Med.* **2023**, *29*, 366–375. [CrossRef]
40. Chutiyami, M.; Salihu, D.; Bello, U.M.; Winser, S.J.; Gambo, A.A.; Sabo, H.; Kolo, A.M.; Jalo, H.A.; Muhammad, A.S.; Mahmud, F.A.; et al. Are Fear of COVID-19 and Vaccine Hesitancy Associated with COVID-19 Vaccine Uptake? A Population-Based Online Survey in Nigeria. *Vaccines* **2022**, *10*, 1271. [CrossRef]
41. Habersaat, K.B.; Jackson, C. Understanding vaccine acceptance and demand—And ways to increase them. *Bundesgesundheitsblatt Gesundheitsforschung Gesundheitsschutz* **2020**, *63*, 32. [CrossRef]
42. Bell, B.P.; Romero, J.R.; Lee, G.M. Scientific and ethical principles underlying recommendations from the advisory committee on immunization practices for COVID-19 vaccination implementation. *JAMA* **2020**, *324*, 2025–2026. [CrossRef]
43. Shimabukuro, T.T. COVID-19 vaccine safety updates. In Proceedings of the Advisory Committee on Immunization Practices Meeting, Atlanta, GA, USA, 12 May 2021.
44. Jarrett, C.; Wilson, R.; O'Leary, M.; Eckersberger, E.; Larson, H.J. Strategies for addressing vaccine hesitancy—A systematic review. *Vaccine* **2015**, *33*, 4180–4190. [CrossRef]
45. Peretti-Watel, P.; Seror, V.; Cortaredona, S.; Launay, O.; Raude, J.; Verger, P.; Fressard, L.; Beck, F.; Legleye, S.; l'Haridon, O. A future vaccination campaign against COVID-19 at risk of vaccine hesitancy and politicisation. *Lancet Infect. Dis.* **2020**, *20*, 769–770. [CrossRef]
46. Neumann-Böhme, S.; Varghese, N.E.; Sabat, I.; Barros, P.P.; Brouwer, W.; van Exel, J.; Schreyögg, J.; Stargardt, T. *Once We Have it, Will We Use it? A European Survey on Willingness to be Vaccinated against COVID-19*; Springer: Berlin/Heidelberg, Germany, 2020; Volume 21, pp. 977–982.
47. Malik, A.A.; McFadden, S.M.; Elharake, J.A.; Genevieve Aguolu, O.; Shafiq, M.; Omer, S.B. COVID-19 risk perception among US adults: Changes from February to may 2020. *medRxiv* **2020**. [CrossRef]
48. Dodd, R.H.; Cvejic, E.; Bonner, C.; Pickles, K.; McCaffery, K.J.; Ayre, J.; Batcup, C.; Copp, T.; Cornell, S.; Dakin, T. Willingness to vaccinate against COVID-19 in Australia. *Lancet Infect. Dis.* **2021**, *21*, 318–319. [CrossRef] [PubMed]
49. Bell, S.; Clarke, R.; Mounier-Jack, S.; Walker, J.L.; Paterson, P. Parents' and guardians' views on the acceptability of a future COVID-19 vaccine: A multi-methods study in England. *Vaccine* **2020**, *38*, 7789–7798. [CrossRef]
50. Skjefte, M.; Ngirbabul, M.; Akeju, O.; Escudero, D.; Hernandez-Diaz, S.; Wyszynski, D.F.; Wu, J.W. COVID-19 vaccine acceptance among pregnant women and mothers of young children: Results of a survey in 16 countries. *Eur. J. Epidemiol.* **2021**, *36*, 197–211. [CrossRef] [PubMed]
51. Dubé, E.; Gagnon, D.; Vivion, M. Public health network: Optimizing communication material to address vaccine hesitancy. *Can. Commun. Dis. Report.* **2020**, *46*, 48. [CrossRef]
52. Goldman, R.D.; Yan, T.D.; Seiler, M.; Cotanda, C.P.; Brown, J.C.; Klein, E.J.; Hoeffe, J.; Gelernter, R.; Hall, J.E.; Davis, A.L. Caregiver willingness to vaccinate their children against COVID-19: Cross sectional survey. *Vaccine* **2020**, *38*, 7668–7673. [CrossRef] [PubMed]
53. Ruiz, J.B.; Bell, R.A. Parental COVID-19 vaccine hesitancy in the United States. *Public. Health Rep.* **2022**, *137*, 1162–1169. [CrossRef]
54. Carcelen, A.C.; Prosperi, C.; Mutembo, S.; Chongwe, G.; Mwansa, F.D.; Ndubani, P.; Simulundu, E.; Chilumba, I.; Musukwa, G.; Thuma, P. COVID-19 vaccine hesitancy in Zambia: A glimpse at the possible challenges ahead for COVID-19 vaccination rollout in sub-Saharan Africa. *Hum. Vaccines Immunother.* **2022**, *18*, 1–6. [CrossRef]
55. Puri, N.; Coomes, E.A.; Haghbayan, H.; Gunaratne, K. Social media and vaccine hesitancy: New updates for the era of COVID-19 and globalized infectious diseases. *Hum. Vaccines Immunother.* **2020**, *16*, 2586–2593. [CrossRef]
56. Bernard, R.; Bowsher, G.; Sullivan, R.; Gibson-Fall, F. Disinformation and epidemics: Anticipating the next phase of biowarfare. *Health Secur.* **2021**, *19*, 3–12. [CrossRef]
57. Wan, X.; Huang, H.; Shang, J.; Xie, Z.; Jia, R.; Lu, G.; Chen, C. Willingness and influential factors of parents of 3–6-year-old children to vaccinate their children with the COVID-19 vaccine in China. *Hum. Vaccines Immunother.* **2021**, *17*, 3969–3974. [CrossRef] [PubMed]
58. Smith, N.; Graham, T. Mapping the anti-vaccination movement on Facebook. *Inf. Commun. Soc.* **2019**, *22*, 1310–1327. [CrossRef]
59. Cascini, F.; Pantovic, A.; Al-Ajlouni, Y.A.; Failla, G.; Puleo, V.; Melnyk, A.; Lontano, A.; Ricciardi, W. Social media and attitudes towards a COVID-19 vaccination: A systematic review of the literature. *EClinicalMedicine* **2022**, *48*, 101454. [CrossRef] [PubMed]
60. Baumel, N.M.; Spatharakis, J.K.; Baumel, L.D.; Sellas, E.I. Disparity in public perception of Pfizer and Moderna COVID-19 vaccines on TikTok. *J. Adolesc. Health* **2022**, *70*, 514. [CrossRef] [PubMed]

medicina

MDPI

Article

Comparative Analysis of COVID-19 Outcomes in Type 1 and Type 2 Diabetes: A Three-Year Retrospective Study

Flavius Cioca [1], Romulus Timar [2], Flavia Ignuta [1,*], Adrian Vlad [2,3], Felix Bratosin [4], Ovidiu Rosca [4], Adelina Maria Jianu [5], Daniela Rosca [1], Susa Septimiu-Radu [1], Sonia-Roxana Burtic [1,6], Ariadna Petronela Fildan [7] and Sorina Maria Denisa Laitin [8]

1 Doctoral School, "Victor Babes" University of Medicine and Pharmacy, Eftimie Murgu Square 2, 300041 Timisoara, Romania; flaviuscioca@yahoo.com (F.C.); daniela.rosca@umft.ro (D.R.)
2 Department of Internal Medicine II, Division of Diabetes, Nutrition and Metabolic Diseases, "Victor Babes" University of Medicine and Pharmacy, Eftimie Murgu Square 2, 300041 Timisoara, Romania; timar.romulus@umft.ro (R.T.)
3 Centre for Molecular Research in Nephrology and Vascular Disease, Faculty of Medicine, "Victor Babes" University of Medicine and Pharmacy, Eftimie Murgu Square 2, 300041 Timisoara, Romania
4 Department of Infectious Diseases, "Victor Babes" University of Medicine and Pharmacy Timisoara, 300041 Timisoara, Romania; felix.bratosin@umft.ro (F.B.); ovidiu.rosca@umft.ro (O.R.)
5 Department of Anatomy and Embryology, "Victor Babes" University of Medicine and Pharmacy Timisoara, 300041 Timisoara, Romania; adelina.jianu@umft.ro
6 Department II, Discipline of Medical Communication, "Victor Babes" University of Medicine and Pharmacy, Eftimie Murgu Square 2, 300041 Timisoara, Romania
7 Department of Pulmonology, Faculty of Medicine, "Ovidius" University of Constanta, 900470 Constanta, Romania
8 Discipline of Epidemiology, "Victor Babes" University of Medicine and Pharmacy Timisoara, 300041 Timisoara, Romania; laitin.sorina@umft.ro
* Correspondence: flavia.ignuta@umft.ro

Abstract: *Background and Objectives*: This comprehensive retrospective study assesses COVID-19 outcomes in type 1 (T1D) and type 2 diabetes (T2D) patients across three years, focusing on how these outcomes varied with the evolving pandemic and changes in diabetes management. The study aims to determine if COVID-19 outcomes, including severity, intensive care unit (ICU) admission rates, duration of hospitalization, and mortality, are significantly different between these diabetes subtypes. *Materials and Methods*: The study analyzed data from patients admitted to the Victor Babes Hospital for Infectious Diseases and Pulmonology with confirmed COVID-19 and pre-existing diabetes, from the years 2020, 2021, and 2022. *Results*: Among 486 patients (200 without diabetes, 62 with T1D, 224 with T2D), T2D patients showed notably higher severity, with 33.5% experiencing severe cases, compared to 25.8% in T1D. Mortality rates were 11.6% in T2D and 8.1% in T1D. T2D patients had longer hospital stays (11.6 ± 7.0 days) compared to T1D (9.1 ± 5.8 days) and were more likely to require ICU admission (OR: 2.24) and mechanical ventilation (OR: 2.46). Hyperglycemia at admission was significantly higher in the diabetes groups, particularly in T2D (178.3 ± 34.7 mg/dL) compared to T1D (164.8 ± 39.6 mg/dL). *Conclusions*: The study reveals a discernible difference in COVID-19 outcomes between T1D and T2D, with T2D patients having longer hospital admissions, mechanical ventilation necessities, and mortality risks.

Keywords: diabetes mellitus; COVID-19; SARS-CoV-2

1. Introduction

Diabetes mellitus, encompassing both type 1 and type 2 variants, represents a significant global health challenge [1]. As of early 2023, the International Diabetes Federation estimated that approximately 537 million adults (20–79 years) were living with diabetes worldwide, with this number projected to rise to 783 million by 2045 [2]. Concurrently, the

COVID-19 pandemic, caused by the novel coronavirus SARS-CoV-2, emerged as a defining global health crisis [3]. By early 2023, the World Health Organization (WHO) reported over 500 million confirmed cases globally, with a significant mortality burden [4].

Emerging evidence has consistently highlighted diabetes, particularly poorly controlled diabetes, as a risk factor for severe COVID-19 outcomes [5,6]. Studies have shown that individuals with diabetes are more likely to experience severe symptoms, require hospitalization, and face a higher risk of mortality from COVID-19 compared to those without diabetes [7,8]. The pathophysiological mechanisms underlying this increased risk involve a confluence of impaired immune response, chronic inflammation, and potentially direct pancreatic damage by the virus, which aggravates hyperglycemia [9,10].

The two primary forms of diabetes, type 1 (T1D) and type 2 diabetes (T2D), exhibit distinct pathophysiological characteristics that could differentially impact COVID-19 outcomes [11]. Type 1 diabetes, an autoimmune condition, leads to the destruction of insulin-producing beta cells in the pancreas, resulting in insulin deficiency [12,13]. In contrast, type 2 diabetes primarily involves insulin resistance and relative insulin insufficiency [14,15]. These differences suggest potential variations in the clinical progression and outcomes of COVID-19 in patients with these two types of diabetes.

The COVID-19 pandemic has also influenced diabetes management, with disruptions in healthcare services, changes in physical activity patterns, and psychological stress affecting glycemic control in patients with diabetes [16,17]. This evolving context underscores the importance of reassessing the interplay between diabetes types and COVID-19 outcomes as the pandemic progressed.

The increased risk and mortality from COVID-19 in individuals with diabetes are partly due to compromised immune responses, heightened chronic inflammatory states, and the possibility of direct viral damage to pancreatic cells [18]. These factors exacerbate hyperglycemia and contribute to the deterioration of clinical outcomes. The differential pathophysiology of type 1 and type 2 diabetes further influences these outcomes, necessitating a deeper examination of their respective impacts on the severity of COVID-19. Therefore, this study aims to conduct a comprehensive retrospective analysis of COVID-19 outcomes in patients with type 1 and type 2 diabetes over a three-year period (2020–2022). It is hypothesized that COVID-19 outcomes, including severity, intensive care unit (ICU) hospitalization rates, and mortality, differ significantly between patients with type 1 and type 2 diabetes. Additionally, we aim to explore how these outcomes have evolved over the course of the pandemic, considering the changing dynamics of both COVID-19 and diabetes management.

2. Materials and Methods

2.1. Study Design and Participants

This retrospective study evaluated COVID-19 outcomes in patients with type 1 and type 2 diabetes, admitted to the Victor Babes Hospital for Infectious Diseases and Pulmonology from 1 January 2020, to 31 December 2022. Patients aged 18 and above were included, with a pre-existing diagnosis of diabetes (type 1 or type 2 as per American Diabetes Association guidelines) [19], and a confirmed COVID-19 diagnosis, as per the Center for Disease Control criteria [20]. Data were extracted from the database and paper records of the Victor Babes Hospital for Infectious Diseases and Pulmonology tertiary care center.

The study protocol was reviewed and approved by the institutional ethics committee of each participating center. Patient confidentiality was strictly maintained, with data anonymized before analysis. The research strictly followed the ethical guidelines and obtained clearance from the Local Commission of Ethics for Scientific Research, ensuring compliance with the EU GCP Directives 2005/28/EC, ICH guidelines, and the tenets of the Declaration of Helsinki.

2.2. Inclusion and Exclusion Criteria

Inclusion criteria comprised the following: (1)—confirmed diagnosis of type 1 or type 2 diabetes, based on ADA criteria (type 1: evidence of autoimmune beta-cell destruction, type 2: evidence of insulin resistance with relative insulin deficiency); (2)—laboratory-confirmed SARS-CoV-2 infection by reverse transcription polymerase chain reaction (RT-PCR); (3)—age 18 years or older at the time of COVID-19 diagnosis; (4)—patients' consent for analysis of their personal medical records.

Exclusion criteria comprised the following: (1)—gestational diabetes or other forms of diabetes; (2)—patients with evidence of high serum glucose levels but without a clear diagnosis of type 1 or type 2 diabetes; (3)—incomplete medical records or missing key data like HbA1c levels, COVID-19 treatment details, or outcome data; (4)—lack of consent.

2.3. Data Collection and Variables

Data were collected from digital and paper records of the patients, and included demographics such as age, gender, place of origin, diabetes type, duration of diabetes, HbA1c levels and laboratory data (with normal ranges according to our laboratory standards), insulin use, comorbidities (cardiovascular disease, neuropathy, kidney disease), Charlson Comorbidity Index (CCI) [21], COVID-19 severity (mild, moderate, severe/critical as per WHO criteria [22]), hospitalization details, patients on dialysis, ICU admissions, mechanical ventilation, and mortality. COVID-19 severity was defined based on symptoms, oxygen requirements, and chest imaging findings. Patients were matched by age, gender, body mass index (BMI), and CCI.

2.4. Statistics

Data were analyzed using SPSS Version 26. Descriptive statistics summarized baseline characteristics. Chi-square tests were used to compare proportions of categorical variables, while independent *t*-tests or analysis of variance (ANOVA) were employed for comparing continuous variables' means and standard deviations. Spearman's correlation was calculated between the significant study variables. Multivariable logistic regression models identified factors associated with severe COVID-19 outcomes, adjusting for age, gender, BMI, comorbidities, and diabetes duration. Kaplan–Meier curves analyzed time-to-event data, and Cox proportional hazards models evaluated mortality risk.

3. Results

Patients' Background Analysis

The retrospective analysis of 486 COVID-19 patients, comprising 200 without diabetes, 62 with type 1 diabetes mellitus, and 224 with type 2 diabetes mellitus, revealed no significant differences in age, gender, body mass index (BMI), smoking habits, frequent alcohol use, place of origin, COVID-19 vaccination status, and Charlson Comorbidity Index greater than 2. The mean age was comparable across groups (no diabetes: 55.3 years; T1D: 53.6 years; T2D: 56.4 years; $p = 0.281$). The gender distribution showed a majority of men in each group, but without statistical significance ($p = 0.586$). Similarly, the average BMI across groups showed no significant difference ($p = 0.234$).

However, significant differences emerged in COVID-19 severity. A higher proportion of severe cases were observed in the T2D group (33.5%) compared to the T1D (25.8%) and no diabetes groups (15.0%), with a p-value of <0.001. This trend was also reflected in higher rates of ICU admissions and mechanical ventilation in the T2D group (31.7% and 35.3%, respectively) compared to T1D (22.6% and 29.0%) and no diabetes groups (17.0% and 18.0%), indicating a more severe clinical course in T2D patients (ICU admissions $p = 0.002$; mechanical ventilation $p \leq 0.001$). Mortality rates were also notably higher in the T2D group (11.6%) compared to patients with T1D (8.1%) and those without diabetes (3.5%, $p = 0.008$).

Regarding diabetes-related complications, there were no significant differences in the prevalence of cardiovascular disease, neuropathy, kidney disease, and other complications among T1D and T2D patients. However, hyperglycemia at admission was significantly more prevalent in the T2D group (51.8%) compared to the T1D group (32.3%) with a *p*-value of 0.006. Insulin use was universal among T1D patients (100%) and significantly lower in the T2D group (17.0%), with a *p*-value of <0.001. Dialysis use did not differ significantly between the two groups of patients with diabetes ($p = 0.377$), as presented in Table 1.

Table 1. Background characteristics of COVID-19 patients with and without diabetes mellitus.

Variables	No Diabetes (*n* = 200)	T1D (*n* = 62)	T2D (*n* = 224)	*p*-Value	*p*-Value *
Age, years (mean ± SD)	55.3 ± 12.5	53.6 ± 11.7	56.4 ± 13.1	0.281	0.129
Gender, men	118 (59.0%)	35 (56.5%)	121 (54.0%)	0.586	0.733
BMI (mean ± SD)	25.8 ± 4.1	24.7 ± 5.0	26.0 ± 6.3	0.234	0.135
Currently smoking	58 (29.0%)	20 (32.3%)	68 (30.4%)	0.878	0.774
Alcohol use (frequent)	19 (9.5%)	4 (6.5%)	12 (5.4%)	0.249	0.739
Place of origin (urban)	126 (63.0%)	40 (64.5%)	144 (64.3%)	0.955	0.973
COVID-19 vaccinated	52 (26.0%)	20 (32.3%)	68 (30.4%)	0.498	0.774
CCI > 2	46 (23.0%)	17 (27.4%)	56 (25.0%)	0.756	0.698
COVID-19 severity				<0.001	0.498
Mild	99 (49.5%)	22 (35.5%)	68 (30.4%)		
Moderate	71 (35.5%)	24 (38.7%)	81 (36.2%)		
Severe	30 (15.0%)	16 (25.8%)	75 (33.5%)		
Duration of diabetes diagnosis, years (mean ± SD)	-	10.9 ± 4.6	9.6 ± 5.1	-	0.071
Diabetes-related complications					
Cardiovascular disease	-	26 (41.9%)	108 (48.2%)	-	0.380
Neuropathy	-	19 (30.6%)	81 (36.2%)	-	0.420
Kidney disease	-	13 (21.0%)	75 (33.5%)	-	0.058
Others	-	9 (14.5%)	36 (16.1%)	-	0.766
Hyperglycemia at admission	-	20 (32.3%)	116 (51.8%)	-	0.006
Insulin use	-	62 (100%)	38 (17.0%)	-	<0.001
Dialysis users	-	5 (8.1%)	27 (12.1%)	-	0.377
ICU admissions	34 (17.0%)	14 (22.6%)	71 (31.7%)	0.002	0.164
Mechanical ventilation	36 (18.0%)	18 (29.0%)	79 (35.3%)	<0.001	0.358
Mortality	7 (3.5%)	5 (8.1%)	26 (11.6%)	0.008	0.427

*—Comparison between T1D and T2D groups; SD—standard deviation; BMI—body mass index; T1D—type 1 diabetes; T2D—type 2 diabetes; CCI—Charlson Comorbidity Index; ICU—intensive care unit.

Blood glucose levels were significantly higher in the diabetes groups (T1D: 164.8 mg/dL, T2D: 178.3 mg/dL) compared to the no diabetes group (95.1 mg/dL), with a *p*-value of <0.001. HbA1c levels also differed markedly, being within the normal range for the no diabetes group (5.6%) and elevated in the T1D (7.7%) and T2D (8.1%) groups, consistent with their diabetic status ($p < 0.001$).

C-reactive protein levels, indicative of inflammation, were significantly higher in the T1D (27.4 mg/L) and T2D (38.2 mg/L) groups compared to the no diabetes group (15.2 mg/L), suggesting more pronounced inflammatory responses in patients with diabetes ($p < 0.001$). Elevated D-dimer levels, suggestive of coagulation abnormalities, were observed in the diabetes groups (T1D: 2.8 µg/mL, T2D: 2.9 µg/mL) compared to the no diabetes group (1.6 µg/mL, $p < 0.001$).

Oxygen saturation, a key indicator of respiratory function, was lower in T1D (91.7%) and T2D (90.8%) groups compared to the no diabetes group (93.9%), with a statistically significant difference ($p = 0.037$). Creatinine levels, reflecting kidney function, were also significantly higher in patients with diabetes (T1D: 1.2 mg/dL, T2D: 1.3 mg/dL) compared to those without diabetes (0.9 mg/dL, $p < 0.001$). Lymphocyte and white blood cell (WBC) counts, however, did not show significant differences across groups, with lymphocytes and WBC counts being similar, as presented in Table 2.

Table 2. Laboratory findings at admission.

Variables	Normal Range	No Diabetes (n = 200)	T1D (n = 62)	T2D (n = 224)	p-Value	p-Value *
Blood Glucose (mg/dL)	70–99	95.1 ± 15.2	164.8 ± 39.6	178.3 ± 34.7	<0.001	0.009
HbA1c (%)	4.0–5.6	5.6 ± 0.5	7.7 ± 1.1	8.1 ± 1.4	<0.001	0.038
C-Reactive Protein (mg/L)	<5.0	15.2 ± 8.9	27.4 ± 13.8	38.2 ± 14.6	<0.001	<0.001
D-Dimer (μg/mL)	<0.5	1.6 ± 1.2	2.8 ± 1.3	2.9 ± 2.0	<0.001	0.798
Oxygen Saturation (%)	95–100	93.9 ± 10.8	91.7 ± 12.9	90.8 ± 13.7	0.037	0.643
Creatinine (mg/dL)	0.7–1.2	0.9 ± 0.4	1.2 ± 0.6	1.3 ± 0.9	<0.001	0.410
Lymphocyte Count ($\times 10^9$/L)	1.0–3.0	3.4 ± 2.5	3.2 ± 2.6	3.1 ± 2.4	0.455	0.775
WBC Count ($\times 10^9$/L)	4.5–11.0	9.0 ± 6.6	10.5 ± 4.8	10.2 ± 5.0	0.052	0.673

*—Comparison between T1D and T2D groups; T1D—type 1 diabetes; T2D—type 2 diabetes; WBC—white blood cell; HbA1c—Hemoglobin A1c.

The analysis of patient outcomes in our study revealed significant differences in the length of hospital stay and the extent of medical interventions among patients with no diabetes, T1D, and type 2 diabetes mellitus. Notably, the length of hospital stay was significantly longer for T2D patients (11.6 days) compared to T1D (9.1 days) and no diabetes groups (7.2 days), with a significant difference ($p < 0.001$), highlighting the increased healthcare burden in T2D patients.

Regarding treatment, the proportion of patients receiving antiviral treatment and steroids was higher in the diabetes groups, particularly in T2D, but these differences were not statistically significant for antiviral treatments ($p = 0.117$). However, the use of steroids was significantly more prevalent in T2D (74.6%) compared to no diabetes group (60.5%, $p = 0.008$), indicating a more aggressive treatment approach in patients with diabetes, especially those with type 2 diabetes.

The requirement for non-invasive ventilation was significantly higher in the T2D group (53.1%) compared to T1D (45.2%) and no diabetes (31.0%) groups ($p < 0.001$), aligning with the observed trend of increased COVID-19 severity in T2D patients. Finally, the discharge status indicated a lower recovery rate in the T2D group (88.4%) compared to the no diabetes (96.5%) and T1D (91.9%) groups, with a statistically significant difference ($p = 0.008$), suggesting the increased risk and complications associated with COVID-19 in patients with type 2 diabetes, as seen in Table 3.

Table 3. Patient outcomes.

Variables	No Diabetes (n = 200)	T1D (n = 62)	T2D (n = 224)	p-Value	p-Value *
Length of hospital stay (days)	7.2 ± 6.6	9.1 ± 5.8	11.6 ± 7.0	<0.001	0.010
Received antiviral treatment (%)	156 (78.0%)	51 (82.3%)	192 (85.7%)	0.117	0.501
Received steroids (%)	121 (60.5%)	43 (69.4%)	167 (74.6%)	0.008	0.412
Non-invasive ventilation (%)	62 (31.0%)	28 (45.2%)	119 (53.1%)	<0.001	0.266
Discharge status (recovered) (%)	193 (96.5%)	57 (91.9%)	198 (88.4%)	0.008	0.427

*—Comparison between T1D and T2D groups; T1D—type 1 diabetes mellitus; T2D—type 2 diabetes mellitus.

The analysis of COVID-19 outcomes over three years revealed a significant evolution in disease severity, hospitalization length, ICU admissions, and mortality among patients with type 1 and type 2 diabetes mellitus (T1D and T2D). In 2020, both groups had moderate COVID-19 severity, but T2D patients experienced slightly higher rates of severe cases (17.0% vs. 14.5% in T1D) and longer hospital stays (10.8 days for T2D vs. 9.0 days for T1D), alongside higher ICU admissions and mortality rates.

The year 2021 marked a peak in severity, particularly for T2D patients, who exhibited a greater proportion of severe cases (25.0% vs. 20.3% in T1D) and the longest hospital stays (12.4 days for T2D vs. 9.9 days for T1D). ICU admissions and mortality rates were notably higher in T2D during this year, aligning with the observed increase in disease severity.

In 2022, a decline in severe cases was observed, yet T2D patients continued to experience higher severity, longer hospital stays, and elevated ICU admissions and mortality rates compared to T1D patients. These findings highlight the disproportionately higher impact of COVID-19 on T2D patients over the years, with 2021 being the most challenging year, as presented in Table 4.

Table 4. Evolution of COVID-19 outcomes over time.

Year	COVID-19 Severity		Length of Hospital Stay		ICU Admissions		Mortality	
	T1D	T2D	T1D	T2D	T1D	T2D	T1D	T2D
2020	Moderate: 30.6%, Severe: 14.5%	Moderate: 33.9%, Severe: 17.0%	9.0 ± 5.8 *	10.8 ± 6.1 *	11.3%	15.2%	4.0%	5.6%
2021	Moderate: 35.5%, Severe: 20.3%	Moderate: 40.2%, Severe: 25.0%	9.9 ± 6.3 *	12.4 ± 6.9 *	19.4%	26.3%	7.7%	11.2%
2022	Moderate: 32.3%, Severe: 16.1%	Moderate: 36.6%, Severe: 21.9%	7.8 ± 4.9 *	9.6 ± 5.6 *	14.5%	20.5%	6.1%	9.4%

*—Statistically significant differences between T1D and T2D groups; T1D—type 1 diabetes; T2D—type 2 diabetes.

A significant negative correlation was observed between BMI and COVID-19 severity (ρ = −0.473, $p < 0.05$), suggesting that higher BMI was associated with less severe COVID-19 outcomes. This finding could imply a protective aspect of higher BMI against COVID-19 severity, which contradicts typical health assumptions. Similarly, a significant correlation between BMI and the requirement for mechanical ventilation (ρ = 0.439, $p < 0.05$) was found, indicating that higher BMI might be linked to an increased need for mechanical support due to respiratory complications. Hyperglycemia at admission showed a significant negative correlation with COVID-19 severity (ρ = −0.528, $p < 0.05$) and mortality (ρ = −0.414, $p < 0.05$), highlighting the impact of initial glucose levels on disease progression and survival. This finding underscores the importance of glycemic control in patients with diabetes during COVID-19 infection.

ICU admissions were significantly correlated with age (ρ = 0.289, $p < 0.05$) and COVID-19 severity (ρ = 0.603, $p < 0.05$), suggesting that older age and higher disease severity were predictive of ICU admission. This outcome aligns with global observations that severe cases of COVID-19 are more likely to require intensive care, particularly among older populations. Notably, the correlation matrix revealed significant relationships involving diabetes type. Diabetes type showed a positive correlation with hyperglycemia at admission (ρ = 0.327), indicating a higher likelihood of elevated blood glucose levels in patients with diabetes, particularly those with type 2 diabetes, as presented in Table 5 and Figure 1.

Table 5. Correlation matrix of COVID-19 outcomes and characteristics.

Variables	Age	BMI	COVID-19 Severity	Hyperglycemia at Admission	ICU Admissions	Mechanical Ventilation	Mortality	Diabetes Type
Age	1	−0.315	0.124	−0.206	0.289 *	−0.148	0.032	−0.178
BMI	−0.315	1	−0.473 *	0.217	−0.356	0.439 *	−0.112	0.264
COVID-19 Severity	0.124	−0.473 *	1	−0.528 *	0.603 *	−0.287	0.456 *	−0.219
Hyperglycemia at Admission	−0.206	0.217	−0.528 *	1	−0.192	0.348	−0.414 *	0.327
ICU Admissions	0.289 *	−0.356	0.603 *	−0.192	1	−0.311	0.279	−0.243
Mechanical Ventilation	−0.148	0.439 *	−0.287	0.348	−0.311	1	−0.253	0.197
Mortality	0.032	−0.112	0.456 *	−0.414 *	0.279	−0.253	1	−0.287
Diabetes Type	−0.178	0.264	−0.219	0.327	−0.243	0.197	−0.287	1

*—Statistically significant differences; ICU—intensive care unit.

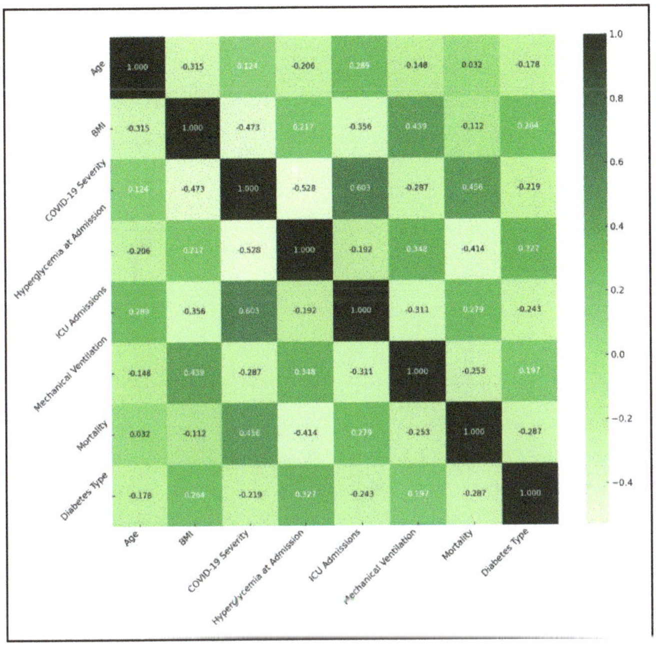

Figure 1. Correlation matrix of COVID-19 outcomes and characteristics.

The ICU admission risk was notably higher in the T2D group at 31.70% compared to 17.00% in the no diabetes group. This significant increase was quantified with an odds ratio (OR) of 2.24, indicating more than double the risk. T2D patients also faced a higher risk of ICU admission than T1D patients (22.60%), with an OR of 1.59, indicating substantially elevated risk of severe COVID-19 complications requiring intensive care among T2D patients.

Similarly, the risk of requiring mechanical ventilation followed a significant trend. For T2D patients, this risk was 35.30%, compared to 18.00% for those with no diabetes. The OR of 2.46 suggested a markedly higher likelihood of needing mechanical respiratory support for T2D patients. The comparison with T1D patients, who had a 29.00% risk, also showed a higher, though less pronounced, risk for T2D individuals.

Mortality rates provided further critical insights. T2D patients exhibited a mortality rate of 11.60%, significantly higher than the 3.50% in the no diabetes cohort. The OR of 3.60 underlined the grave impact of T2D on COVID-19 fatality rates. The mortality rate for T1D patients was also higher than for those without diabetes, but the relative increase was lower compared to T2D patients. The duration of hospitalization further mirrored these trends. T2D patients had an average hospital stay of 11.6 days, longer than the 7.2 days observed in the no diabetes group, with an OR of 1.61, as seen in Figure 2 and Table 6.

In the analysis, patients with no diabetes (represented by the light green curve) exhibit the highest survival probability over the observed period. This group's curve descends most gradually, indicating a lower rate of mortality compared to the diabetes groups. The survival probability for this group remains relatively high throughout the time frame, affirming the less severe impact of COVID-19 on patients without diabetes.

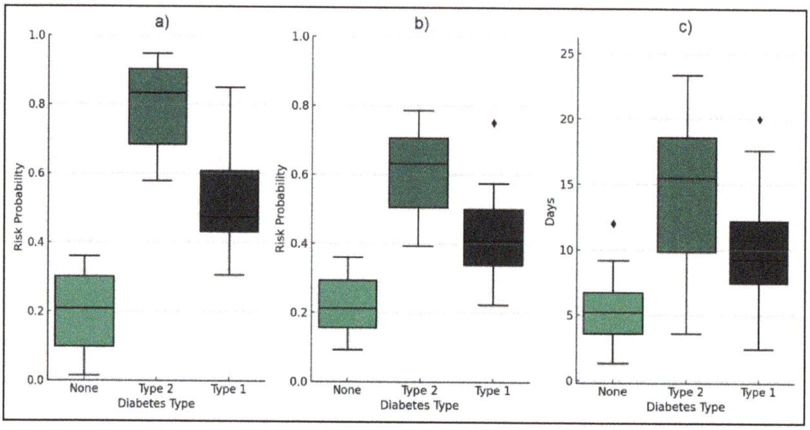

Figure 2. Comparative analysis of COVID-19 clinical outcomes across diabetes and no diabetes groups; (**a**)—ICU admission risk; (**b**)—mechanical ventilation risk; (**c**)—hospitalization duration.

Table 6. COVID-19 outcomes by diabetes status.

Variables	No Diabetes (n = 200)	T1D (n = 62)	T2D (n = 224)	OR (T2D vs. None) (95% CI)	OR (T2D vs. T1D) (95% CI)
ICU admission risk	17.00%	22.60%	31.70%	2.24 (1.40–3.57) *	1.59 (1.09–2.83) *
Mechanical Ventilation Risk	18.00%	29.00%	35.30%	2.46 (1.55–3.90) *	1.37 (0.81–2.30)
Mortality	3.50%	8.10%	11.60%	3.60 (1.08–8.20) *	1.48 (0.58–3.76)
Hospitalization Duration (Days)	7.2 ± 6.6	9.1 ± 5.8	11.6 ± 7.0	1.61 (1.25–2.08) *	1.28 (1.07–1.68) *

*—Statistically significant differences (p-value < 0.05); T1D—type 1 diabetes; T2D—type 2 diabetes; ICU—intensive care unit; odds ratios (OR) with 95% confidence intervals (CI) compare type 1 and type 2 diabetes to the control group (no diabetes). The logistic regression model was controlled for age, gender, BMI, and comorbidities. Model fit statistics: Hosmer–Lemeshow test p = 0.320, indicating a good fit.

Patients with type 1 diabetes, denoted by the medium sea green curve, show a moderately decreased survival probability compared to the no diabetes group. The curve for T1D descends at a faster rate than that of the no diabetes group, but not as rapidly as the type 2 diabetes group. The log-rank test between T1D and no diabetes yields a p-value of 0.068, which is marginally above the typical threshold for statistical significance, suggesting a trend towards but not definitively indicating higher mortality in the T1D group compared to those without diabetes.

The most notable observation comes from the survival curve for patients with T2D, depicted in dark green. This curve shows a significantly steeper decline, especially in the initial phase, reflecting a higher mortality rate. The rapid descent of the T2D curve underscores the severe impact of type 2 diabetes on COVID-19 outcomes. The log-rank p-values corroborate this observation, with a highly significant difference (p < 0.001) in survival when compared to the no diabetes group, and a significant difference (p = 0.033) when compared to the T1D group, as seen in Figure 3. These results indicate that T2D is a significant risk factor for poorer outcomes in COVID-19 patients.

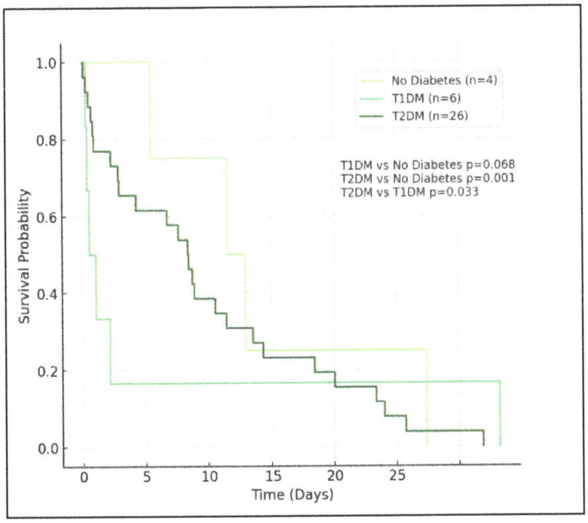

Figure 3. Kaplan–Meier survival analysis curves.

4. Discussion

The current study observed distinct patterns in COVID-19 severity and outcomes between patients with type 1 and type 2 diabetes mellitus, findings that are critical in understanding the impact of the pandemic on diabetic populations and aligns with emerging global data indicating an increased diabetes risk post-COVID-19 infection. There was a higher rate of severe COVID-19 cases in T2D patients (33.5%) compared to T1D (25.8%). This disparity is reflected in the hospitalization duration, which was longer for T2D (11.6 days) than T1D (9.1 days). These results are consistent with the observed global trend where COVID-19 has been associated with a 66% higher risk of death in patients with diabetes, underscoring the severity of the disease in patients with diabetes [23,24].

Our study also revealed more elevated blood glucose levels at admission in T2D (178.3 mg/dL) compared to T1D (164.8 mg/dL), highlighting the distinct pathophysiological mechanisms of these diabetes types, indicating that SARS-CoV-2 can exacerbate glucose metabolism disorders, as patients without diabetes had a serum glucose level of 95.1 mg/dL. The modest increase in diabetes risk due to COVID-19, as evidenced in our study and global data, suggests an impending rise in global diabetes diagnoses, calling for vigilant monitoring of glucose dysregulation in COVID-19 patients and survivors, especially in countries with high diabetes prevalence [25,26]. The pronounced hyperglycemia observed during stress and infection, a common response in individuals, is notably more severe in patients with type 2 diabetes, as reflected by elevated HbA1c levels. This indicates that these patients often experience poorly controlled diabetes, exacerbating their body's response to stress and infection.

In our study, T2D patients showed a higher mortality rate (11.6%) compared to T1D (8.1%), and significantly higher than patients with no diabetes (3.5%), which may be indicative of the generally more severe clinical presentation and comorbidities associated with T2D. This aligns with a systematic review that found no significant differences in disease severity but a potentially lower mortality rate in T1D COVID-19 patients [27]. Thus, our study contributes to the limited information on how COVID-19 affects T1D patients. The prevalence of T1D in our COVID-19 cohort was 31% compared to global reports ranging from 0.15% to 28.98%, illustrating the diverse clinical presentations and outcomes in this patient population [28].

In a study covering the initial three waves of the COVID-19 pandemic, researchers observed a significantly higher likelihood of severe COVID-19 outcomes, including hospitalization, intensive care unit admission, and mortality, in individuals with type 2 diabetes, which corroborates our findings that compared three consecutive years of the pandemic [28]. Notably, younger individuals with type 2 diabetes exhibited disproportionately higher odds for these severe outcomes compared to their older counterparts and the general non-diabetic population. For those with type 1 diabetes, the study found a moderate increase in hospitalization rates due to COVID-19, but no significant rise in ICU admissions or mortality was observed. Moreover, the authors emphasized the influence of age and socioeconomic factors in predicting severe COVID-19 outcomes across both types of diabetes.

There was also an elevated risk for severe COVID-19 in individuals under 55 with T2D, probably attributed to fewer competing risks in this younger demographic. The study also shed light on the delicate balance needed in managing type 2 diabetes during the pandemic, especially considering the negative impacts of reduced mobility and the significant role of obesity in worsening COVID-19 outcomes. The findings also underscored the relevance of hypertension and renal disease in the context of SARS-CoV-2 infections [16,29]. In our study the observed negative correlation between BMI and COVID-19 severity appears counterintuitive, given the established health risks associated with higher BMI. However, it echoes emerging evidence suggesting a protective role of higher BMI in the context of COVID-19, also known as the "obesity paradox" phenomenon [30]. One hypothesis for this phenomenon could be that patients with higher BMI receive respiratory support earlier in the course of infection, which may prevent the escalation of severity.

In the context of diabetes management, maintaining controlled glucose levels and avoiding hyperglycemia are crucial for reducing severe COVID-19 risks [31]. Diabetes can lead to inflammatory responses, hypercoagulation, and severe pneumonia, exacerbated by elevated D-dimer and fibrinogen levels. While 2020 data indicated increased risks of ICU care and death post-COVID-19 infection in patients with type 1 diabetes, the current study did not find a significant excess risk of ICU care or death in this group, but mostly in the T2D group [32]. This finding is consistent with other research, despite a longer observation period allowing for more outcomes. Interestingly, the majority of deaths in T1D patients were among those older than 75 years, and after adjusting for comorbidities, there was no increase in odds. This suggests that younger and middle-aged individuals with uncomplicated type 1 diabetes may not face increased risks of severe COVID-19 outcomes compared to their non-diabetic peers [33].

The lesser severity of COVID-19 observed in patients with type 1 diabetes compared to those with type 2 may be partially attributed to the general blood sugar control maintained by insulin therapy. Individuals with T1D often have regimented treatment protocols, including insulin administration, that could result in a more stable glycemic state prior to COVID-19 infection [34]. This contrasts with the varied management effectiveness in T2D, where insulin resistance and other metabolic complications might predispose individuals to worse outcomes when infected. Therefore, the disciplined glycemic control inherent to type 1 diabetes management might confer a relative protective advantage against the severity of COVID-19.

Regarding hospitalization rates, another study found a significant independent increase in the odds of hospitalization for COVID-19 in patients with type 1 diabetes, as opposed to ICU care and death, which was significantly higher in T2D patients, and similar to our study's findings [35]. This could be attributed to a higher propensity for admitting these patients due to perceived risks. Despite potential reductions in physical hospital visits, there is evidence indicating that glycemic control in T1D patients might not have been significantly affected by the pandemic [36]. The observed low odds of hospitalization and death could also be due to precautionary measures taken by these patients, such as working from home; however, tendencies of increased ICU care and death were observed in the overall analyses.

The elevated white blood cell count in patients with type 2 diabetes, despite a typically suppressed immune response, may reflect a complex interplay of factors during COVID-19 infection. The heightened WBC count could indicate an acute inflammatory response triggered by the virus, countering the expected immunosuppressive state of T2D. While lymphocyte counts remain similar across groups, the increased WBC count in T2D patients could signify a compensatory mechanism or an atypical immune response to infection, as a previous study indicated that WBCs are more significant among patients with diabetes [37].

In our study, several limitations should be acknowledged, such as the retrospective nature of the study at the Victor Babes Hospital for Infectious Diseases and Pulmonology, which inherently limits our ability to establish causal relationships. Secondly, our patient cohort, comprising 486 individuals, may not fully represent the broader population, particularly given the specific healthcare setting and regional demographics. Thirdly, the reliance on existing medical records might have introduced biases related to documentation accuracy and completeness. Furthermore, the exclusion of patients with incomplete records or those lacking consent could have led to selection bias. Finally, the study's findings may not be generalizable beyond the context of the Romanian healthcare system and the specific period of the COVID-19 pandemic studied.

5. Conclusions

Conclusions: This extensive retrospective study provides critical insights into the differential impacts of COVID-19 on patients with type 1 and type 2 diabetes mellitus. Analyzing data from the Victor Babes Hospital for Infectious Diseases and Pulmonology over three years, the study identifies that T2DM patients faced notably harsher outcomes from COVID-19. These individuals experienced higher rates of severe cases, increased mortality, and a greater likelihood of requiring intensive care and mechanical ventilation compared to their T1D counterparts. Additionally, T2D patients had longer hospital stays and presented with higher levels of hyperglycemia upon admission. These findings underscore the importance of targeted strategies in managing T2D patients with COVID-19, considering their elevated risk profile. The study highlights the evolving nature of the pandemic's impact on different diabetic subtypes, emphasizing the need for continuous monitoring and tailored healthcare approaches for patients with diabetes.

Author Contributions: Conceptualization, F.C., A.V. and R.T.; methodology, F.C., S.-R.B. and R.T.; software, F.I., S.S.-R. and F.B.; validation, F.I. and F.B.; formal analysis, O.R., A.V. and S.S.-R.; investigation, O.R., A.V. and S.S.-R.; resources, A.M.J., S.-R.B. and A.P.F.; data curation, A.M.J. and S.-R.B.; writing—original draft preparation, F.C. and F.I.; writing—review and editing, D.R. and A.P.F.; visualization, S.M.D.L. and D.R.; project administration, S.M.D.L. and R.T.; supervision, S.M.D.L. and R.T. All authors have read and agreed to the published version of the manuscript.

Funding: This research received no external funding.

Institutional Review Board Statement: The Local Commission of Ethics for Scientific Research from the Timis County Emergency Clinical Hospital "Pius Brinzeu" from Timisoara, Romania, operates under article 167 provisions of Law no. 95/2006, art. 28, chapter VIII of order 904/2006; with EU GCP Directives 2005/28/EC, International Conference of Harmonisation of Technical Requirements for Registration of Pharmaceuticals for Human Use (ICH); and with the Declaration of Helsinki—Recommendations Guiding Medical Doctors in Biomedical Research Involving Human Subjects (approved on 28 February 2022, with the approval number 05).

Informed Consent Statement: Informed consent was obtained from all subjects involved in the study.

Data Availability Statement: The data presented in this study are available on request from the corresponding author.

Conflicts of Interest: The authors declare no conflicts of interest.

References

1. Kharroubi, A.T.; Darwish, H.M. Diabetes mellitus: The epidemic of the century. *World J. Diabetes* **2015**, *6*, 850–867. [CrossRef]
2. Magliano, D.J.; Boyko, E.J. IDF Diabetes Atlas 10th Edition Scientific Committee. In *IDF Diabetes Atlas [Internet]*, 10th ed.; International Diabetes Federation: Brussels, Belgium, 2021. Available online: https://www.ncbi.nlm.nih.gov/books/NBK581934/ (accessed on 25 October 2023).

3. Allan, M.; Lièvre, M.; Laurenson-Schaefer, H.; de Barros, S.; Jinnai, Y.; Andrews, S.; Stricker, T.; Formigo, J.P.; Schultz, C.; Perrocheau, A.; et al. The World Health Organization COVID-19 surveillance database. *Int. J. Equity Health* **2023**, *22* (Suppl. S3), 95, Erratum in *Int. J. Equity Health* **2023**, *22*, 95. [CrossRef]
4. Nguyen, N.T.H.; Ou, T.-Y.; Huy, L.D.; Shih, C.-L.; Chang, Y.-M.; Phan, T.-P.; Huang, C.-C. A global analysis of COVID-19 infection fatality rate and its associated factors during the Delta and Omicron variant periods: An ecological study. *Front. Public Health* **2023**, *11*, 1145138. [CrossRef] [PubMed]
5. Seiglie, J.; Platt, J.; Cromer, S.J.; Bunda, B.; Foulkes, A.S.; Bassett, I.V.; Hsu, J.; Meigs, J.B.; Leong, A.; Putman, M.S.; et al. Diabetes as a Risk Factor for Poor Early Outcomes in Patients Hospitalized With COVID-19. *Diabetes Care* **2020**, *43*, 2938–2944. [CrossRef] [PubMed]
6. Pelle, M.C.; Zaffina, I.; Provenzano, M.; Moirano, G.; Arturi, F. COVID-19 and diabetes—Two giants colliding: From pathophysiology to management. *Front. Endocrinol.* **2022**, *13*, 974540. [CrossRef]
7. Mantovani, A.; Byrne, C.D.; Zheng, M.-H.; Targher, G. Diabetes as a risk factor for greater COVID-19 severity and in-hospital death: A meta-analysis of observational studies. *Nutr. Metab. Cardiovasc. Dis.* **2020**, *30*, 1236–1248. [CrossRef]
8. Khunti, K.; Valabhji, J.; Misra, S. Diabetes and the COVID-19 pandemic. *Diabetologia* **2023**, *66*, 255–266. [CrossRef]
9. Zaccardi, F.; Webb, D.R.; Yates, T.; Davies, M.J. Pathophysiology of type 1 and type 2 diabetes mellitus: A 90-year perspective. *Postgrad. Med. J.* **2016**, *92*, 63–69. [CrossRef] [PubMed]
10. Narasimhulu, C.A.; Singla, D.K. Mechanisms of COVID-19 pathogenesis in diabetes. *Am. J. Physiol. Heart Circ. Physiol.* **2022**, *323*, H403–H420. [CrossRef]
11. Bedoya, J.P.P.; Muñoz, A.M.; Barengo, N.C.; Valencia, P.A.D. Type 1 and type 2 diabetes mellitus: Clinical outcomes due to COVID-19. Protocol of a systematic literature review. *PLoS ONE* **2022**, *17*, e0271851. [CrossRef]
12. Simmons, K.M. Type 1 diabetes: A predictable disease. *World J. Diabetes* **2015**, *6*, 380–390. [CrossRef] [PubMed]
13. Toren, E.; Burnette, K.S.; Banerjee, R.R.; Hunter, C.S.; Tse, H.M. Partners in Crime: Beta-Cells and Autoimmune Responses Complicit in Type 1 Diabetes Pathogenesis. *Front. Immunol.* **2021**, *12*, 756548. [CrossRef] [PubMed]
14. Wondmkun, Y.T. Obesity, Insulin Resistance, and Type 2 Diabetes: Associations and Therapeutic Implications. *Diabetes Metab. Syndr. Obes.* **2020**, *13*, 3611–3616. [CrossRef] [PubMed]
15. Olokoba, A.B.; Obateru, O.A.; Olokoba, L.B. Type 2 diabetes mellitus: A review of current trends. *Oman Med. J.* **2012**, *27*, 269–273. [CrossRef] [PubMed]
16. Sutkowska, E.; Marciniak, D.M.; Sutkowska, K.; Biernat, K.; Mazurek, J.; Kuciel, N. The impact of lockdown caused by the COVID-19 pandemic on glycemic control in patients with diabetes. *Endocrine* **2022**, *76*, 273–281. [CrossRef] [PubMed]
17. Khunti, K.; Aroda, V.R.; Aschner, P.; Chan, J.C.N.; Del Prato, S.; Hambling, C.E.; Harris, S.; Lamptey, R.; McKee, M.; Tandon, N.; et al. The impact of the COVID-19 pandemic on diabetes services: Planning for a global recovery. *Lancet Diabetes Endocrinol.* **2022**, *10*, 890–900. [CrossRef] [PubMed]
18. Lim, S.; Bae, J.H.; Kwon, H.-S.; Nauck, M.A. COVID-19 and diabetes mellitus: From pathophysiology to clinical management. *Nat. Rev. Endocrinol.* **2021**, *17*, 11–30. [CrossRef]
19. American Diabetes Association. Standards of Medical Care in Diabetes—2021 Abridged for Primary Care Providers. *Clin. Diabetes* **2021**, *39*, 14–43. [CrossRef]
20. Cascella, M.; Rajnik, M.; Aleem, A.; Dulebohn, S.C.; Di Napoli, R. Features, Evaluation, and Treatment of Coronavirus (COVID-19) [Updated 2023 Aug 18]. In *StatPearls [Internet]*; StatPearls Publishing: Treasure Island, FL, USA, 2023. Available online: https://www.ncbi.nlm.nih.gov/books/NBK554776/ (accessed on 25 October 2023).
21. Charlson, M.E.; Carrozzino, D.; Guidi, J.; Patierno, C. Charlson Comorbidity Index: A Critical Review of Clinimetric Properties. *Psychother. Psychosom.* **2022**, *91*, 8–35. [CrossRef]
22. Zayed, N.E.; Abbas, A.; Lutfy, S.M. Criteria and potential predictors of severity in patients with COVID-19. *Egypt. J. Bronchol.* **2022**, *16*, 11. [CrossRef]
23. Ssentongo, P.; Zhang, Y.; Witmer, L.; Chinchilli, V.M.; Ba, D.M. Association of COVID-19 with diabetes: A systematic review and meta-analysis. *Sci. Rep.* **2022**, *12*, 20191. [CrossRef] [PubMed]
24. Tabrizi, F.M.; Rasmi, Y.; Hosseinzadeh, E.; Rezaei, S.; Balvardi, M.; Kouchari, M.R.; Ebrahimi, G. Diabetes is associated with increased mortality and disease severity in hospitalized patients with COVID-19. *EXCLI J.* **2021**, *20*, 444–453. [CrossRef]
25. Barbosa, M.; Marques-Sá, J.; Carvalho, C.; Fernandes, V. Is elevated blood glucose at admission associated with poor outcomes in hospitalized COVID-19 patients? *Arch. Endocrinol. Metab.* **2023**, *67*, e000649. [CrossRef]
26. Beshbishy, A.M.; Oti, V.B.; Hussein, D.E.; Rehan, I.F.; Adeyemi, O.S.; Rivero-Perez, N.; Zaragoza-Bastida, A.; Shah, M.A.; Abouelezz, K.; Hetta, H.F.; et al. Factors Behind the Higher COVID-19 Risk in Diabetes: A Critical Review. *Front. Public Health* **2021**, *9*, 591982. [CrossRef]
27. Shafiee, A.; Athar, M.M.T.; Nassar, M.; Seighali, N.; Aminzade, D.; Fattahi, P.; Rahmannia, M.; Ahmadi, Z. Comparison of COVID-19 outcomes in patients with Type 1 and Type 2 diabetes: A systematic review and meta-analysis. *Diabetes Metab. Syndr. Clin. Res. Rev.* **2022**, *16*, 102512. [CrossRef] [PubMed]
28. Edqvist, J.; Lundberg, C.; Andreasson, K.; Björck, L.; Dikaiou, P.; Ludvigsson, J.; Lind, M.; Adiels, M.; Rosengren, A. Severe COVID-19 Infection in Type 1 and Type 2 Diabetes During the First Three Waves in Sweden. *Diabetes Care* **2023**, *46*, 570–578. [CrossRef] [PubMed]

29. Elith, J.; Leathwick, J.R.; Hastie, T. A working guide to boosted regression trees. *J. Anim. Ecol.* **2008**, *77*, 802–813. [CrossRef] [PubMed]
30. Jennings, M.; Burova, M.; Hamilton, L.G.; Hunter, E.; Morden, C.; Pandya, D.; Beecham, R.; Moyses, H.; Saeed, K.; Afolabi, P.R.; et al. Body mass index and clinical outcome of severe COVID-19 patients with acute hypoxic respiratory failure: Unravelling the "obesity paradox" phenomenon. *Clin. Nutr. ESPEN* **2022**, *51*, 377–384. [CrossRef] [PubMed]
31. Holman, N.; Knighton, P.; Kar, P.; O'Keefe, J.; Curley, M.; Weaver, A.; Barron, E.; Bakhai, C.; Khunti, K.; Wareham, N.J.; et al. Risk factors for COVID-19-related mortality in people with type 1 and type 2 diabetes in England: A population-based cohort study. *Lancet Diabetes Endocrinol.* **2020**, *8*, 823–833. [CrossRef] [PubMed]
32. McGurnaghan, S.J.; Weir, A.; Bishop, J.; Kennedy, S.; Blackbourn, L.A.K.; McAllister, D.A.; Hutchinson, S.; Caparrotta, T.M.; Mellor, J.; Jeyam, A.; et al. Risks of and risk factors for COVID-19 disease in people with diabetes: A cohort study of the total population of Scotland. *Lancet Diabetes Endocrinol.* **2021**, *9*, 82–93. [CrossRef] [PubMed]
33. Demeterco-Berggren, C.; Ebekozien, O.; Rompicherla, S.; Jacobsen, L.; Accacha, S.; Gallagher, M.P.; Alonso, G.T.; Seyoum, B.; Vendrame, F.; Haw, J.S.; et al. Age and Hospitalization Risk in People With Type 1 Diabetes and COVID-19: Data From the T1D Exchange Surveillance Study. *J. Clin. Endocrinol. Metab.* **2022**, *107*, 410–418. [CrossRef]
34. Hamilton, K.; Stanton-Fay, S.H.; Chadwick, P.M.; Lorencatto, F.; de Zoysa, N.; Gianfrancesco, C.; Taylor, C.; Coates, E.; Breckenridge, J.P.; Cooke, D.; et al. Sustained type 1 diabetes self-management: Specifying the behaviours involved and their influences. *Diabet. Med.* **2021**, *38*, e14430. [CrossRef]
35. Sen, S.; Chakraborty, R.; Kalita, P.; Pathak, M.P. Diabetes mellitus and COVID-19: Understanding the association in light of current evidence. *World J. Clin. Cases* **2021**, *9*, 8327–8339. [CrossRef] [PubMed]
36. Patel, S.Y.; McCoy, R.G.; Barnett, M.L.; Shah, N.D.; Mehrotra, A. Diabetes Care and Glycemic Control During the COVID-19 Pandemic in the United States. *JAMA Intern. Med.* **2021**, *181*, 1412–1414. [CrossRef] [PubMed]
37. Atwah, B.; Iqbal, M.S.; Kabrah, S.; Kabrah, A.; Alghamdi, S.; Tabassum, A.; Baghdadi, M.A.; Alzahrani, H. Susceptibility of Diabetic Patients to COVID-19 Infections: Clinico-Hematological and Complications Analysis. *Vaccines* **2023**, *11*, 561. [CrossRef] [PubMed]

medicina

MDPI

Article

Oropharyngeal Manifestations in Patients with HIV from Northeastern Romania

Amelia Elena Surdu [1], Isabela Ioana Loghin [2,3,*], Victor Daniel Dorobăţ [4], Vlad Hârtie [5], Şerban Alin Rusu [3], Ion Cecan [3], Amelia Andreea Mihăescu [3], Otilia Eva [3,6] and Carmen Mihaela Dorobăţ [3]

1 Department of Implantology, Removable Prostheses and Technology, Faculty of Dental Medicine, "Grigore T. Popa" University of Medicine and Pharmacy, 700115 Iasi, Romania; amelia.surdu@dentesse.ro

2 Department of Infectious Diseases, Faculty of Medicine, "Grigore T. Popa" University of Medicine and Pharmacy, 700115 Iasi, Romania

3 Department of Infectious Diseases, "St. Parascheva" Clinical Hospital of Infectious Diseases, 700116 Iasi, Romania; rususerbanalin@yahoo.com (Ş.A.R.); ion11cecan@gmail.com (I.C.); ameliamihaescu@gmail.com (A.A.M.); evaotilia@yahoomail.com (O.E.); carmendorobat@yahoo.com (C.M.D.)

4 Department of Intensive Care, University Hospital of Emergency, 050098 Bucharest, Romania; victordorobat@yahoo.com

5 Department of Intensive Care, Clinical Hospital of Emergency "Prof. Dr. Nicolae Oblu", 700309 Iasi, Romania; vladhartie@yahoo.com

6 Department of Otolaryngology, Faculty of Medicine, Apollonia University, 700511 Iasi, Romania

* Correspondence: isabelabegezsan@yahoo.com

Abstract: *Backgrounds and objective*: Disorders in the stomatognathic system and otorhinolaryngologic manifestations are frequently observed in individuals living with HIV. Ear, neck, and throat (ENT) signs and symptoms often serve as critical markers of treatment failure, particularly in the advanced stages of HIV infection. This article aims to evaluate and consolidate recent developments in the treatment and management of otorhinolaryngological manifestations in HIV-positive patients. *Materials and methods*: We carried out a retrospective clinical investigation of patients admitted with HIV/AIDS in the northeastern region of Romania, hospitalized in the "St. Parascheva" Clinical Hospital of Infectious Diseases in Iasi. We followed the viro-immunological status correlated with patients' otolaryngology and dental symptomatology, aiming to emphasize the comorbidities of HIV/AIDS cases. The study period spanned from 1 January 2020 to 30 November 2024. *Results*: There were a total of 552 recorded cases of oropharyngeal manifestations in patients with HIV. They were more frequent in men (358 cases, 64.85%) than women (194 cases, 35.15%). The majority of cases were young adults, aged 30 to 39 years, comprising 255 patients (46.19%), and most cases (36.85%) had CD4+ T-lymphocyte values between 200 and 499 cells/μL. The most frequent diagnosis was oral candidiasis, recorded in 335 male and 174 female cases (509, 92.21% total). Other notable conditions included gingivitis/periodontitis, sinusitis/rhinosinusitis, mastoiditis, and dental abscesses, albeit at lower frequencies. Notably, antifungal therapy with fluconazole was the most frequently employed treatment, followed by aminopenicillins and fluoroquinolones. With respect to the antiretroviral treatment, 83.69% of cases were prescribed a single-pill regimen. *Conclusions*: The key to the management of HIV-positive patients is a multidisciplinary approach, including an ENT specialist and access to antiretroviral therapy.

Keywords: stomatognathic system; ENT manifestations; dental diagnosis; HIV infection; oral disease

1. Introduction

Human immunodeficiency virus (HIV) and acquired immunodeficiency syndrome (AIDS) have emerged as a global pandemic, affecting approximately 40 million individuals worldwide. This widespread health crisis underscores the critical need for effective prevention, diagnosis, and treatment strategies to mitigate its impact on public health and reduce the global disease burden [1].

Human immunodeficiency virus (HIV) is a persistent viral infection that progressively undermines the immune system by selectively infecting and depleting CD4+ T-lymphocytes, which are crucial in orchestrating immune responses. If left untreated, HIV can advance to acquired immunodeficiency syndrome (AIDS), a stage marked by profound immunosuppression and increased susceptibility to opportunistic infections and various malignancies. HIV primarily disseminates to lymphoid tissues through the bloodstream after crossing mucosal barriers. The progression from HIV to AIDS is typically characterized by a significant decline in the CD4+ T cell count, accompanied by the emergence of clinical conditions that are rare in individuals with intact immune systems [1–3].

According to the World Health Organization (WHO), HIV remains a major global health concern, ranking as the ninth leading cause of mortality in low-income countries and the sixth leading cause of death among communicable diseases. Despite its significant burden, there has been substantial progress in reducing HIV-related mortality. Between 2000 and 2019, HIV-related deaths decreased by 59%, reflecting advancements in prevention, diagnosis, and treatment. Furthermore, scaling up the AIDS response in low- and middle-income countries could prevent an estimated 28 million new HIV infections and 21 million AIDS-related deaths between 2015 and 2030, underscoring the critical need for sustained efforts to combat the epidemic [4].

Since the introduction of antiretroviral therapy (ART), the prognosis for individuals living with HIV has significantly improved, transforming the condition from a fatal illness into a manageable chronic disease for many. ART effectively suppresses viral replication and prevents the progression of AIDS. However, despite advancements in viral control, HIV-positive individuals remain at an elevated risk for various non-AIDS-defining conditions, such as cardiovascular diseases, neurocognitive impairments, and malignancies. This continued risk is attributed to persistent immune activation and chronic inflammation, which are hallmarks of HIV infection even in individuals with well-controlled viral loads [5].

Disorders in the stomatognathic system and otorhinolaryngologic manifestations are frequently observed in individuals living with HIV. A thorough understanding of the disease's progression is crucial for accurate diagnosis and effective management. Ear, neck, and throat (ENT) signs and symptoms often serve as critical markers of treatment failure, particularly in the advanced stages of HIV infection [6].

Oropharyngeal manifestations, as part of opportunistic infections, are well recognized in individuals living with HIV and play a significant role in the clinical staging of the disease. These manifestations, which include infections of the oral cavity, sinuses, throat, and ears, are indicative of immune system deterioration and are commonly observed as HIV progresses. The World Health Organization includes these opportunistic infections in its clinical staging system, highlighting their importance in monitoring the progression of HIV and guiding treatment decisions. These manifestations often signal a compromised immune response, necessitating early intervention to prevent further complications and improve patient outcomes [6,7].

Oral lesions associated with HIV infection may result from fungal, viral, or bacterial pathogens, as well as neoplastic or idiopathic processes. These lesions are indicative of the immunosuppressed state induced by HIV, rendering patients more susceptible to severe presentations of conventional periodontal conditions. This increased severity underscores the need for vigilant oral health monitoring in this population to facilitate the timely diagnosis and management of underlying systemic and opportunistic infections [8].

Romania is home to one of the largest pediatric HIV cohorts in Europe, largely resulting from nosocomial transmission events during the late 1980s and early 1990s. A significant proportion of these patients were infected with the F1 HIV-1 subtype, a genetic variant predominantly found in Romania, which continues to impact long-term clinical outcomes. Additionally, disparities in healthcare access between urban and rural populations may delay the diagnosis and treatment of HIV-related complications. This unique combination of historical, virological, and socioeconomic factors underscores the clinical importance of this regional dataset [9].

This study aims to evaluate and consolidate recent developments in the treatment and management of otorhinolaryngological manifestations in HIV-positive patients. In the context of pathological changes in the stomatognathic system observed in patients with HIV/AIDS, it is essential to have a thorough understanding of these pathologies, allowing other specialties to respond appropriately and refer patients promptly to HIV/AIDS departments. We hypothesize that lower CD4+ T cell counts, smoking status, rural residence, and periodontal disease are significantly associated with the presence of oral candidiasis in this population.

2. Materials and Methods

2.1. Study Design and Database Information

To highlight the characteristics and ENT-related comorbidities of HIV/AIDS cases, we conducted a retrospective clinical investigation of patients with HIV/AIDS in the northeastern region of Romania who were admitted to the Clinical Hospital of Infectious Diseases in Iasi, based on hospital medical data. The study period spanned from 1 January 2020 to 30 November 2024.

Patients over the age of 18 who were hospitalized during the study period at our Regional HIV/AIDS Center in northeastern Romania were included in this study if they tested positive for HIV via an enzyme-linked immunosorbent assay (ELISA) and had their diagnosis confirmed via Western blot (WB). HIV plasma viral loads and CD4+ T cell counts were measured for all confirmed cases. The serological testing process involved two ELISA tests for initial screening, followed by a confirmatory Western blot performed by the regional public health management network's epidemiologists. Following confirmation, patients were referred to the local HIV/AIDS facility for comprehensive evaluation and management.

2.2. Ethical Approval

The "St. Parascheva" Clinical Hospital of Infectious Diseases in Iasi, Romania, cleared this study (Febr. 2025; Approval No. 3/12 February 2025). At admission, every individual signed documentation indicating informed consent.

2.3. Study Variables

Demographic data, stratified by age and sex, were systematically documented alongside detailed anamnesis and clinical characteristics. The dataset encompassed extensive viro-immunological assessments, including serological testing for opportunistic pathogens such as *Toxoplasma gondii*, *Cytomegalovirus*, hepatitis B and C viruses, and *Candida* spp. infections. HIV infection stages were determined following established immunological and clinical criteria, while the initiation of antiretroviral therapy (ART) and the longitudinal progression of the disease were meticulously recorded to ensure comprehensive patient profiling and outcome analysis. We also focused on viro-immunological evaluation to monitor the status of immunosuppression.

To ensure consistent treatment outcomes, all patients were routinely assessed by an ENT specialist and a dentist, addressing the high prevalence of ENT and stomatognathic complications in this population. Clinical examination—tongue scraping, followed by microscopic examination and fungal cultures (for oral candidiasis)—and imagistic evaluation (sinus X-ray) were used to confirm the diagnosis. The collected data, encompassing both retrospective and current clinical findings, were analyzed to identify trends and correlations in disease progression. In one case, we used a histological tissue biopsy for the diagnosis.

Of the patients admitted to our hospital, some were not included in this study based on the following exclusion criteria: positive viro-immunological status, adherence to treatment, and absence of symptoms in the ENT and dental fields. Patients were also excluded from this study if they had a CD4+ T-lymphocyte count greater than 200 cells/mm^3; an HIV viral load below 40 copies/mL, or an undetectable load; and no ENT or stomatognathic manifestations at the time of evaluation. These criteria were applied to ensure that the study population consisted of individuals with clinically significant immunosuppression who were at risk for HIV-related ENT and oral complications. This approach allowed for a more focused analysis of predictors associated with these manifestations.

The FACS (fluorescence-activated cell sorting) count technique was used to measure and quantify cell subpopulations, particularly CD4+ and CD8+ T-lymphocytes in the blood. A FACS count analyzer uses flow cytometry, where cells pass through a laser beam. Based on fluorescent cellular markers (fluorescently labeled monoclonal antibodies), the device detects and counts different types of cells. It relies on monoclonal antibodies tagged with fluorochromes that specifically bind to CD4 or CD8 molecules on the cell surface. Normal LyT CD4 values were recorded between 500 cells/mm^3 and 1400 cells/mm^3.

Cepheid's GeneXpert® system (Sunnyvale, CA, USA) was used for HIV viral load testing. It utilizes real-time polymerase chain reaction (PCR) technology for the rapid and accurate detection of HIV RNA, making it a crucial tool for monitoring viremia in HIV patients. The GeneXpert system amplifies and detects HIV RNA using a cartridge-based PCR assay. A viral load below 40 copies/mL was deemed undetectable; a load above 40 copies/mL was deemed detectable.

The Centers for Disease Control and Prevention (CDC), located in Atlanta, states that the specific CD4+ T-lymphocyte count or the CD4+ T-lymphocyte percentage of the total T-lymphocyte cells is used to define the HIV infection stage. There are three phases of HIV infection and AIDS: stage 1 occurs when the CD4+ T-lymphocyte counts exceed 500 cells/µL, stage 2 occurs when they fall between 200 and 499 cells/µL, and stage 3 occurs when they fall below 200 cells/µL. Stages 1 and 2 signify HIV infection, and stage 3 denotes AIDS.

2.4. Study Setting

The "St. Parascheva" Clinical Hospital of Infectious Diseases in Iasi serves as the main referral hospital for the Moldova area of Romania. There are six pavilions within it. An Infectious Diseases and HIV/AIDS Regional Center is located in Pavilion V, where patients are routinely assessed following CDC and EACS guidelines.

All blood tests were performed at the hospital's central laboratory, and the molecular biology lab was used to assess the patients' HIV plasma viral loads and CD4+ T cell counts. Cepheid's GeneXpert® system was used in conjunction with RT-PCR for HIV-1 to measure viral load levels and assess HIV viremia. Viral loads were considered undetectable if they were below 40 copies/mL, and detectable otherwise.

The Regional HIV/AIDS Center in Iasi maintains comprehensive medical records for its 1724 active patients, facilitating continuous care and monitoring. Each patient's medical file includes detailed information about their immunological and virological status, comorbid conditions, and adherence to ART regimens.

2.5. Statistical Analysis

The correlation between the results, clinical data, and demographic variables was assessed using a Pearson test in the XLSTAT program, version 2019, and the correlation coefficients of Kendall's Tau were determined. Statistical analysis was performed using Statistical Software for Excel (XLSTAT), version 2019.4.

3. Results

The active records of the Regional HIV/AIDS Center from Iasi covered 1724 patients. From 1st January 2020 to 31st November 2024, among the patients admitted at the Iasi Regional HIV/AIDS Center who visit periodically for viro-immunological evaluation, 552 were selected based on their presentation of acute lesions of the stomatognathic and otorhinolaryngologic system. Admissions were lowest in 2020, with only 281 admissions and 3 cases (1.1%) with stomatognathic lesions, due to the COVID-19 pandemic. The highest number of admissions was recorded in 2024, with 1239 cases, including 165 involving stomatognathic lesions (Table 1).

Table 1. Study group patients with lesions of the stomatognathic system by the year of admission.

Year of Admission	Number of HIV/AIDS Infection Cases Admitted to Our Hospital (n)	Number of HIV/AIDS Infection Cases Admitted to Our Hospital with Lesions of the Stomatognathic System (n)
2020	281	3
2021	379	104
2022	774	141
2023	1223	139
2024	1239	165

Young adults made up the majority of cases, with 255 patients (46.19%) between the ages of 30 and 39, followed by patients in the 40–49 age range (23.91%), those in the 50–59 age group (10.86%), those in the 18–29 age group (10.68%), and those over 60 years old (41 patients, 7.42%) (Table 1). The study group's average age was 37.31 years old. Men were more likely to be infected (358 cases, 64.85%) than women (194 cases, 35.15%) (Table 2). The remaining 359 cases (65%) were from rural areas, while 193 patients (35%) were from northeastern Romania's urban area.

Table 2. Distribution of new HIV/AIDS cases by age and gender.

Age (Years)	Total Patients (n, %)	Male (n)	Female (n)
18–29	59 (10.68%)	38	21
30–39	255 (46.19%)	165	90
40–49	132 (23.91%)	84	48
50–59	60 (10.86%)	36	24
Over 60	41 (7.42%)	35	6
Total	552 (100%)	358	194

Considering the route of transmission, all cases reported a possible cause. The most common was the sexual transmission route, with a total of 529 cases (95.83). Perinatal transmission was recorded in 17 cases (3.07%), and intravenous drug use was recorded in 6 cases (1.08%). Young adult males (ages 21 to 50) were the most afflicted group in terms of the sexual route of transmission (heterosexual men and MSM—men who have sex with men—accounting for 36.21% of cases) (Table 3).

Table 3. The route of transmission of the study group.

Route of Transmission	n	%
Sexual transmission Heterosexual MSM	331 198	59.96 36.21
Intravenous drug use	6	1.08
Perinatal	17	3.07

The study group from the Iasi HIV/AIDS Regional Center was virologically and immunologically evaluated.

The average CD4+ T-lymphocyte level was 372.34 cells/µL: 32.52% of cases had levels between 1 and 199 cells/µL, 36.85% of cases had values between 200 and 499 cells/µL, and 30.63% had values exceeding 500 cells/µL (Table 4, Figure 1). Males were primarily affected, exhibiting a decreased total CD4+ T-lymphocyte level, according to the gender–lymphocyte correlation. According to Table 4 and Figure 1, the average HIV viral load was 429.271 copies/m.

Table 4. Distribution of cases by CD4+ T-lymphocyte level and gender.

CD4+ T-Lymphocyte Level	Male		Female		Total	
	n	%	n	%	n	%
0–199 cells/µL	108	19.66	71	12.86	179	32.52
200–499 cells/µL	123	22.18	81	14.67	204	36.85
>500 cells/µL	127	23	42	7.63	169	30.63

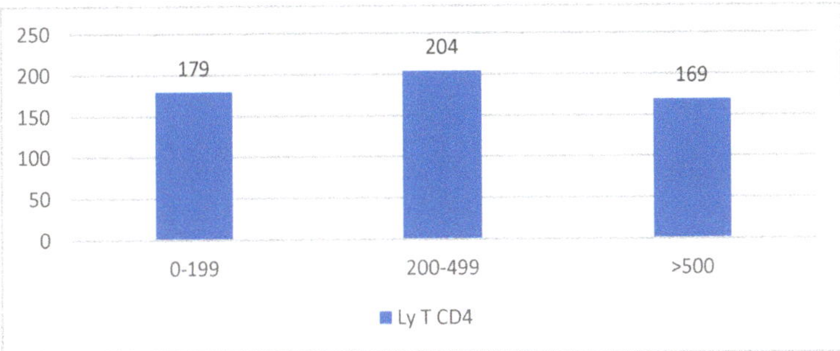

Figure 1. Distribution of cases by CD4+ T-lymphocyte level (cells/µL).

The study group was screened for the most prevalent co-infections linked to HIV/AIDS. The findings demonstrate that various opportunistic infections were present in over half (96.04%) of the patients admitted to our clinic during the study period.

The results show that the most frequent co-infections were oral candidiasis (92.21% of patients); hepatitis B (19.91%); tuberculosis, either recent-onset or recorded in past admissions (14.84%); and hepatitis C (4.88%). Males were more affected than females, exhibiting a higher percentage of co-infections (Table 5).

Table 5. Distribution of new HIV/AIDS cases by co-infections.

Co-infections	Men		Women		Total	
	n	%	n	%	n	%
Oral Candidiasis	335	60.68	174	31.52	509	92.21
HBV	76	13.76	34	6.15	110	19.91
HCV	15	2.71	12	2.17	27	4.88
Tuberculosis	49	8.87	33	5.97	82	14.84

The ENT manifestations observed in this study, with oral candidiasis being the most frequent diagnosis, were recorded in 335 male and 174 female cases (509, 92.21% total). Sinusitis/rhinosinusitis was the second most common condition, affecting 9 females and 8 males, with an additional case associated with temporomandibular arthritis in a female patient (18 cases, 3.26% total). Ethmoiditis was noted in four females (0.72%) and two males (0.36%), while dental abscesses and rhinosinusitis occurred in five male patients (0.90%). Mastoiditis was equally distributed, with three cases each in males and females (six cases, 1.08% total). Nasal septum deviation was reported in one female, and in two males in combination with sinusitis/rhinosinusitis (three cases, 0.54%). Otitis occurred exclusively in males (two cases, 0.36%), and temporomandibular arthritis was observed in one female (0.18%). This distribution highlights the predominance of oral candidiasis and sinusitis/rhinosinusitis, with certain conditions exhibiting gender-specific trends. In a few cases, dental abscesses were also diagnosed. Gingivitis and periodontitis were found in 552 patients with HIV. Gingivitis was diagnosed in 32% (n = 177) of patients, while periodontitis was observed in 36% (n = 199). The high prevalence of periodontal diseases in this cohort suggests a significant burden of oral inflammatory conditions, which may be exacerbated by immunosuppression, poor oral hygiene, and smoking (Table 6). One case recorded upper lip verrucous carcinoma, diagnosed via tissue biopsy.

Multivariable regression analysis was used to evaluate the predictors of oral candidiasis in HIV-positive patients. The dependent variable was the presence of oral candidiasis, while the independent variables included the CD4+ T-lymphocyte count, HIV viral load, gender, ART adherence, co-infections (HBV, HCV, and tuberculosis), sociodemographic characteristics, smoking status, and periodontal conditions (gingivitis and periodontitis) (Table 7).

The CD4+ T-lymphocyte count emerged as the most significant predictor, with a coefficient of −0.30 ($p < 0.001$), indicating a 26% reduction in candidiasis risk per 100-cell/μL increase (OR = 0.74). Among patients with CD4+ counts below 200 cells/μL, the prevalence of candidiasis exceeded 90%, confirming the role of severe immunodeficiency as a major risk factor.

Smoking was another highly significant predictor, with a coefficient of +1.25 ($p < 0.001$), corresponding to a 3.5-fold increased risk of candidiasis among smokers compared to non-smokers. Given that 60% of smokers in this study were diagnosed with *Candida* spp., this finding underscores the role of tobacco use in promoting fungal colonization and infection.

Sociodemographic characteristics (urban vs. rural) also played a significant role (B = −1.36, $p < 0.001$, OR = 0.26), indicating that patients from rural areas had a fourfold increased risk of developing candidiasis compared to urban residents. Notably, 65% of the study population resided in rural areas, further reinforcing healthcare access disparities as a critical determinant of opportunistic infections.

Table 6. Dental and ENT manifestations were recorded in our study.

Diagnosis	Gender	Total Patients (n, %)
Ethmoiditis	Female Male	4 cases, (0.72%) 2 cases, (0.36%)
Dental Abscesses/Rhinosinusitis	Male	5 cases, (0.90%)
Mastoiditis	Female Male	3 cases (0.54%) 3 cases (0.54%)
Nasal Septum Deviation	Female	1 case (0.18%)
Nasal Septum Deviation, Sinusitis/Rhinosinusitis	Male	2 cases (0.36%)
Otitis	Male	2 cases (0.36%)
Sinusitis/Rhinosinusitis	Female Male	9 cases (1.63%) 8 cases (1.44%)
Sinusitis/Rhinosinusitis, Temporomandibular Arthritis	Female	1 case (0.18%)
Temporomandibular Arthritis	Female	1 case (0.18%)
Oral Candidiasis	Male Female	335 cases, 60.68% 174 cases, 31.52%
Gingivitis	Male Female	100 cases, 18.2% 76 cases, 13.77%
Periodontitis	Male Female	123 cases, 22.28% 75 cases, 13.59%

Table 7. Regression analysis results for oral candidiasis predictors.

Variable	Coefficient (B)	*p*-Value	Odds Ratio (OR)	95% Confidence Interval (CI)
CD4+ T-Lymphocyte Count (per 100 cells/μL)	−0.30	<0.001	0.74	0.66–0.83
HIV Viral Load (log10 copies/mL)	−0.05	0.82	NS°	—
Gender (Male vs. Female)	0.09	0.80	NS	—
ART Adherence (Good vs. Poor)	−0.22	0.55	NS	—
HBV Co-infection	−0.39	0.33	NS	—
HCV Co-infection	−0.92	0.15	NS	—
Tuberculosis Co-infection	−0.54	0.20	NS	—
Sociodemographic Characteristics (Urban vs. Rural)	−1.36	<0.001	0.26	0.14–0.47
Smoking (Smoker vs. Non-Smoker)	+1.25	<0.001	3.5	2.30–5.40
Gingivitis (Present vs. Absent)	+0.85	0.004	2.35	1.30–4.25
Periodontitis (Present vs. Absent)	+1.10	0.002	3.02	1.50–6.00

°NS: Not Significant.

In terms of periodontal conditions, gingivitis (B = +0.85, $p = 0.004$, OR = 2.35) and periodontitis (B = +1.10, $p = 0.002$, OR = 3.02) were significant predictors, demonstrating that patients with these conditions were more likely to develop oral candidiasis. In this cohort, 32% of patients had gingivitis, while 36% had periodontitis, suggesting that periodontal disease is prevalent in HIV-positive individuals and contributes to higher candidiasis rates.

In contrast, HIV viral load, gender, ART adherence, and co-infections (HBV, HCV, and tuberculosis) were not statistically significant predictors ($p > 0.15$), suggesting that their impact on candidiasis is mediated primarily through CD4+ depletion rather than direct effects. Despite this, patients with detectable HIV viremia had higher overall candidiasis rates.

Candida spp. diagnosis among smokers and non-smokers was based on lingual swab results from patients with HIV/AIDS in our cohort. Among 442 smokers (80% of patients), 60% (n = 265) were diagnosed with *Candida* spp., indicating a strong association between smoking and fungal colonization. In contrast, among 110 non-smokers (20% of patients), only 20% (n = 22) tested positive for *Candida* spp. after lingual swab (Table 8).

Table 8. *Candida* spp. diagnosis among smokers and non-smokers.

Smoking Status	Total Patients	Patients with *Candida* spp. Diagnosis	Percentage (%)
Smokers	442	265	60%
Non-Smokers	110	22	20%

For every patient diagnosed with an oropharyngeal manifestation and dental abscesses, empirical antibiotic/antifungal treatment was initiated with favorable outcomes. Aminopenicillins, specifically amoxicillin–clavulanate, were used in 2.35% of patients for 7–10 days. Second-generation cephalosporins, represented by cefuroxime, and third-generation cephalosporins, such as ceftriaxone and ceftazidime, were administered to 0.90% and 1.44% of patients, respectively, for a treatment duration of 7 days. Fluoroquinolones, particularly ciprofloxacin, were used in 2.17% of cases, with treatment lengths ranging from 7 to 14 days. Notably, antifungal therapy with fluconazole was the most frequently employed treatment, accounting for 92.21% of patients, with a standard duration of 3 days (Table 9).

Table 9. Treatment used for ENT manifestations and dental abscesses.

Treatment	Patients (n, %)	Number of Days
Aminopenicillin: Amoxicillin–Clavulanate	13 (2.35%)	7–10 days
Second-Generation Cephalosporin: Cefuroxime	5 (0.90%)	7 days
Third-Generation Cephalosporin: Ceftriaxone	5 (0.90%)	7 days
Third-Generation Cephalosporin: Ceftazidime	8 (1.44%)	7 days
Fluoroquinolone: Ciprofloxacin	12 (2.17%)	7–14 days
Antifungal: Fluconazole	509 (92.21%)	3 days

The patients diagnosed with *Candida* spp. infection received fluconazole 150 mg per day as the primary antifungal therapy. At the follow-up assessment, 80% (n = 407) of treated patients had a negative tongue swab for *Candida* spp., indicating successful resolution of the infection. The remaining 20% (n = 102) of patients exhibited persistent colonization or infection, which may suggest fluconazole resistance, suboptimal adherence, or severe immunosuppression (Table 10).

Antiretroviral therapy was prescribed for every patient identified at the Iasi HIV/AIDS Regional Center. Consequently, a single-pill regimen was administered in 83.69% of instances, while a regimen that considered their comorbidities and adhered to guidance from www.hiv-druginteractions.org accessed on 20 March 2025, was prescribed to the remaining 16.31% of cases (Table 11).

Table 10. Fluconazole treatment outcome in HIV patients with oropharyngeal candidiasis.

Parameter	n	%
Total Patients with Oropharyngeal Candidiasis	509	100
Patients Treated with Fluconazole 150 mg/oral/per day/3 days	509	100
Patients with Negative Follow-up Tongue Swab (after treatment)	407	80

Table 11. The antiretroviral regimen that was used.

Antiretroviral Regimen	n	%
Single-pill regimen	462	83.69
Multi-pill regimen	90	16.31

Integrase inhibitor-based antiretroviral regimens were the most commonly used (309 patients, 55.97%), followed by nucleoside reverse transcriptase inhibitor (NRTI)-based regimens with non-nucleoside reverse transcriptase inhibitors (NNRTIs), which were used in 200 patients (36.23%), and protease inhibitor-based regimens (29 patients, 5.25%). Fourteen patients (2.53%) were treated with other antiretroviral regimens, such as CCR5 inhibitors, NRTIs + integrase inhibitors, or protease inhibitors + integrase inhibitors (Table 12).

Table 12. Distribution of HIV/AIDS cases by ART regimen.

ART Regimen	n	%
Integrase inhibitors	309	55.97
Protease inhibitors	29	5.25
NRTIs + 2 NNRTIs	200	36.23
Other	14	2.53

4. Discussion

This study highlights the significant burden of oropharyngeal manifestations among people living with HIV in northeastern Romania, emphasizing their correlation with advanced stages of immunosuppression. Oral candidiasis emerged as the most prevalent condition, affecting 92.21% of patients, reflecting its role as a primary marker of disease progression. Other notable conditions included gingivitis/periodontitis, sinusitis/rhinosinusitis, mastoiditis, and dental abscesses, albeit at lower frequencies. Gender differences were evident, with males exhibiting higher rates of co-infections and oropharyngeal complications.

Oral lesions, often accompanied by nonspecific symptoms, are among the earliest clinical manifestations of HIV infection and serve as critical markers for disease progression to AIDS. These lesions are reported in approximately 30% of individuals with HIV and up to 80% of patients diagnosed with AIDS, highlighting their prevalence and diagnostic significance in the context of immunosuppression and disease advancement [10–12]. Among the patients admitted, 552 patients (14.19%) were selected based on their reported presentation of acute lesions of the stomatognathic and otorhinolaryngologic systems.

The Oral Manifestations of Human Immunodeficiency Virus, as classified by the EC–Clearinghouse and the World Health Organization (WHO), categorize oral lesions based on their relationship with HIV infection into three groups: those strongly associated with HIV, those less commonly associated, and those observed in individuals with HIV [13].

We observed a predominance of oral candidiasis and gingivitis/periodontitis, with certain conditions exhibiting gender-specific trends. In a few cases, dental abscesses were also diagnosed.

In alignment with the EC–Clearinghouse–WHO classification, common oral manifestations in HIV/AIDS patients, such as candidiasis, oral hairy leukoplakia, periodontal disease, and Kaposi sarcoma, continue to be frequently reported. Additionally, conditions such as oral mucosal hyperpigmentation, HIV-related salivary gland disorders, and potentially HIV-associated oral ulcerations are increasingly recognized, suggesting that improved access to antiretroviral therapy (ART) in recent years has influenced the prevalence and presentation of these manifestations. Furthermore, variations in the frequency of HIV-related oral conditions between developed and developing regions are evident, likely reflecting disparities in socioeconomic, cultural, and healthcare accessibility factors [13–16]. Our findings support these observations, as oral candidiasis was the most common manifestation in the study group.

In their study, Dongo M. et al. observed that in a total of 750 men and 237 women, oral manifestations were less prevalent in females than in males [17,18]. Similarly, we recorded that stomatognathic system oral lesions were more frequent in men (358 cases, 64.85%) than in women (194 cases, 35.15%).

Sex-based differences appear to influence the prevalence of oral manifestations associated with HIV/AIDS. Research indicates that oral hairy leukoplakia and Kaposi sarcoma are more commonly observed in men, whereas conditions such as linear gingival erythema and aphthous ulcers are more frequently reported in women. These findings highlight potential variations in clinical presentation that may be influenced by biological or environmental factors, emphasizing the need for personalized approaches to diagnosis and management [19–21]. We did not, however, record any cases of oral hairy leukoplakia or Kaposi sarcoma.

Candidiasis is the most prevalent opportunistic fungal infection in HIV-positive individuals, with a prevalence of 17–75%, primarily caused by *Candida albicans*, but also involving other species like *C. glabrata* and *C. tropicalis*. Oral candidiasis is commonly one of the first clinical manifestations observed during the acute phase of HIV infection, indicating early immune system involvement. It is a significant indicator of immune system compromise and can precede a formal HIV diagnosis [10,13]. Its prevalence exhibits significant variability across different studies. In agreement with previous findings, oral candidiasis was observed in 92.21% of the cases in our study.

Key risk factors include severe immunosuppression (CD4+ T cell count <200 cells/μL), tobacco use, broad-spectrum antibiotics, corticosteroids, and local contributors such as partial dentures, reduced saliva flow, and nutritional deficiencies. Clinically, it presents as pseudomembranous candidiasis, erythematous candidiasis, or angular cheilitis, necessitating prompt diagnosis and management to prevent complications in immunocompromised individuals [22,23]. In our study, oral candidiasis was the most frequent diagnosis; in some cases, it was associated with low immunological status.

Based on the disease topography in 552 patients, Keita A. et al. found rhinitis (80.2%), rhinosinusitis (18.9%), and epistaxis (0.9%) to be present in 55.7% of cases with ENT involvement. A total of 50.9% of cases involved the oral cavity and oropharynx, including tonsillitis (37.2%), oral thrush (3.8%), and candidiasis (54.3%) [24]. Our study found that oral candidiasis was the most frequent diagnosis, recorded in 335 male and 174 female cases (509, 92.21% total). Gingivitis was the second most common condition, affecting 374 cases (67.75%).

Variations in the prevalence of oral lesions among different anatomical sites appear to correlate with educational level, with regions such as the floor of the mouth and buccal mucosa being more frequently affected in individuals with informal education. This disparity may reflect differences in oral hygiene practices. Previous studies, such as those by Johnson and Tirwomwe et al., suggest that the increased frequency of oral lesions in patients with HIV/AIDS is linked to poor dietary and oral hygiene habits, discomfort during tooth brushing, and difficulties with chewing or swallowing. These observations underscore the influence of educational and behavioral factors on the manifestation of oral conditions in HIV-positive individuals [25,26]. This aligns with our findings, as 65% of the cases in our study were rural residents with a deficit in access to otolaryngology and dental care.

The Romanian pediatric HIV/AIDS cohort emerged during the late 1980s and early 1990s due to unsafe medical practices, including the reuse of needles and contaminated blood transfusions, primarily affecting children under three years of age, many from institutionalized care settings. Most infections were linked to HIV-1 subtype F1, unique to Romania.

As of 30 June 2024, Romania has recorded 28,273 HIV/AIDS cases, with 18,605 progressing to AIDS and 9668 remaining HIV-positive without AIDS. HIV/AIDS-related deaths have reached 8651, and 1263 patients have been lost to follow-up. Currently, 18,359 people are living with HIV/AIDS [27].

In the first half of 2024, 321 new HIV/AIDS cases were reported (186 HIV cases and 135 AIDS cases), and 95 AIDS-related deaths occurred. Heterosexual transmission remains dominant (61%), followed by transmission by MSM (31.15%) and injection drug use (4.67%). Among tested populations, HIV contacts had an 11.6% positivity rate; MSM, 1.68%; and prisoners, 13.64% [27].

ART coverage was estimated at 80–90%, but 42% of new cases were already at the AIDS stage, highlighting the urgent need for earlier diagnosis, prevention efforts, and adherence support [27].

The most common transmission route in the study group was sexual transmission, as with other regions from our country [27]. At the national level, heterosexual transmission remains the primary mode of HIV infection, followed by injection drug use and MSM-associated transmission [28,29].

We reflect on the changes in the stomatognathic system to raise awareness among colleagues from other medical fields and specialties. HIV/AIDS infection occurs and must be recognized in various medical domains.

The limitations of this study were caused by restricted access to other medical services, such as otolaryngology and dental care, during the COVID-19 pandemic. This reduced access may have delayed the diagnosis of HIV-related manifestations in the stomatognathic system. Consequently, early detection and interdisciplinary collaboration remain crucial for the timely management of HIV/AIDS cases. Another limitation is the lack of long-term follow-up data, which restricted our ability to conclude the progression and long-term outcomes of ENT and dental conditions in our HIV-positive patients.

Another limitation of this study lies in its retrospective design, which may be affected by the quality and completeness of the available data. Challenges such as incomplete medical records and the inability to account for all confounding factors at the time of data collection are inherent to retrospective analyses. Additionally, recall bias may impact the accuracy of self-reported symptoms or medical history.

Furthermore, the absence of a control group limits our ability to determine whether the observed outcomes—such as the high incidence of oropharyngeal manifestations—are specific to the HIV-positive population or are also prevalent in HIV-negative individuals or other demographic groups. This restricts the generalizability of this study's findings and highlights the need for future comparative studies.

The key to the management of HIV-positive patients is a multidisciplinary approach, with the aid of different specialists (including ENT specialists and dentists) and access to antiretroviral therapy. We must find and eliminate obstacles affecting patients and the healthcare system in order to increase ART uptake [30–32]. Regular screening for oral and ENT manifestations can lead to earlier diagnosis of opportunistic infections and improved quality of life. Additionally, enhancing communication between primary care providers and specialists is essential for delivering comprehensive and continuous care [33].

Although oral candidiasis is a well-known and widely reported opportunistic infection in immunosuppressed patients with HIV, our findings contribute novel insight by analyzing this manifestation in a uniquely structured regional cohort from northeastern Romania. Romania remains home to one of the largest pediatric HIV populations in Europe, primarily infected with HIV-1 subtype F1—a globally rare but locally endemic variant with long-term clinical implications [9].

In contrast to most Western European datasets, our cohort included a high proportion of patients from rural areas (65%), where access to dental and ENT specialists remains limited. This disparity likely contributes to diagnostic delays and more advanced presentations at the time of hospital admission. Additionally, gender differences were noted: male patients showed a higher prevalence of co-infections and more severe ENT involvement, findings consistent with previous Eastern European studies [34].

When compared to other regional reports, such as the EuroAIDS cohort, which shows higher AIDS-related mortality in Eastern Europe, our data reinforce the need for improved early detection strategies and integrated care models tailored to local realities. These regional differences underscore the importance of continuing to document and analyze HIV-related complications in underrepresented settings.

5. Conclusions

This study's findings underscore the critical role of the early diagnosis and management of oropharyngeal manifestations in improving patient outcomes. Integrating routine otorhinolaryngological assessments into the standard care for HIV-positive individuals is imperative, especially for those with CD4+ T cell counts below 200 cells/μL. Antifungal treatments, particularly fluconazole, demonstrated high efficacy, underscoring their importance in clinical management.

Additionally, we must improve access to HIV testing, with community outreach initiatives being especially valuable, and always provide counseling and fast referrals to medical facilities to start ART to support these outreach initiatives. Finally, to complete the management plan for people living with HIV/AIDS infection to support their quality of life, a complete evaluation must be conducted by both a dentist and an ENT specialist.

Author Contributions: Conceptualization, I.I.L., A.E.S. and C.M.D.; methodology, Ș.A.R. and A.A.M.; software, Ș.A.R., I.C. and A.A.M.; validation, I.I.L., C.M.D. and A.E.S.; formal analysis, V.D.D. and V.H.; investigation, I.I.L., Ș.A.R., O.E. and I.C.; resources, I.I.L. and Ș.A.R.; data curation, A.E.S. and A.A.M.; writing—original draft preparation, I.I.L. and Ș.A.R.; writing—review and editing, A.E.S., V.D.D. and V.H.; visualization, I.I.L., A.E.S. and O.E.; supervision, C.M.D.; project administration, A.E.S.; funding acquisition, C.M.D. All authors have read and agreed to the published version of the manuscript.

Funding: This research received no external funding.

Institutional Review Board Statement: This study was conducted following the Declaration of Helsinki and approved by the Ethics Committee of the "St. Parascheva" Clinical Hospital of Infectious Diseases, Iasi, Romania (Febr. 2025; Approval No. 3/12 February 2025).

Informed Consent Statement: This was a retrospective study, and written informed consent was obtained from the patients when they were admitted to our hospital, according to the hospital's policy.

Data Availability Statement: All data generated or analyzed during this study are included in this published article.

Conflicts of Interest: The authors declare no conflicts of interest.

Abbreviations

The following abbreviations are used in this manuscript:

ENT	Ear, neck, and throat;
OHL	Oral hairy leukoplakia;
HIV	Human immunodeficiency virus;
AIDS	Acquired immunodeficiency syndrome;
ART	Antiretroviral therapy;
WHO	World Health Organization;
NS	Not significant.

References

1. Iacovou, E.; Vlastarakos, P.V.; Papacharalampous, G.; Kampessis, G.; Nikolopoulos, T.P. Diagnosis and treatment of HIV-associated manifestations in otolaryngology. *Infect. Dis. Rep.* **2012**, *4*, e9. [CrossRef] [PubMed]
2. Hines, L.R.; Jones, B.S. Stoelting's Anesthesia and Co-Existing Disease. In *Diseases Related to Immune System Dysfunction*, 8th ed.; Elsevier Inc.: Amsterdam, The Netherlands, 2022; pp. 87–113.
3. Nayyar, A.S.; Ratnam, M.; Reddy, D.S.; Ruparani, B.; Chalapathi, K.; Azmi, S. CD4 cell counts and oral manifestations in HIV infected and AIDS patients. *J. Oral. Maxillofac. Pathol.* **2018**, *22*, 282. [CrossRef] [PubMed]
4. UNAIDS/WHO. On the Fast Track to End AIDS. 2016–2021 Strategy United Nations Programme on HIV/AIDS. Available online: https://www.unaids.org/en/resources/documents/2015/UNAIDS_PCB37_15-18 (accessed on 16 March 2025).
5. European AIDS Clinical Society: EACS Guidelines Version 12.0. October 2023. Available online: https://www.eacsociety.org/media/guidelines-12.0.pdf (accessed on 4 March 2025).
6. Shah, F.A. ENT Manifestations of HIV Infection. *Acta Sci. Otolaryngol.* **2022**, *4*, 1–3.
7. Tanzania Commission for AIDS (TACAIDS) Dar es Salaam T; Zanzibar ZAC (ZAC); National Bureau of Statistics (NBS) Dar es Salaam T; Zanzibar O of CGS (OCGS). ICF International Calverton MU. HIV/AIDS and Malaria Indicator Survey 2011–2012. History of AIDS. 2011. Available online: https://dhsprogram.com/pubs/pdf/SR196/SR196.pdf (accessed on 16 March 2025).
8. *WHO Case Definitions of HIV for Surveillance and Revised Clinical Staging and Immunological Classification of HIV-Related Disease in Adults and Children*; World Health Organization Library Cataloguing-in-Publication Data: Geneva, Switzerland, 2007.
9. Preda, M.; Manolescu, L.C.S. Romania, a Harbour of HIV-1 Subtype F1: Where Are We after 33 Years of HIV-1 Infection? *Viruses* **2022**, *14*, 2081. [CrossRef]
10. Ayyagari, K.R.; Karra, K.K.; Birra, V.; STriveni, V.V.; Sreedevi, J.; Peela, P. "Oral manifestations of HIV in accordance with CD4 count"—A cross-sectional study. *Indian J. Dent. Res.* **2022**, *33*, 408–412. [CrossRef]
11. Pakfetrat, A.; Falaki, F.; Delavarian, Z.; Dalirsani, Z.; Sanatkhani, M.; Zabihi Marani, M. Oral manifestations of human immunodeficiency virus-infected patients. *Iran. J. Otorhinolaryngol.* **2015**, *27*, 43–54.
12. Sridevi, K.; Malathi, S.; Kv, C.; G, C.N.; Gayathri, M.; Chand, G.E.; Nayyar, A.S. CD4 Cell Counts, Lipid Profile, and Oral Manifestations in HIV-Infected and AIDS Patients. *Front. Dent.* **2019**, *16*, 436–449. [CrossRef]
13. Tappuni, A.R. The global changing pattern of the oral manifestations of HIV. *Oral Dis.* **2020**, *26* (Suppl. S1), 22–27. [CrossRef]
14. Greenspan, J.S.; Challacombe, S.J. The impact of the world Workshops on oral health and disease in HIV and AIDS (1988–2020). *Oral. Dis.* **2020**, *26* (Suppl. S1), 3–8. [CrossRef]
15. Challacombe, S.J. Global inequalities in HIV infection. *Oral. Dis.* **2020**, *26*, 16–21. [CrossRef]
16. Khoury, Z.H.; Meeks, V. The influence of antiretroviral therapy on HIV-related oral manifestations. *J. Natl. Med. Assoc.* **2021**, *113*, 449–456. [CrossRef] [PubMed]
17. Dongo, M.; Gonçalves, L.S.; Ferreira, S.M.; Noce, C.W.; Dias, E.P.; Júnior, A.S. Gender differences in oral manifestations among HIV-infected Brazilian adults. *Int. Dent. J.* **2013**, *63*, 189–195. [CrossRef] [PubMed]
18. Chen, Y.; Zhao, J.; Sun, P.; Cheng, M.; Xiong, Y.; Sun, Z.; Zhang, Y.; Li, K.; Ye, Y.; Shuai, P.; et al. Estimates of the global burden of non-Hodgkin lymphoma attributable to HIV: A population attributable modeling study. *EClinicalMedicine* **2023**, *67*, 102370. [CrossRef] [PubMed] [PubMed Central]

19. Ferreira, S.; Noce, C.; Júnior, A.S.; Gonçalves, L.; Torres, S.; Meeks, V.; Luiz, R.; Dias, E. Prevalence of oral manifestations of HIV infection in Rio De Janeiro, Brazil from 1988 to 2004. *AIDS Patient Care STDS* **2007**, *21*, 724–731. [CrossRef] [PubMed]
20. Ranganathan, K.; Umadevi, M.; Saraswathi, T.R.; Kumarasamy, N.; Solomon, S.; Johnson, N. Oral lesions and conditions associated with human immunodeficiency virus infection in 1000 South Indian patients. *Ann. Acad. Med. Singap.* **2004**, *33* (Suppl. S4), 37–42. [CrossRef] [PubMed]
21. Sharma, G.; Pai, K.M.; Suhas, S.; Ramapuram, J.T.; Doshi, D.; Anup, N. Oral manifestations in HIV/AIDS infected patients from India. *Oral. Dis.* **2006**, *12*, 537–542. [CrossRef] [PubMed]
22. El Howati, A.; Tappuni, A. Systematic review of the changing pattern of the oral manifestations of HIV. *J. Investig. Clin. Dent.* **2018**, *9*, e12351. [CrossRef] [PubMed]
23. Berberi, A.; Noujeim, Z. Epidemiology and Relationships between CD4+ Counts and Oral Lesions among 50 Patients Infected with Human Immunodeficiency Virus. *J. Int. Oral. Health* **2015**, *7*, 18–21.
24. Keita, A.; Rigaill, J.; Pillet, S.; Sereme, Y.; Coulibaly, S.; Diallo, F.; Verhoeven, P.; Pozzetto, B.; Thiero, T.A.; Bourlet, T. Evidence of HIV-1 Genital Shedding after One Year of Antiretroviral Therapy in Females Recently Diagnosed in Bamako, Mali. *Microorganisms* **2021**, *9*, 2164. [CrossRef] [PubMed] [PubMed Central]
25. Tirwomwe, J.F.; Rwenyonyi, C.M.; Muwazi, L.M.; Besigye, B.; Mboli, F. Oral manifestations of HIV/AIDS in clients attending TASO clinics in Uganda. *Clin. Oral. Investig.* **2007**, *11*, 289–292. [CrossRef] [PubMed]
26. Johnson, N.W. The mouth in HIV/AIDS: Markers of disease status and management challenges for the dental profession. *Aust. Dent. J.* **2010**, *55* (Suppl. S1), 85–102. [CrossRef] [PubMed]
27. Department for Monitoring and Evaluation of HIV/AIDS infection in Romania, National Institute of Infectious Diseases "Prof. dr. Matei Balș". Available online: https://www.cnlas.ro/images/doc/31122022_rom.pdf (accessed on 18 March 2025).
28. Johnson, B.T.; Buzducea, D. HIV-positive Romanian adolescents: Acquisition routes, risk behaviors, and psychological correlates. *AIDS Behav.* **2007**, *11*, 716–725. [CrossRef] [PubMed]
29. Hohan, R.; Paraschiv, S.; Nicolae, I.; Oțelea, D. Estimating the Current Routes of Transmission in HIV-1 F1 Subtype Infected Persons in Romania: Differences Between Self-Reporting and Phylogenetic Data. *Pathogens* **2024**, *13*, 960. [CrossRef] [PubMed] [PubMed Central]
30. Cobaschi, M.; Loghin, I.I.; Dorobăț, V.D.; Silvaș, G.; Rusu, Ș.A.; Hârtie, V.; Aramă, V. Ophthalmological Manifestations in People with HIV from Northeastern Romania. *Medicina* **2023**, *59*, 1605. [CrossRef] [PubMed] [PubMed Central]
31. Richards, G.A.; Zamparini, J.; Kalla, I.; Laher, A.; Murray, L.W.; Shaddock, E.J.; Stacey, S.; Venter, W.F.; Feldman, C. Critical illness due to infection in people living with HIV. *Lancet HIV.* **2024**, *11*, e406–e418. [CrossRef] [PubMed]
32. Juta, P.M.; Jansen van Vuuren, J.M.; Mbaya, K.J. A multidisciplinary approach for people with HIV failing antiretroviral therapy in South Africa. *South Afr. J. HIV Med.* **2024**, *25*, 1579. [CrossRef] [PubMed] [PubMed Central]
33. Apetroaei, M.M.; Velescu, B.Ș.; Nedea, M.I.I.; Dinu-Pîrvu, C.E.; Drăgănescu, D.; Fâcă, A.I.; Udeanu, D.I.; Arsene, A.L. The Phenomenon of Antiretroviral Drug Resistance in the Context of Human Immunodeficiency Virus Treatment: Dynamic and Ever Evolving Subject Matter. *Biomedicines* **2024**, *12*, 915. [CrossRef] [PubMed] [PubMed Central]
34. Pleșca, V.Ș.; Miron, V.D.; Marinescu, A.G.; Drăgănescu, A.C.; Pleșca, A.D.; Săndulescu, O.; Voiosu, C.; Hainăroșie, R.; Streinu-Cercel, A. Hospitalizations for Acute Otitis and Sinusitis in Patients Living with HIV: A Retrospective Analysis of a Tertiary Center in Romania. *J. Clin. Med.* **2024**, *13*, 3346. [CrossRef] [PubMed] [PubMed Central]

MDPI AG
Grosspeteranlage 5
4052 Basel
Switzerland
Tel.: +41 61 683 77 34

Medicina Editorial Office
E-mail: medicina@mdpi.com
www.mdpi.com/journal/medicina

MDPI

www.ingramcontent.com/pod-product-compliance
Lightning Source LLC
Chambersburg PA
CBHW061847210926
51850CB00006B/994